SpringerWienNewYork

Sponsored by the
European Association of Neurosurgical Societies

# Advances and Technical Standards in Neurosurgery

Vol. 33

Edited by
J. D. Pickard, Cambridge (Editor-in-Chief),
N. Akalan, Ankara, C. Di Rocco, Roma,
V. V. Dolenc, Ljubljana, J. Lobo Antunes, Lisbon,
J. J. A. Mooij, Groningen, J. Schramm, Bonn,
M. Sindou, Lyon

SpringerWienNewYork

With 74 Figures (thereof 51 coloured)



SpringerWienNewYork is part of Springer Science Business Media
springer.at



Printed on acid-free and chlorine-free bleached paper

ISSN 0095-4829

ISBN 978-3-211-99902-8 e-ISBN 978-3-211-72283-1

## Preface

As an addition to the European postgraduate training system for young neurosurgeons, we began to publish in 1974 this series of *Advances and Technical Standards in Neurosurgery* which was later sponsored by the European Association of Neurosurgical Societies.

This series was first discussed in 1972 at a combined meeting of the Italian and German Neurosurgical Societies in Taormina, the founding fathers of the series being Jean Brihaye, Bernard Pertuiset, Fritz Loew and Hugo Krayenbuhl. Thus were established the principles of European co-operation which have been born from the European spirit, flourished in the European Association, and have been associated throughout with this series.

The fact that the English language is now the international medium for communication at European scientific conferences is a great asset in terms of mutual understanding. Therefore we have decided to publish all contributions in English, regardless of the native language of the authors.

All contributions are submitted to the entire editorial board before publication of any volume for scrutiny and suggestions for revision.

Our series is not intended to compete with the publications of original scientific papers in other neurosurgical journals. Our intention is, rather, to present fields of neurosurgery and related areas in which important recent advances have been made. The contributions are written by specialists in the given fields and constitute the first part of each volume.

In the second part of each volume, we publish detailed descriptions of standard operative procedures and in depth reviews of established knowledge in all aspects of neurosurgery, furnished by experienced clinicians. This part is intended primarily to assist young neurosurgeons in their postgraduate training. However, we are convinced that it will also be useful to experienced, fully trained neurosurgeons.

We hope therefore that surgeons not only in Europe, but also throughout the world, will profit by this series of *Advances and Technical Standards in Neurosurgery*.

*The Editors*

## Contents



## Advances

**Tumor-biology and current treatment of skull-base chordomas.** M. N. PAMIR and K. ÖZDUMAN, Marmara University Faculty of Medicine, Department of Neurosurgery, Marmara University Institute of Neurological Sciences, Istanbul, Turkey

**Management of brachial plexus injuries.** G. Blaauw[1], R. S. Muhlig[2], and J. W. Vredeveld[3], [1] Department of Neurosurgery, University Hospital, Maastricht, The Netherlands, [2] Rehabilitation Out-Patient Clinic, S.G.L., Heerlen, The Netherlands, [3] Department of Neurophysiology, Atrium Medical Centre, Heerlen, The Netherlands

**Surgical anatomy of the jugular foramen.** P.-H. Roche[1], P. Mercier[2], T. Sameshima[3], and H.-D. Fournier[2], [1] Service de Neurochirurgie, Hôpital Sainte Marguerite, CHU de Marseille, Marseille, France, [2] Service de Neurochirurgie et Laboratoire d'anatomie de la faculté de Médecine d'Angers, France, [3] Carolina Neuroscience Institute, Raleigh, NC, USA

## List of contributors

Blaauw, G., Department of Neurosurgery, University Hospital, Maastricht, The Netherlands

Cappabianca, P., Division of Neurosurgery, Department of Neurological Sciences, Università degli Studi di Napoli Federico II, Naples, Italy

Cavallo, L. M., Division of Neurosurgery, Department of Neurological Sciences, Università degli Studi di Napoli Federico II, Naples, Italy

de Divitiis, E., Division of Neurosurgery, Department of Neurological Sciences, Università degli Studi di Napoli Federico II, Naples, Italy

de Divitiis, O., Division of Neurosurgery, Department of Neurological Sciences, Università degli Studi di Napoli Federico II, Naples, Italy

Duffau, H., Department of Neurosurgery, Hôpital Gui de Chauliac, CHU de Montpellier, Montpellier Cedex, France and Laboratoire de Psychologie et Neurosciences Cognitives (CNRS FRE 2987/Université de Paris V René Descartes), Institut de Psychologie, Boulogne Billancourt, France

Esposito, F., Division of Neurosurgery, Department of Neurological Sciences, Università degli Studi di Napoli Federico II, Naples, Italy

Fournier, H.-D., Service de Neurochirurgie et Laboratoire d'anatomie de la faculté de Médecine d'Angers, France

Krischek, B., Department of Neurosurgery, University of Tuebingen, Tuebingen, Germany

Mercier, P., Service de Neurochirurgie et Laboratoire d'anatomie de la faculté de Médecine d'Angers, France

Messina, A., Division of Neurosurgery, Department of Neurological Sciences, Università degli Studi di Napoli Federico II, Naples, Italy

Muhlig, R. S., Rehabilitation Out-Patient Clinic, S.G.L., Heerlen, The Netherlands

Özduman, K., Marmara University Faculty of Medicine, Department of Neurosurgery, Marmara University Institute of Neurological Sciences, Istanbul, Turkey

Pamir, M. N., Marmara University Faculty of Medicine, Department of Neurosurgery, Marmara University Institute of Neurological Sciences, Istanbul, Turkey

Roche, P.-H., Service de Neurochirurgie, Hôpital Sainte Marguerite, CHU de Marseille, Marseille, France

Sameshima, T., Carolina Neuroscience Institute, Raleigh, NC, USA

Tatagiba, M., Department of Neurosurgery, University of Tuebingen, Tuebingen, Germany

Vredeveld, J. W., Department of Neurophysiology, Atrium Medical Centre, Heerlen, The Netherlands

## Advances

# Brain plasticity and tumors

H. DUFFAU

Department of Neurosurgery, Hôpital Gui de Chauliac, CHU de Montpellier, Montpellier Cedex, France and Laboratoire de Psychologie et Neurosciences Cognitives (CNRS FRE 2987/Université de Paris V René Descartes), Institut de Psychologie, Boulogne Billancourt, France

With 6 Figures

## Contents

## Abstract

Brain plasticity is the potential of the nervous system to reshape itself during ontogeny, learning or following injuries. The first part of this article reviews the pathophysiological mechanisms underlying plasticity at different functional levels. Such plastic potential means that the anatomo-functional organization of the brain in humans, both physiological and pathological, has flexibility. Patterns of reorganization may differ according to the time-course of cerebral damage, with better functional compensation in more slowly growing lesions. The second part of this review analyzes the interactions between tumor growth and brain reshaping, using non-invasive (neuroimaging) and invasive (electrophysiological) methods of functional mapping. Finally, the therapeutic implications provided by a greater understanding of these mechanisms of cerebral redistribution are explored from a surgical point of view. Enhanced preoperative prediction of an individual's potential for reorganization might be integrated into surgical planning and preserving quality of life through tailored rehabilitation programmes to optimize functional recovery following resection of a brain tumor.

*Keywords:* Brain plasticity; sensorimotor; language; functional neuroimaging; electrical stimulation mapping; brain tumor; neuro-oncology; low-grade glioma.

## Introduction

As early as the beginning of the XIX$^{th}$ century, two opposing concepts of the functioning of the central nervous system were suggested. First, the theory of "equipotentiality" hypothesized that the entire brain, or at least one complete hemisphere, was involved in the performance of a functional task. In contrast, the theory of "localizationism", supposed that each part of the brain corresponded to a specific function, so called "phrenology". Reports of lesion studies led to an intermediate view, namely a brain organized (1) into highly specialized functional areas called "eloquent" regions (such as the central, Broca's and Wernicke's areas), in which any lesion gives rise to major irrevocable neurological deficits, and (2) into "non-functional" structures, with no apparent clinical consequence when injured.

Based on these initial anatomo-functional correlations and despite the description by some pioneers of several examples of post-lesional recovery [9, 138], the dogma of a static functional organization of the brain was secure for a long time, with no ability to compensate for any injury involving the so-called eloquent areas. However, through regular reports of improvement of the functional status following damage to cortical and/or subcortical structures considered as "critical", this view of a "fixed" central nervous system has been called into question. In particular, slow-growing cerebral tumors such as low grade gliomas (LGG), have demonstrated that large amounts of cerebral tissue may be removed, inside or outside the so-called eloquent areas, with impressive recovery and often no detectable permanent functional consequences [37]. This finding parallels some old reports in humans and animals. In humans, for instance, it was shown that large brain tumors did not prevent patients from living a normal life [69, 138]. As a consequence, a growing number of investigations have recently been performed, not only in vitro and in animals, but also in humans since the development of non-invasive neuroimaging methods, in order to study the mechanisms underlying these compensatory phenomena: the concept of cerebral plasticity was born.

The goal of this article is to link enhanced understanding of the pathophysiology of cerebral plasticity (at sub-cellular, cellular, up to the topographical level) to the possible use of this dynamic potential for clinical applications in neuro-oncology.

## Cerebral plasticity: fundamental considerations

### *Definitions*

Cerebral plasticity is a continuous process allowing short-term, middle-term and long-term remodelling of the neural organization, with the aim of optimizing the functioning of brain networks [49]. Plastic changes constitute fundamental events which underly various kinds of brain development (1) during phylogenesis, with structural and functional cerebral maturation throughout evolution of the species; (2) during ontogeny and ageing, with the elaboration of new circuits induced by learning, and also with the maintenance of neural networks in adults into old age [63]: these physiological processes constitute "natural plasticity"; (3) after injury of the peripheral or central nervous system, with functional reshaping underlying a partial or complete clinical recovery: this is the "post-lesional plasticity" [146]. In all cases, these dynamic phenomena have to be stabilized in order to allow the functioning of the system: these mechanisms of regulation represent "homeostatic plasticity" [133].

### *Pathophysiological mechanisms subserving cerebral plasticity*

Several mechanisms underlying brain plasticity have been reported, from the ultrastuctural to the topographical levels [14, 47] (Table 1).

At the ultrastructural scale, beyond the processing involved in development [66] and potentiated by learning according to Hebbian's concept [22], the other mechanisms advocated are: modifications of synaptic weight [15, 87], synchrony [75], unmasking of latent connections and networks [70, 81], glial modulation [52, 61], regulation by the extracellular matrix [26], phenotypic changes [74, 102, 134] and neurogenesis [57, 60, 79, 112] – which might also play a role in glioma genesis [114].

**Table 1.** *Mechanisms subserving brain plasticity at ultrastructural and macroscopic levels*

| Microscopic level | Map level |
|---|---|
| Modification of synaptic weight | Resolution of diaschisis |
| Synchrony | within-area reshaping via recruitment of functional redundancies |
| Unmasking of latent connections and networks | Redistribution within eloquent network |
| Glial modulation | Cross-modal plasticity |
| Phenotypic changes | Macroscopic changes |
| Neurogenesis | Compensatory strategies |

These ultrastructural changes may lead to a functional reorganization at a macroscopic scale, via the following mechanisms: resolution of diaschisis [121]; within-area reshaping via recruitment of functional redundancies [29, 31], redistribution within eloquent network [104] – especially through the recruitment of contralateral homologue areas [72] – cross-modal plasticity [6, 54, 93], compensatory strategies [107] and macroscopic structural changes [28, 80, 97].

Moreover, numerous experiments over the past twenty years in animals have demonstrated that functional cortical organization could be modulated not only by experience, but also by lesions of the peripheral [117, 144] and central nervous system [94]. This plastic potential was observed within the visual, auditory, and above all, sensorimotor cortex [78, 108]. Furthermore, the possibility that functional recovery is modulated by the kinetics of the lesion inflicted on the brain has been addressed in a series of animal studies [1, 53, 89, 96, 105, 125, 139]. Such factors are very important in order to better understand the variability with regard to the functional compensation in humans with cerebral lesions, according to the time-course of the injury (acute versus slow-growing lesions) – thus to adapt the therapeutic strategy, as will be detailed later [25]. In addition to studies showing that the cortical motor map could be modulated by skill acquisition with specific learning-dependent enlargement of cortical representation, animal studies suggested that, after local damage to the motor cortex, rehabilitative training such as constraint-therapy could shape subsequent reorganization in the adjacent intact cortex and could favor the recruitment of the undamaged motor cortex, which might play an important role in motor recovery [94]. These first results in animals have provided the basis for the elaboration of specific retraining in humans following nervous system injury (see below). Potentiation of post-lesional plasticity using pharmacological agents was also tested in animals, especially with the demonstration of a neuroprotective effect on the somatotopic map with chronic treatments such as piracetam [146].

In summary, the better understanding of the pathophysiological mechanisms underlying the functional and morphological changes (and their stabilization) at the microscopic and macroscopic levels, as studied in vitro, in vivo in animals and also in silico, have provided the basis for analyzing the behavioural plasticity in humans.

## Natural plasticity in humans

Despite a static "point by point" view of the somatotopic organization of the homonculus since its description by Penfield in humans [100], recent studies in healthy volunteers have demonstrated the existence of multiple represention of movements within the primary sensorimotor cortex [115], with an overlap and a likely hierarchical organization of the functional redundancies [65]. It has been advocated that some cortical sites within the primary motor area could correspond to a representation of muscle, while other sites might rather correspond to a representation of postures, and even of more complex movements [56, 59]. Moreover, this cortical representation of the muscles and movements seems to be organized as a "mosaic" [118], which may facilitate an intrinsic reshaping of this primary area during learning and following an injury (see below). These concepts are in accordance with neurofunctional imaging studies performed in healthy volunteers during skill learning [10]: extension of activation was observed, most likely corresponding to a recruitment of adjacent sites in order to favor the acquisition of new motor sequences. Interestingly, this phenomenon can be durable, particularly in musicians [92].

In addition to this "spatial" distribution based on multiple functional representations, the "temporal" organization of this mosaic must also be considered. Numerous electrophysiological recording studies, notably using magnetoencephalography in humans, have shown changes in neural activity in the sensorimotor cortex following skill learning, and changes in oscillations of neural activity in this same region during motor action [111]. These oscillations could reflect the synchronous cortical activity of many neurons, and might allow the rapid modification of the ensemble of neurons involved in the execution of a motor task, through a modulation of their temporal relationships [75]. Therefore, these mechanisms could contribute to sensorimotor plasticity.

Beyond this dynamic organization of the primary sensorimotor cortex with its ability to reshape, such plasticity mechanisms also imply possible changes (a) in activity within the other "non-primary" structures implicated in the sensorimotor network, and (b) in the effective connectivity within this whole network – as revealed by measurement of the coherence of the activity between the distinct areas involved in the sensorimotor function [2].

Finally, this recent progress in human brain mapping methods has also led to a revised view of the neural basis of language, i.e. a spatio-temporal functioning of parallel distributed cortico-cortical and cortico-subcortical networks, with the simultaneous and/or successive involvement of a mosaic of hierarchically organized areas, some of them essential and others compensatable, with an inter-individual variability [136].

## Plasticity in acute brain lesions

### *Post-lesional sensorimotor plasticity*

In cases of acute cerebral lesions, especially stroke, plasticity mechanisms frequently include both intrinsic reorganization of the primary sensorimotor cortex, and also the recruitment of other "non-primary" regions implicated in the functional network. Indeed, remodelling of the primary sensorimotor area was first observed following damage to the corticospinal pathway, in particular in cases of deep stroke: the cortical representation of the paretic hand expanded laterally, within the face representation [141]. Second, due to the fact that reorganization within the primary sensorimotor cortex is often insufficient to insure a (complete) functional compensation, numerous neurofunctional studies performed in patients who recovered following a lesion of the sensorimotor network showed activations of other ipsi-hemispheric regions – such as the premotor areas [18], supplementary motor area [16], retrocentral areas including the posterior parietal cortex [32], and the insula [19]. Furthermore, the participation of the contralateral hemisphere, in particular the "mirror" primary sensorimotor area was also suggested [16, 84, 98, 104]. In the same way, in cases of damage involving the primary somatosensory area, several works showed the recruitment of the contralateral homologue [57], in addition to the ipsilateral posterior insula and to the secondary somatosensory areas bilaterally [32]. However, it is worth noting that, in recent longitudinal studies following stroke, with repeated neurofunctional imaging performed in the same patients throughout their recovery, the exact role of the contralateral homologue was questioned [51, 86].

### *Post-lesional language plasticity*

In cases of acute brain lesions involving the language network, as for the sensorimotor function, plasticity mechanisms seem to be based: first on intrinsic reorganisation within injured language areas (indice of favorable outcome) [62, 64, 106]; second, when this reshaping is insufficient, other regions implicated in the language circuits will be recruited, in the ipsilateral hemisphere (close and even remote to the damaged area) then in the contralateral hemisphere [142] – even in this case however, the functional recovery is usually poor [122].

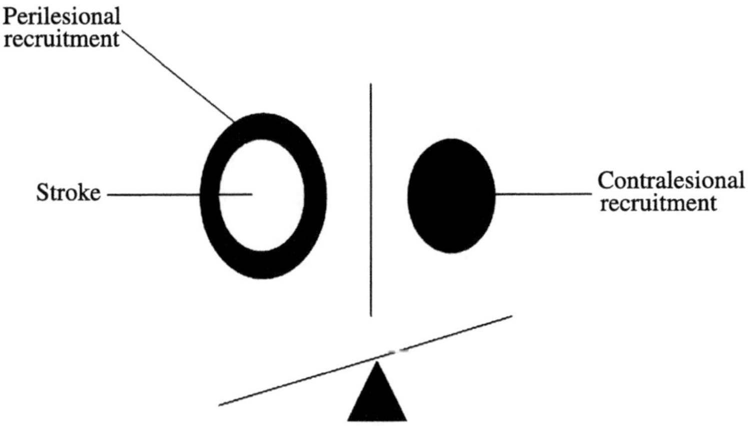


**Fig. 1.** Hierarchical model of functional compensation following acute stroke, with a recruitment of ipsilesional (especially peri-lesional) areas before the recruitment of contralateral homologous. Remote compensations are a marker of poor recovery

In summary, numerous observations of functional improvement following acute brain lesions have been reported, most of the time in stroke studies, underlining the existence of a post-lesional plasticity. Moreover, recent advances in non-invasive neurofunctional imaging has allowed a better understanding of the mechanisms of cerebral remapping. These data suggest that functional recovery is better when occurring within the limits of the original (non lesioned) network. The best outcome is found when plastic neural reorganizations take place within the regions adjacent to the infarct zone. A poor level of recovery is usually observed when neural reorganizations involve the intact (contralateral) hemisphere (Fig. 1).

Nevertheless, due to the acute nature of this kind of lesion, it was impossible to compare the redistributed maps to the functional organization before the damage – because of the lack of neuroimaging examination in the patient before the brain injury. Furthermore, the recovery was incomplete in many patients. As a consequence, it seems that stroke represents a limited model of the study of cerebral plasticity. Interestingly, more recently, researches have been performed in slow-growing brain tumors, especially in low-grade gliomas (LGG): these works have provided new insights into the brain's capacity of functional compensation.

## Plasticity in slow-growing brain tumors: the example of low-grade glioma

LGG – gliomas WHO grade II – are slow-growing primary tumors of the central nervous system, which represent approximately 15% of gliomas [140]. They can evolve in three ways: (1) local growth (2) invasion (3) anaplastic transformation. First, recent works demonstrated that before any anaplastic degeneration, LGG showed a continuous, constant growth of it mean tumor diameter over time, with an average of around 4 mm per year [82]. Second, invasion of LGG along the main white matter pathways within the lesional hemisphere or even contralaterally via the corpus callosum has also been extensively described [83]. Third, it is currently well-known that LGG systematically changes its biological nature and evolves to a high grade glioma, with a median of anaplastic transformation of around 7 to 8 years, a process which proves fatal (median survival around 10 years) [143].

Interestingly, during the long stage before the transformation of the tumor, in spite of some possible slight cognitive disorders (in particular involving working memory) found only using extensive neuropsychological assessments [127, 129], the patient presents most of the time with a normal neurological examination and has a normal socio-professional life. Indeed, more than 80% of LGG are revealed by seizures, usually efficiently treated by antiepileptic drugs [23]. Thus, due to the recent advances in the field of functional mapping, many authors have studied brain plasticity in patients harboring a LGG, with the goal (1) to better understand the mechanisms of cerebral reorganization induced by these slow-growing tumors, explaining the frequent lack of deficit despite an invasion of the so-called "eloquent areas" and (2) to try to use this dynamic potential in order to improve the functional and neurooncological result in treatment of LGG, especially surgical resection [25, 42].

## *Functional reorganization induced by LGG*

Numerous preoperative neurofunctional imaging studies have recently shown that LGG induced a progressive redistribution of the eloquent sites, explaining why most of these patients have a normal neurological examination or only a slight deficit [37].

Interestingly, the patterns of reorganization may differ between patients [42] (Fig. 2).

In the first one, due to the infiltrative feature of gliomas, function still persists within the tumor. This LGG invasion to functional sensorimotor and language cortices was reported as possibly occurring in up to 36% of cases in some recent series using magnetoencephalography [55].

In the second possible pattern of reshaping, eloquent areas are redistributed immediately around the tumor, according to a mechanism of "within-area" reorganization. With reference to sensorimotor function, preoperative neuroimaging showed that the activated areas on the tumor side could be broader than in normal volunteers and/or could be displaced compared with that in the normal contralateral hemisphere – with a functional shift which cannot be explained by the anatomical deformation of the central sulcus [3]. As

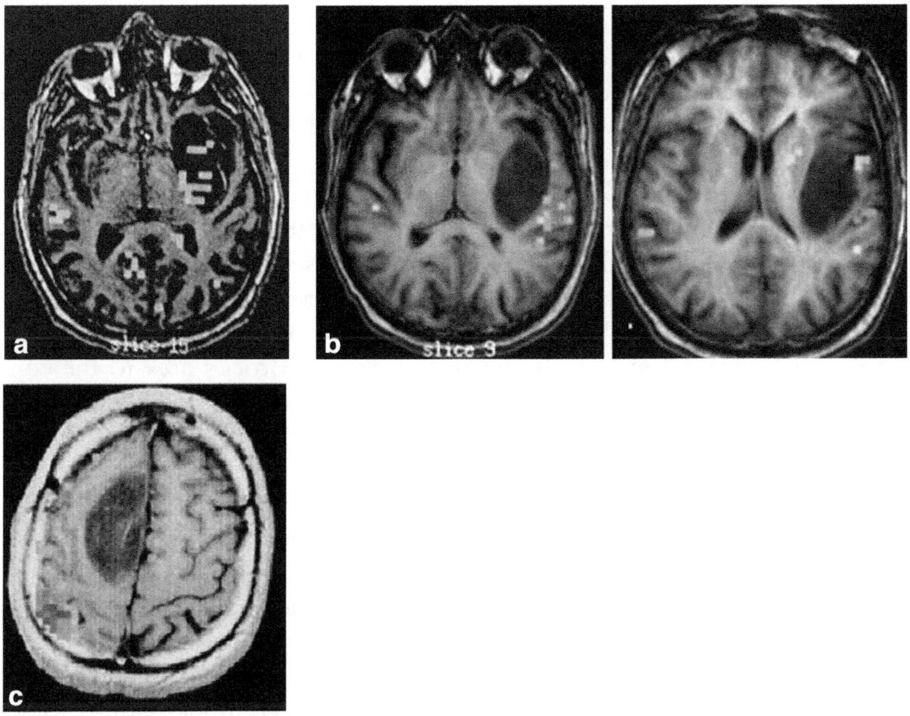


**Fig. 2.** Different patterns of remapping induced by slow-growing LGG, as shown by preoperative fMRI (a) intralesional activations during fluency task in a patient with no deficit harboring a left insular LGG (b) perilesional language reshaping during fluency task in a patient with no deficit harboring a left insular LGG (c) recruitment of contralateral homologous, with activation of the left contrahemispheric SMA during movement of the left hand (in addition to the activation of the right primary motor cortex), in a patient with no deficit harboring a right mesio-premotor LGG

regards language, activation of the adjacent left inferior frontal cortex was demonstrated for patients without aphasic symptoms harboring glioma located within the classical Broca's area [90].

In the third pattern of compensation, there is a recruitment of a widely distributed network within the lesion hemisphere. Typically, concerning motor function, activation of thc "secondary motor areas", including the supplemen tary motor area, the premotor cortex and even the superior parietal lobe was frequently observed in patients performing a simple (and not complex) motor task [3, 73]. Concerning the recruitment of the other regions implicated in the language circuit, activation of the left superior temporal gyrus was shown for a glioma within Broca's area [62, 90], while an activation of the Broca's area was observed in left temporoparietal tumor [90]. Moreover, patients with slowly evolving gliomas regularly recruited frontolateral regions other than "classic" language areas, such as left BA 46, BA 47, supplementary motor area (and left cerebellum) [90, 131]. Finally, the left insula, a structure known to be involved in the complex planning of speech, when invaded by a LGG, was demonstrated to be compensated for by the recruitment of a network involving not only Broca's area and the left superior temporal gyrus, but also the left putamen [33].

There is also possible compensation by the contralateral hemisphere, likely due to a decrease of the transcallosal inhibition on the opposite homologous area. In glioma located within the rolandic region, several reports found activations within the contralesional primary motor cortex [5, 109], the contralesional premotor area [50] and contralateral supplementary motor area [72]. Concerning language function, both translocation of Broca's area to the contralateral hemisphere as the result of the growth of left inferior frontal glioma [67] and translocation of Wernicke's area to the right hemisphere in left temporo-parietal glioma [101] have been demonstrated.

Finally, association of different patterns was reported, in particular with combination of peritumoral and contra-hemispheric activations, both for sensorimotor [50] and language [62, 90] functions. In the largest activation study to date in patients with gliomas of the left hemisphere, in addition to left activations, right inferior frontal activations were reported in 60% of patients [131].

Therefore, sensorimotor and language plasticity mechanisms in slow-growing LGG seem to be based on an hierarchically organized model, similar to the one previously described in stroke, i.e.: first, with intrinsic reorganization within injured areas, the perilesional structures playing a major role in the functional compensation [62, 131]; when this reshaping is not sufficient, with recruitment of other regions implicated in the functional network, in the ipsilateral hemisphere (remote to the damaged area) then in the contralateral hemisphere. Indeed, some works even stated that in cases of bilateral activations, langage performances could be worse than after possible regression of the right activations [62]. However, the debate concerning the actual role of the recruitment of the contralateral homologuous area through a decrease of the transcallosal inhibition [123] – inhibition essential during language learning – is still open [67, 104]. The use of new techniques such as TMS might provide further information [132], in particular taking account of additional parameters such as the inter-individual variability of the hemispheric specialization for language [136] and the timing of occurrence of the lesion during language acquisition [91]. In this way, a recent combined PET and TMS study in right-handed patients with a left glioma, showed that all subjects had a significant activation of the left inferior frontal gyrus, and that they were all susceptible to TMS over this left IFG. Moreover, 50% had an associated right IFG activity during verb generation: these patients had also significantly longer language latencies during TMS over the right IFG. These results have indicated that in all patients, but especially in those with left IFG activation only, the residual language function

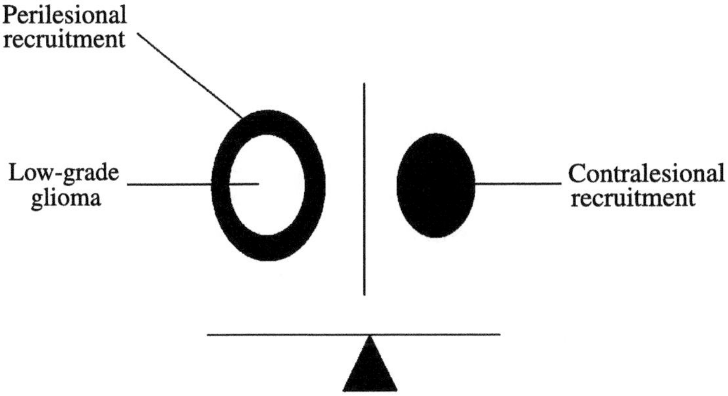


**Fig. 3.** Hierarchical model of functional compensation in case of slow-growing LGG, with a recruitment of ipsilesional (especially peri-lesional) areas before the recruitment of contralateral homologous. However, in this pathology, remote compensations are not a marker of poor recovery. Thus, bilateral recruitments are frequent in patients with a normal clinical examination

of the left hemisphere was responsible for maintenance of language function – reinforcing the hypothesis which emphasized the importance of the residual language capacity of the left hemisphere for quality of language compensation. However, this study also demonstrated relevant language function of the right IFG in right-handed patients with gliomas of the left hemisphere [132].

In summary, the data above suggest that different plastic processes compensate for LGG invasion. These processes seem to follow a hierarchical model similar to the one previously discussed in the context of acute strokes: local compensations take place before the occurrence of remote recruitments. Beyond this analogy, however, LGG recovery presents two major specificities. First, compensations can involve areas that are not part of the typical functional network (e.g. BA 46, BA 47, for speech [131]). Second, remote compensations in the intact or lesioned hemisphere are not a marker of poor recovery (Fig. 3). Concerning this latter point, one may argue that LGG resections would be impossible if this was not the case. Indeed, if efficient plastic compensations were only possible within and around the glioma, it would be impossible to resect the tumoral tissue without generating major functional deficits. With respect to this point, it may be noticed that neurosurgeons usually tend to remove a small layer of tissue around the tumor to increase the likelihood of obtaining a more complete resection [44].

## *Functional reorganization induced by LGG resection*

While controversial for a long time, maximal resection of brain glioma, especially LGG, when possible, appears currently to be a valuable treatment to influence the natural history of this tumor [7, 21, 44]. Thus, the double goal of surgery is to maximize the quality of resection while minimizing the operative risk [46]. Nonetheless, due to the frequent location of supratentorial gliomas near or within so-called "eloquent" areas [40], and due to their infiltrative feature previously mentioned, it was considered that the chances to perform an extensive glioma removal were low, whereas the risk of inducing post-operative sequelae was high. Indeed, many surgical series have reported a rate of permanent and severe deficit between 13% and 27.5% following removal of intra-axial tumors [12, 119, 137]. Therefore, to optimize the benefit to risk ratio of surgery, functional mapping methods have been used extensively in the last decade. We have already detailed that slow-growing LGG induced brain reshaping with a considerable interindividual anatomofunctional variability [42]. It is thus mandatory to study for each patient the cortical functional organization, the effective connectivity and the brain plastic potential, in order to tailor the resection according to both oncological and also cortico-subcortical functional boundaries.

## Methodological considerations

The knowledge of such a preoperative functional reorganization is very important for both surgical indication and planning [55]. Indeed, if function still persists within the tumor, there is very limited chance to perform a good resection without inducing postoperative sequelae [120]. Conversely, if eloquent areas are redistributed around the tumor [90], there is a reasonable chance of performing a near-total resection despite a likely immediate transient deficit – but with secondary recovery within some weeks to some months (see below). Finally, if there is already a preoperative compensation by ispsilesional remote areas [62] and/or by the contra-hemispheric homologuous area [5, 67, 72, 109], the chances to perform a real total resection are high, with only a slight and very transient deficit.

Nevertheless, accumulating evidence seems to indicate that the BOLD response in the vicinity of brain tumors does not reflect the neuronal signal as accurately as it does in healthy tissue, – with the sensitivity still too low [110]. Although poorly understood, the mechanisms seem not to result from reduced neuronal activity, but rather from an alteration of neurovascular and metabolic coupling [4]. Consequently, glioma-induced neurovascular uncoupling may cause reduced fMRI signal in perilesional eloquent cortex, in conjunction with normal or increased activity in homologous brain regions: this phenomenon can simulate a pseudo-reorganization of the function, namely can mimic a false functional transfer to the opposite side of the lesion preoperatively [135].

This is the reason why the additional use of intraoperative direct electrical stimulation (DES) has been widely advocated, under general or local anesthesia, during surgery of glioma in eloquent areas [8, 44]. DES allows the mapping of motor function (possibly under general anesthesia, by inducing involuntary movement if stimulation of a motor site), somatosensory function (by eliciting dysesthesia described by the patient himself), and also cognitive functions such as language (spontaneaous speech, object naming, comprehension, etc. . . .), calculation, memory, reading or writing, performed in these cases on awake patients – by generating transient disturbances if DES is applied at the level of a functional "epicenter" [95].

Furthermore, DES also permits the study of the anatomo-functional connectivity by directly stimulating the white matter tracts all along the resection [43, 46]. A speech therapist must be present in the operative room, in order to interpret accurately the kind of disorders induced by the cortical and subcortical stimulations, e.g. speech arrest, anarthria, speech apraxia, phonological disturbances, semantic paraphasia, perseveration, anomia, and so on [45]. Such on-line intraoperative anatomo-functional correlations give a unique opportunity to study the individual connectivity, as demonstrated concerning (1) motor pathways and their somatotopy from the corona radiata to the internal capsule and the mesencephalic peduncles [38], (2) thalamo-cortical somatosensory pathways [37], (3) subcortical visual pathways [43], (4) pathway subserving the spatial cognition, that is, the superior fronto-occipital fasciculus [130] and right superior longitudinal fasciculus [124], as well as (5) and language pathways – concerning loco-regional connectivity, cortico-cortical connections such as the phonological loop, striato-cortical loop such as the subcallosal medialis fasciculus, as well as long-distance association language bundles such as the arcuate fasciculus [34] or the inferior fronto-occiptal fasciculus involved in the semantic connectivity [45].

Therefore, DES represents an accurate, reliable and safe technique for the on-line detection of the cortical and subcortical regions essential for the function, at each place and each moment of the resection. Consequently, any functional disturbance induced by DES with reproducibility must lead to interruption of the resection at this level, both for cortical and subcortical structures. The tumor removal is then performed according to functional boundaries, in order to optimize the quality of resection while minimizing the risk of postoperative permanent deficit [44].

## Intra-operative plasticity

Thus, DES during surgery for LGG within or near the sensorimotor areas, has allowed the study of brain plasticity in humans. In this way, cortical stimulation after brain exposure and before any resection confirmed the frequent existence of a peri-lesional redistribution of the eloquent areas, due to the slow-growing LGG, as suggested by preoperative neurofunctional imaging [37, 42].

These observations were also confirmed using DES under local anesthesia during resection of LGG within language areas, in patients with no or slight previous deficit. Indeed, as preoperative functional neuroimaging, stimulations also found essential language sites (i.e. eliciting language disturbances when stimulated) preferentially located in the immediate vicinity of the lesion, sup-

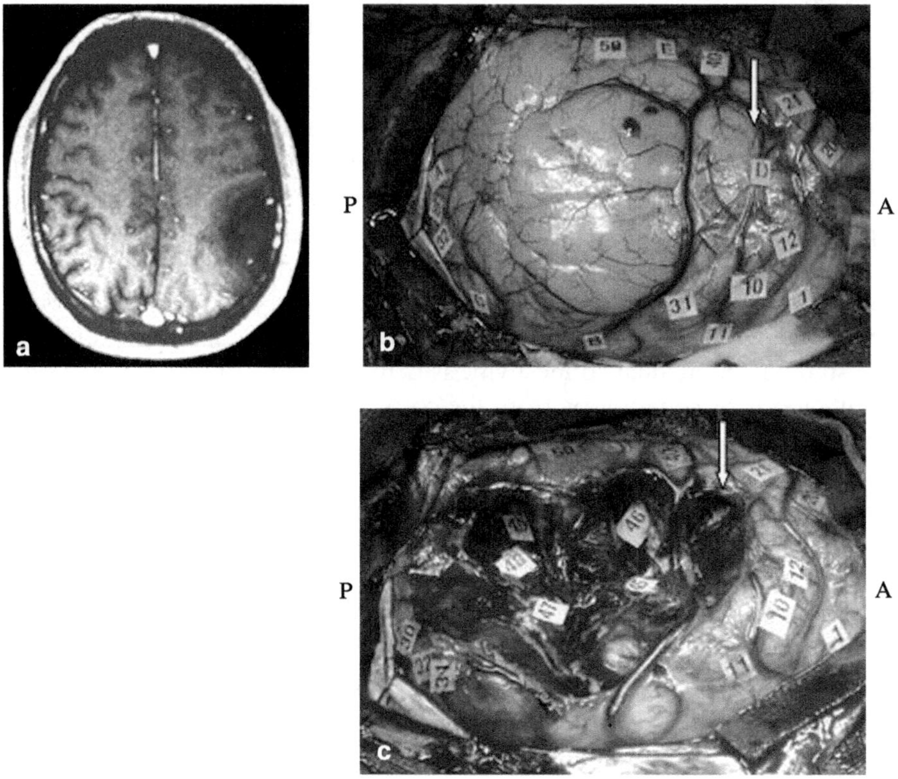


**Fig. 4.** Language reorganization induced by a LGG located within the left supramarginal gyrus (a) Preoperative axial T1-weighted enhanced MRI (b) Intraoperative view before resection of the tumor, delineated by letter tags. Electrical cortical mapping shows a reshaping of the eloquent maps, with a recruitment of perilesional language sites, i.e. the rolandic operculum (tags 20 and 21), angular gyrus (tags 30 and 32) and posterior part of the superior temporal gyrus (tags 40 and 50). The straight arrow shows the lateral part of the retrocentral sulcus. (c) Intraoperative view after resection of the tumor. Electrical subcortical mapping has enabled to study the individual anatomo-functional language connectivity. Indeed, deeply and posteriorly, the posterosuperior loop of the arcuate fasciculus was identified, by eliciting phonological paraphasia during each stimulation (tag 40, 47 and 49). More anteriorly, the lateral part of the superior longitudinal fasciculus was detected, by inducing speech apraxia (articulatory disturbances) (tag 45 and 46). It is worth noting that in the depth, the resection was continued up to the contact of these language pathways, in order to optimize the quality of resection while preserving the eloquent white matter tracts. The arrow shows the lateral part of the retrocentral sulcus. The straight arrow shows the lateral part of the retrocentral sulcus. *A* Anterior, *P* posterior

porting the hypothesis of the major contribution of the intrinsic reshaping mechanisms [25, 37, 42]. For instance, reshaping of the language sites was observed around the Broca's area invaded by a LGG, with a functional compensation related to recruitment of adjacent regions such as the left ventral premotor cortex, the middle frontal gyrus (BA 46) and the pars orbitaris of the IFG (BA 47). Also, the compensation of left insular involvement by LGG, owing to the recruitment of Broca's area, the left superior temporal gyrus and the putamen, was demonstrated intraoperatively by DES [33]. In addition, DES showed a language reshaping of the left supramarginal gyrus, with a recruitment of perilesional sites, i.e. the rolandic operculum, angular gyrus and posterior part of the superior temporal gyrus (Fig. 4). These results fit very well with those reported using neurofunctional imaging previously reviewed.

Furthermore, the persistence of structures still functional within LGG was equally confirmed using DES [46]. Indeed, paresthesias were induced during stimulation of the primary somatosensory cortex despite its tumoral invasion, and motor face responses were elicited during stimulation of the primary motor area involved by LGG [37]. Also, DES regurlarly induced speech disorders when applied over the left insular cortex, even when invaded [30].

It is worth noting that because brain exposure is performed only around the invaded area, DES is generally not relevant for investigating distant compensations.

Regarding intra-surgical plasticity, a very puzzling observation concerns the existence of acute functional remapping triggered by the resection itself that takes place within 15 to 60 minutes of beginning the surgical act. This type of acute reorganization has been very well documented in the motor system (for areview [32]). For instance, it was reported in a 39 old patient with a left precentral lesion and normal pre-operative neurological evaluation [29]. Intraoperative DES performed caudally to the lesion, prior to any resection, allowed identification of three functional sites in M1: one for the forearm, one for the wrist and one for the fingers. No other response was found. Cortical stimulations performed during and after resection replicated the three motor responses identified intraoperatively (of course stimulation parameters were kept constant throughout surgery). Interestingly, two new functional sites were also detected in regions that did not show any response before resection. These sites induced hand and arm movements. They were located in the precentral gyrus, in front of the three original sites. Identical observations were reported in other patients in a subsequent study [31]. Similar acute reorganizations were also found after postcentral resections [32]. The origin of these changes remains poorly understood. The most likely hypothesis suggests that a local increase of cortical excitability allows an acute unmasking of latent functional redundancies (i.e. multiple cortical representation of the same function), via a decrease of intracortical inhibition [29, 31]. In agreement with this idea, animal models have shown that focal brain damages induce large zones of enhanced cortical excitability in both the lesioned and the intact hemisphere [13]. Likewise, human studies have provided evidence that the level of intracortical inhibition is reduced in the damaged hemisphere in stroke patients [20]. Whether or not this hypothesis of increased excitability is true, it is tempting to speculate that the latent redundant networks revealed by the resection process participate in functional recovery. This idea fits well with the importance of adjacent reorganizations for behavioral recuperation.

## Post-operative plasticity

While mechanisms of post-stroke recuperation have been thoroughly investigated during the last 50 years, the processes of post-resection recovery in slow growing lesions have emerged only recently as a major subject of research. This explains why data associated with this topic remain scarce. However, this scarcity is counterbalanced by the existence of a relative consensus among studies. The post-operative literature reinforces the pre-surgical observations by suggesting that functional recovery involves a large array of complementary mechanisms. For instance, using Magneto-Encephalography (MEG), it has been reported that resections of the somatosensory cortex (S1) caused perilesional sites to be recruited around the cavity, within the postcentral gyrus [88]. In addition to this local remapping, contributions of S2, the posterior parietal cortex, and the primary motor cortex were also reported using post-operative DES [32]. Similar combinations of local and remote reorganizations were found in the language domain, after resections of Broca's area. In this case, DES performed right at the end of the resection showed that plasticity involved a reorganization of the neural networks within the premotor cortex, the pars orbitaris of the inferior frontal gyrus, and the insula [37].

Probably, the best evidence for efficient postoperative compensations in remote structures comes from SMA resections. Ablation of this area usually produces an SMA syndrome, due to the removal of the SMA-proper [71]. This syndrome regresses spontaneously within 10 days. Postoperative fMRI images taken after the regression of this surgically-induced SMA syndrome suggest that plastic functional compensations involve the contralesional SMA, the controlesional premotor cortex [72] and, potentially, the ipsilesional primary motor cortex [37]. Unfortunately, to date, no study has tried to directly investigate the functional role of these structures using, for instance, TMS. This direct approach was however exercised in a recent study involving two patients with a large resection of the posterior parietal cortex [11]. In these patients, TMS delivered over the intact parietal cortex did impair the accuracy and kinematic characteristics of reaching movements performed without vision of the arm. No TMS-related effect was observed for healthy subjects, as had already been reported in a previous study [24].

## *Therapeutic implications for LGG*

It was recently proposed to incorporate such better understanding of the individual plastic potential in the surgical strategy for LGG, with the goal (1) to extent the indications for resection in eloquent structures so far considered as "inoperable" (2) to maximize the quality of glioma removal, by performing the resection according to (not fixed) functional boundaries (3) while minimizing the risk of postoperative permanent neurological deficit [44] (Fig. 5).

Consequently, several surgical series showed that it was possible to remove LGG invading the following "eloquent" brain structures:

- SMA resection: it induces the occurrence of an SMA syndrome [148], spatially and temporally due to the removal of the SMA-proper [71]. As previously mentioned, postoperative fMRI after such a surgical SMA syndrome recovery argue in favor of a compensation by the controlateral SMA and premotor cortex [72], and also by the ipsilesional primary motor cortex [37].
- Insular resection: despite a hemiparesis after right insula removal, likely because this region is a non-primary motor area, and transient speech disturbances following left dominant insula resection, all patients recovered [147] – except in rare cases of deep stroke [30, 48]. Moreover, it was possible in right non-dominant fronto-temporo-insular LGG involving the deep grey nuclei, to remove the clautrum without any cognitive disorders (despite its role suggested in consciousness), and to also to remove the invaded striatum without inducing any motor deficit not movement disorders [35].
- S1 resection: the first results using pre- and post-operative MEG suggest the possible recruitment of 'redundant' eloquent sites around the cavity, within the postcentral gyrus [88]. It is in accordance with the DES data, showing unmasking of redundant somatosensory sites during resection, likely explained by the decrease of the cortico-cortical inhibition [31]. The recruitment of the second somatosensory area or posterior parietal cortex, M1 (due to strong anatomo-functional connections between the pre- and retrocentral gyri), and the controlateral S1 are also possible (for a review, see [32]). These plastic phenomena likely explain the recovery of the frequent transient postoperative sensory deficit.
- In addition, the resection of the (dominant) parietal posterior lobe can be performed without inducing any sequelae, and even with a possible improvement in comparaison to the preoperative status, especially using pointing task [11].
- Resection of non-dominant M1 of the face: the recovery of the usual transient central facial palsy [76], with a potential Foix-Chavany-Marie syndrome when the insula is also involved [39], is likely explained by the disinhibition of the contralateral homologous sites, via the transcallosal pathways.

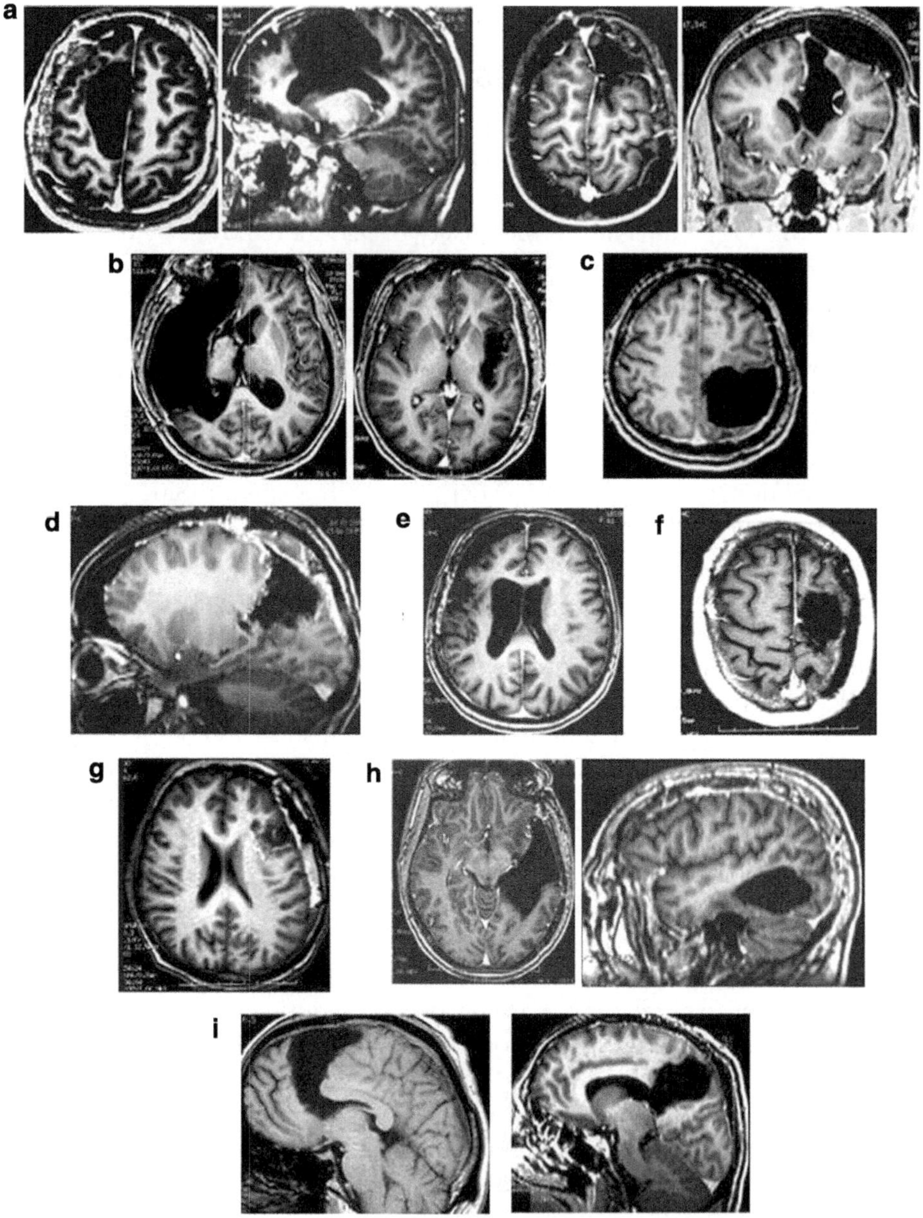


**Fig. 5.** Examples of complete resections of LGG (according to MRI criteria) within classical ''eloquent'' areas, with preservation of the quality of life, owing to the mechanisms of brain plasticity (a) resection involving the right and left supplementary motor areas (b) resection involving the right paralimbic system with the claustrum as well as the striatum (left) and involving the left insula (right) (c) resection involving the primary somatosensory area and the parietal posterior lobe (d) resection involving the left inferior parietal lobule (e) resection involving the primary sensorimotor cortex of the face (f) resection involving the primary motor area of the hand (g) resection involving Broca's area (h) resection involving the anterior and mid- (left) and posterior (right) left dominant temporal lobe (i) resection involving the corpus callosum

- Resection of M1 of the upper limb: on the basis of the existence of multiple cortical motor representations in humans using fMRI [116], and DES [31], the compensation of the motor function could be explained by the recruitment of parallel networks within M1 – allowing the superior limb area removal, eventually using two consecutive surgeries in order to induce durable remapping following the first one [36] (see below).
- Broca's area resection: any language compensation may reflect the recruitment of adjacent regions, in particular BA 46, BA 47 and the insula [42, 90, 131].
- Temporal language area resection: language compensation following left dominant temporal resection could be explained by the fact that this function seems to be organized with multiple parallel networks [136]. Consequently, beyond the recruitment of areas adjacent to the surgical cavity, the long term reshaping could be related to progressive involvement of first remote regions within the left dominant hemisphere – such as the posterior part of the superior temporal gyrus, the pars triangularis of inferior frontal gyrus or other left frontolateral regions (BA 46 and BA 47) [131] – second the contralateral right non-dominant hemisphere due to a transcallosal disinhibition phenomenon [62].
- Finally, a recent study showed that the resection of a part of the corpus callosum invaded by a LGG is possible without motor, language or cognitive deficit [41].

## Improvement of the functional and oncological results of LGG surgery

–Functional results

Thus, the integration of the study of individual plasticity provided by preoperative functional neuroimaging and intraoperative DES in the surgical decision and planning has enabled firstly extention of the indications for surgery for gliomas located in areas considered until now as "inoperable" [44]. Moreover, despite a frequent but transient immediate postoperative functional worsening (due to the attempt to perform a maximal tumor removal according to cortico-subcortical functional limits using IES), in a delay of 3 months following the surgery, more than 95% of patients recovered a normal neurological examination, even with a possible improvement in comparison with their preoperative status – and also with a significant decrease of seizures in 80% of patients with preoperative chronic epilepsia. It is important to underline that all patients returned to a normal socio-professional life, and have been extensively evaluated by repeated neurological examinations, combined with language assessment (in particular using the Boston Diagnostic Aphasia Examination) and neuropsychological assessment [38, 129]. This rate of less than 5% of sequelae is very reproducible among the teams using DES worlwide (for a review, see Ref. [44]).

Interestingly, in comparison, in series which did not use DES, the rate of sequelae ranged from 13 to 27.5%, with a mean of around 19% [12, 119, 137].

–Neuro-oncological results

Since DES allows identification of the cortical and subcortical eloquent structures individually, it seems logical to perform a resection according to *functional boundaries.* Indeed, it has been suggested to continue the resection until the functional structures are detected by DES, *and not before*, in order to optimize the quality of resection – without increasing the risk of permanent deficit [46]. This surgical strategy enables a significative improvement of the quality of glioma removal, despite a higher number of surgeries within critical areas, and a parallel decrease of the rate of sequelae. Indeed, in a recent study comparing LGG resected without or with DES in the same institution, it was demonstrated on control MRI that (1) 62% of gliomas selected for surgery were located within eloquent area with the use of DES, instead of only 35% without IES (2) only 37% of resections were subtotal (less than 10 cc of residue according to the classification from Ref. [7]) and 6% total (with no signal abnormality) without DES, whereas 50.8% of resections were subtotal and 25.4% subtotal with the use of DES ($p < 0.001$) [44].

Moreover, while extensive resection is still controversial in neuro-oncology, especially concerning LGG, current surgical results support the positive impact of such a "maximal" treatment strategy, i.e. with a benefit on the natural history of the tumors which seems to be directly related to the quality of resection. Indeed, it was recently shown in a consecutive series of low-grade gliomas operated on according to functional boundaries using DES that the mortality rate was 20.6% in cases of partial resection, instead of 8% in cases of subtotal resection and 0% in cases of total resection (follow-up 48 months) ($p = 0.02$) [44].

## Conclusions

The current view of the spatio-temporal functioning of the nervous system has dramatically changed. Indeed, the brain is now considered as a morphological and functional dynamic structure, influenced by the environment, and constituted of interactive distributed glio-neunoro-synaptic networks. Each of them comprises several essential and/or modulatory epicenters, with behavioral consequences depending on their effective connectivity, itself modulated by their synchrony. Moreover, this whole dynamic system is stabilized by a homeostatic plasticity.

The better understanding of these phenomena enables us to begin to guide this plastic potential, in order to favorably regulate the dynamic of the eloquent networks – with the aim of facilitating functional recovery following brain damage. Such a linkage between an improved knowledge of the pathophysiological mechanisms underlying cerebral plasticity and its focussed use opens now a large field of new therapeutic perspectives, applied to the functional restoration and the optimization of the quality of life in patients with brain tumors.

## Perspectives

Individual plastic potential could be better understood using repeated intraoperative mappings combined with post-surgical neurofunctional imaging, and *guided by specific post-operative rehabilitation program* in order to optimize the quality of functional recovery. Indeed, functional rehabilitation can be matched to specific (re-)training based on the repetition of the tasks, with the goal of facilitating plasticity phenomena leading to positive reinforcement while inhibiting the others. With regard to sensorimotor rehabilitation, functional neuroimaging studies have shown that (re-)activations of the brain structures may be induced by the mental imagery of the movement alone, by its observation, or by passive training [17]. In addition, a single session of physiotherapy seems to produce a use-dependent enlargement of motor cortex representations paralleled by an improvement in motor function in stroke patients, but with variable durability [77]. The principle of constraint-induced movement therapy is currently extensively used [128]. This method seems to generate (re-)expansion of the cortical motor areas, correlated to the functional recovery, on condition that such therapy is performed 6 hours instead of 3 hours per day [126]. Conversely, immobilization induces a decrease of the size of the cortical motor area. Finally, the timing of rehabilitation following the damage is still controversial, since some studies have suggested that 'precocious' physiotherapy might exacerbate brain injury due to an early postlesional vulnerable period.

With regard to aphasia therapy, while some randomized works have not demonstrated any significant difference between groups of patients with and without training, other trials have shown a favorable impact of language therapy [27]. This discrepancy may be due to differences in the intensity of training. Indeed, aphasia therapy has given strong arguments in favor of its efficacy on condition that the program comprised at least one hour of training per day in the three months following the lesion, namely a minimum of 90 hours (i.e. "constraint-induced therapy") [103]. Furthermore, recent neurofunctional imaging studies performed before and after training have shown a reshaping of the language map, in particular with a re-activation of the Broca's area and left supramarginal gyrus, and even with possible recruitment of the right non-dominant hemisphere [99]. Currently it is proposed that intensive language therapy should be specifically adapted to each aphasic symptom. For instance, semantic training seems more efficient than phonological therapy in patients with a semantic or mixed aphasia.

In patients with LGG, the functional status is now more systematically assessed using extensive neurological and neuropsychological examinations

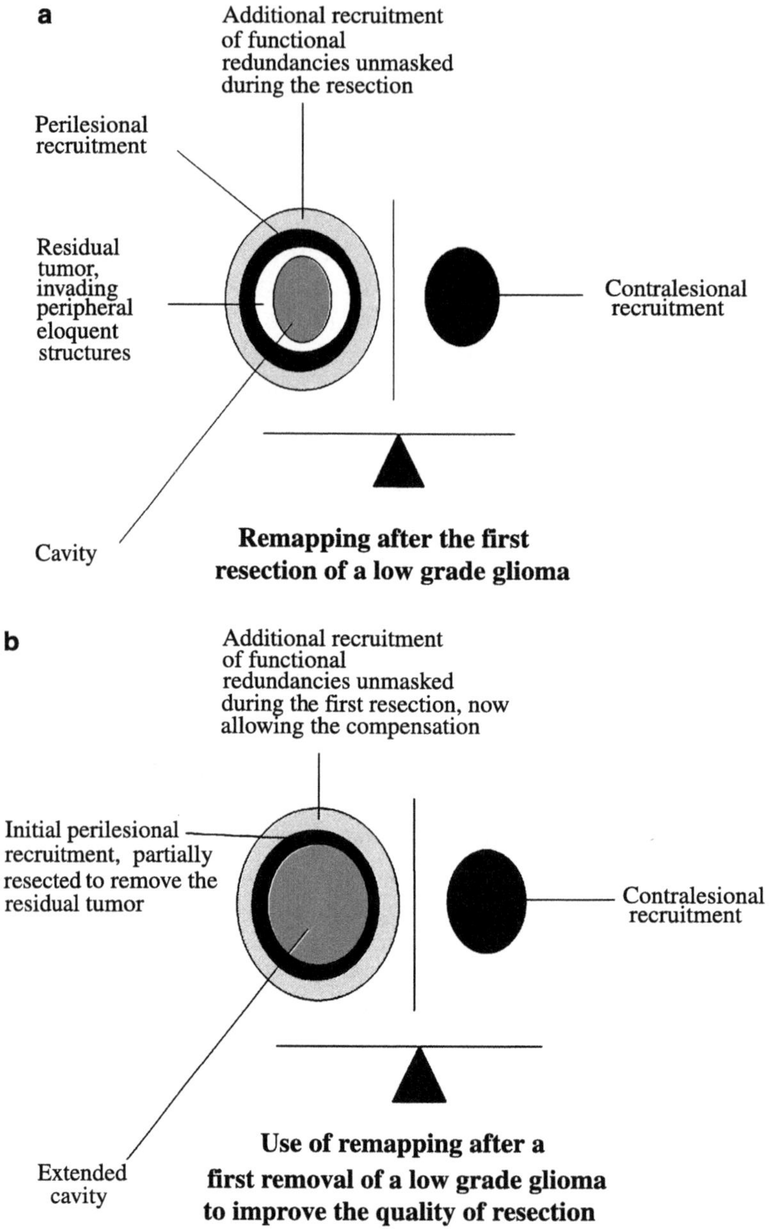


**Fig. 6.** (a) Model of acute plasticity induced by a first surgical resection, underlied by unmasking of additional perilesional functional redundancies (b) use of this remapping, once stabilized, in order to increase the quality of tumor removal while preserving the function, even if the residue involves the areas which have initially been implicated in the compensation of the slow-growing LGG

as well as using subjective scales – with the goal to precisely evaluate the quality of life. Such studies have demonstrated that specific rehabilitation was able to improve the postoperative functional status in comparison to the preoperative one, in particular with regard to cognitive functions such as working memory – in spite of frequent immediate postsurgical deterioration [129].

Long-term functional reorganization might be integrated into a dynamic surgical schedule [25], that is, by considering a second operation in order to increase the quality of resection, when LGG removal was not possible during the first surgery – on the basis of the reshaping of eloquent areas. Indeed, in cases of second surgery in patients with tumor regrowth, a novel intraoperative electrical mapping demonstrated the occurrence of a long-term reshaping of the sensorimotor and language regions [36]. These observations support the fact that the short-term plasticity induced by the first surgical resection can lead to a durable remapping, with an actual functional value, thereby allowing the subsequent removal of the residual tumor without sequelae [42]. Thus, there is the possibility of "dynamic planning" of surgery, by performing multiple resections if the complete removal of the LGG was not initially possible due to the involvement of essential eloquent areas, by eliciting plastic phenomena through the first operation itself [36] (Fig. 6) in addition to a specific rehabilitation program. As a consequence, it may prove possible to provide a more reliable and comprehensive pre-operative prediction of the potential for reorganization and its limitation for each patient using a biomethamatical model based on non-invasive neurofunctional imaging [85] to be integrated into the surgical strategy.

Such advances may enable optimization of the risk/benefit ratio of surgery for brain tumor surgery maximizing the impact on the natural history of the tumor while preserving the quality of life. It is nevertheless mandatory to validate all these new concepts via extensive multi-centre prospective studies.

## References

1. Adametz J (1959) Rate of recovery of functioning in cats with rostral reticular lesions: an experimental study. J Neurosurg 16: 85–97
2. Andres FG, Gerloff C (1999) Coherence of sequential movements and motor learning. J Clin Neurophysiol 16: 520–527
3. Atlas SW, Howard RS, Maldjian J, Alsop D, Detre JA, Listerud J, D'Esposito M, Judy KD, Zager E, Stecker M (1996) Functional magnetic resonance imaging of regional brain activity in patients with intracerebral gliomas: findings and implications for clinical management. Neurosurgery 38: 329–338
4. Aubert A, Costalat R, Duffau H, Benali H (2001) Modeling of pathophysiological coupling between brain electrical activation, energy metabolism and hemodynamics: insights for the interpretation of intracerebral tumor imaging. Acta Biotheor 50: 281–295
5. Baciu M, Le Bas JF, Segebarth C, Benabid AL (2003) Presurgical fMRI evaluation of cerebral reorganization and motor deficit in patients with tumors and vascular malformations. Eur J Radiol 46: 139–146

6. Bavelier D, Neville HJ (2002) Cross-modal plasticity: where and how? Nat Rev Neurosci 3: 443–452
7. Berger MS, Deliganis AV, Dobbins JD, Keles GE (1994) The effect of extent of resection on recurrence in patients with low grade cerebral hemisphere gliomas. Cancer 74: 1784–1791
8. Berger MS, Rostomily RC (1997) Low grade gliomas: functional mapping resection strategies, extent of resection, and outcome. J Neurooncol 34: 85–101
9. Bethe A, Fischer E (1931) Die Anpassungsfähigkeit (Plastizität) des Nervensystems. In: Bethe A, von Bergmann G, Emden G, Ellinger A (eds) Handbuch der normalen und pathologischen Physiologie. Springer, Berlin, Bd 15/2, pp 1045–1130
10. Bischoff-Grethe A, Goedert KM, Willingham DT, Grafton ST (2004) Neural substrates of response-based sequence learning using fMRI. J Cogn Neurosci 16: 127–138
11. Bonnetblanc F, Baraduc P, Duffau H, Desmurget M (2006) Visually-directed movements in slow lesions invading the posterior parietal cortex. TMS based evidence for plastic compensation by the controlesional homologue. NeuroImage 31 Suppl 1: S149
12. Brell M, Ibanez J, Caral L, Ferrer E (2000) Factors influencing surgical complications of intra-axial brain tumours. Acta Neurochir (Wien) 142: 739–750
13. Buchkremer-Ratzmann I, August M, Hagemann G, Witte OW (1996) Electrophysiological transcortical diaschisis after cortical photothrombosis in rat brain. Stroke 27: 1105–1109
14. Buonomano DV, Merzenich MM (1998) Cortical plasticity: from synapses to maps. Ann Rev Neurosci 21: 149–186
15. Byrne JH (1997) Synapses. Plastic plasticity. Nature 389: 791–792
16. Cao Y, D'Olhaberriague L, Vikingstad EM, Levine SR, Welch KM (1998) Pilot study of functional MRI to assess cerebral activation of motor function after poststroke hemiparesis. Stroke 29: 112–122
17. Carel C, Loubinoux I, Boulanouar K, Manelfe C, Rascol O, Celsis P, Chollet F (2000) Neural substrate for the effects of passive training on sensorimotor cortical representation: a study with functional magnetic resonance imaging in healthy subjects. J Cereb Blood Flow Metab 20: 478–484
18. Chassoux F, Devaux B, Landre E, Chodkiewicz JP, Talairach J, Chauvel P (1999) Postoperative motor deficits and recovery after cortical resections. Adv Neurol 81: 189–199
19. Chollet F, DiPiero V, Wise RJ, Brooks DJ, Dolan RJ, Frackowiak RS (1991) The functional anatomy of motor recovery after stroke in humans: a study with positron emission tomography. Ann Neurol 29: 63–71
20. Cicinelli P, Pasqualetti P, Zaccagnini M, Traversa R, Oliveri M, Rossini PM (2003) Interhemispheric asymmetries of motor cortex excitability in the postacute stroke stage: a paired-pulse transcranial magnetic stimulation study. Stroke 34: 2653–2658
21. Claus EB, Horlacher A, Hsu L, Schwartz RB, Dello-Iacono D, Talos F, Jolesz FA, Black PM (2005) Survival rates in patients with low-grade glioma after intraoperative magnetic resonance image guidance. Cancer 103: 1227–1233
22. Cruikshank SJ, Weinberger NM (1996) Evidence for the Hebbian hypothesis in experience-dependent physiological plasticity of neocortex: a critical review. Brain Res Rev 22: 191–228
23. DeAngelis LM (2001) Brain tumors. N Engl J Med 344: 114–123
24. Desmurget M, Epstein CM, Turner RS, Prablanc C, Alexander GE, Grafton ST (1999) Role of the posterior parietal cortex in updating reaching movements to a visual target. NatNeurosci 2: 563–567

25. Desmurget M, Bonnetblanc F, Duffau H (2007) Contrasting acute and slow-growing lesions: a new door to brain plasticity. Brain 130: 898–914
26. Dityatev A, Schachner M (2003) Extracellular matrix molecules and synaptic plasticity. Nat Rev Neurosci 4: 456–468
27. Doesborgh SJ, van de Sandt-Koenderman MW, Dippel DW, van Harskamp F, Koudstaal PJ, Visch-Brink EG (2004) Effects of semantic treatment on verbal communication and linguistic processing in aphasia after stroke: a randomized controlled trial. Stroke 35: 141–146
28. Draganski B, Gaser C, Busch V, Schuierer G, Bogdahn U, May A (2004) Changes in grey matter induced by training. Nature 427: 311–312
29. Duffau H, Sichez JP, Lehéricy S (2000) Intraoperative unmasking of brain redundant motor sites during resection of a precentral angioma. Evidence using direct cortical stimulations. Ann Neurol 47: 132–135
30. Duffau H, Capelle L, Lopes M, Faillot T, Sichez JP, Fohanno D (2000) The insular lobe: physiopathological and surgical considerations. Neurosurgery 47: 801–810
31. Duffau H (2001) Acute functional reorganisation of the human motor cortex during resection of central lesions: a study using intraoperative brain mapping. J Neurol Neurosurg Psychiatry 70: 506–513
32. Duffau H, Capelle L (2001) Functional recuperation following lesions of the primary somatosensory fields. Study of compensatory mechanisms. Neurochirurgie 47: 557–563
33. Duffau H, Bauchet L, Lehericy S, Capelle L (2001) Functional compensation of the left dominant insula for language. Neuroreport 12: 2159–2163
34. Duffau H, Capelle L, Sichez N, Denvil D, Lopes M, Sichez JP, Bitar A, Fohanno D (2002) Intraoperative mapping of the subcortical language pathways using direct stimulations. An anatomo-functional study. Brain 125: 199–214
35. Duffau H, Denvil D, Capelle L (2002) Absence of movement disorders after surgical resection of glioma invading the right striatum. J Neurosurg 97: 363–369
36. Duffau H, Denvil D, Capelle L (2002) Long term reshaping of language, sensory, and motor maps after glioma resection: a new parameter to integrate in the surgical strategy. J Neurol Neurosurg Psychiatry 72: 511–516
37. Duffau H, Capelle L, Denvil D, Sichez N, Gatignol P, Lopes M, Mitchell MC, Sichez JP, van Effenterre R (2003) Functional recovery after surgical resection of low grade gliomas in eloquent brain: hypothesis of brain compensation. J Neurol Neurosurg Psychiatry 74: 901–907
38. Duffau H, Capelle L, Denvil D, Sichez N, Gatignol P, Taillandier L, Lopes M, Mitchell MC, Roche S, Muller JC, Bitar A, Sichez JP, van Effenterre R (2003) Usefulness of intraoperative electrical subcortical mapping during surgery for low-grade gliomas located within eloquent brain regions: functional results in a consecutive series of 103 patients. J Neurosurg 98: 764–778
39. Duffau H, Karachi C, Gatignol P, Capelle L (2003) Transient Foix-Chavany-Marie syndrome after surgical resection of a right insulo-opercular low-grade glioma: case report. Neurosurgery 53: 426–431
40. Duffau H, Capelle L (2004) Preferential brain locations of low-grade gliomas. Cancer 100: 2622–2626
41. Duffau H, Khalil I, Gatignol P, Denvil D, Capelle L (2004) Surgical removal of corpus callosum infiltrated by low-grade glioma: functional outcome and oncological considerations. J Neurosurg 100: 431–437

42. Duffau H (2005) Lessons from brain mapping in surgery for low-grade glioma: insights into associations between tumour and brain plasticity. Lancet Neurol 4: 476–486
43. Duffau H (2005) Intraoperative cortico-subcortical stimulations in surgery of low-grade gliomas. Expert Rev Neurother 5: 473–485
44. Duffau H, Lopes M, Arthuis F, Bitar A, Sichez JP, van Effenterre R, Capelle L (2005) Contribution of intraoperative electrical stimulations in surgery of low grade gliomas: a comparative study between two series without (1985–1996) and with (1996–2003) functional mapping in the same institution. J Neurol Neurosurg Psychiatry 76: 845–851
45. Duffau H, Gatignol P, Mandonnet E, Peruzzi P, Tzourio-Mazoyer B, Capelle L (2005) New insights into the anatomo-functional connectivity of the semantic system: a study using cortico-subcortical electrostimulations. Brain 128: 797–810
46. Duffau H (2006) New concepts in surgery of WHO grade II gliomas: functional brain mapping, connectionism and plasticity – a review. J Neurooncol 79: 77–115
47. Duffau H (2006) Brain plasticity: from pathophysiological mechanisms to therapeutic applications. J Clin Neurosci 13: 885–897
48. Duffau H, Taillandier L, Gatignol P, Capelle L (2006) The insular lobe and brain plasticity: lessons from tumor surgery. Clin Neurol Neurosurg 108: 543–548
49. Duffau H (in press) Contribution of cortical and subcortical electrostimulation in brain glioma surgery: methodological and functional considerations. Neurophysiol Clin
50. Fandino J, Kollias SS, Wieser HG, Valavanis A, Yonekawa Y (1999) Intraoperative validation of functional magnetic resonance imaging and cortical reorganization patterns in patients with brain tumors involving the primary motor cortex. J Neurosurg 91: 238–250
51. Feydy A, Carlier R, Roby-Brami A, Bussel B, Cazalis F, Pierot L, Burnod Y, Maier MA (2002) Longitudinal study of motor recovery after stroke: recruitment and focusing of brain activation. Stroke 33: 1610–1617
52. Fields RD, Stevens-Graham B (2002) New insights into neuron-glia communication. Science 298: 556–562
53. Finger S, Marshak RA, Cohen M, Scheff S, Trace R, Niemand D (1971) Effects of successive and simultaneous lesions of somatosensory cortex on tactile discrimination in the rat. J Comp Physiol Psychol 77: 221–227
54. Finney E, Fine I, Dobkins K (2001) Visual stimuli activate auditory cortex in the deaf. Nat Neurosci 4: 1171–1173
55. Ganslandt O, Buchfelder M, Hastreiter P, Grummich P, Fahlbusch R, Nimsky C (2004) Magnetic source imaging supports clinical decision making in glioma patients. Clin Neurol Neurosurg 107: 20–26
56. Georgopoulos AP (1999) News in motor cortical physiology. News Physiol Sci 14: 64–68
57. Gould E, Reeves AJ, Graziano MS, Gross CG (1999) Neurogenesis in the neocortex of adult primates. Science 286: 548–552
58. Graveline CJ, Mikulis DJ, Crawley AP, Hwang PA (1998) Regionalized sensorimotor plasticity after hemispherectomy fMRI evaluation. Pediatr Neurol 19: 337–342
59. Graziano MS, Taylor CS, Moore T, Cooke DF (2002) The cortical control of movement revisited. Neuron 36: 349–362
60. Gross CG (2000) Neurogenesis in the adult brain: death of a dogma. Nat Rev Neurosci 1: 67–73
61. Haydon PG (2001) GLIA: listening and talking to the synapse. Nat Rev Neurosci 2: 185–193

62. Heiss WD, Thiel A, Kessler J, Herholz K (2003) Disturbance and recovery of language function: correlates in PET activation studies. Neuroimage 20 Suppl 1: S42–S49
63. Hetten T, Gabrieli JDE (2004) Insights into ageing mind: a view from cognitive neuroscience. Nat Rev Neurosci 5: 87–96
64. Herholz K, Heiss WD (2000) Functional imaging correlates of recovery after stroke in humans. J Cereb Blood Flow Metab 20: 1619–1631
65. Hlustik P, Solodkin A, Gullapalli RP, Noll DC, Small SL (2001) Somatotopy in human primary motor and somatosensory hand representations revisited. Cereb Cortex 11: 312–321
66. Holmes GL, McCabe B (2001) Brain development and generation of brain pathologies. Int Rev Neurobiol 45: 17–41
67. Holodny AI, Schulder M, Ybasco A, Liu WC (2002) Translocation of Broca's area to the contralateral hemisphere as the result of the growth of a left inferior frontal glioma. J Comput Assist Tomogr 26: 941–943
68. Ivanco TL, Greenough WT (2000) Physiological consequences of morphologically detectable synaptic plasticity: potential uses for examining recovery following damage. Neuropharmacology 39: 765–776
69. Jackson JH (1879) On affections of speech from disease of the brain. Brain 1879: 323–356
70. Jacobs KM, Donoghue JP (1991) Reshaping the cortical motor map by unmasking latent intracortical connections. Science 251: 944–947
71. Krainik A, Lehéricy S, Duffau H, Capelle L, Chainay H, Cornu P, Cohen L, Boch AL, Mangin JF, Le Bihan D, Marsault C (2003) Postoperative speech disorder after medial frontal surgery: role of the supplementary motor area. Neurology 60: 587–594
72. Krainik A, Duffau H, Capelle L, Cornu P, Boch AL, Mangin JF, Le Bihan D, Marsault C, Chiras J, Lehéricy S (2004) Role of the healthy hemisphere in recovery after resection of the supplementary motor area. Neurology 62: 1323–1332
73. Krings T, Topper R, Willmes K, Reinges MH, Gilsbach JM, Thron A (2002) Activation in primary and secondary motor areas in patients with CNS neoplasms and weakness. Neurology 58: 381–390
74. Lamprecht R, LeDoux J (2004) Structural plasticity and memory. Nat Rev Neurosci 5: 45–54
75. Laubach M, Wessberg J, Nicolelis MA (2000) Cortical ensemble activity increasingly predicts behaviour outcomes during learning of a motor task. Nature 405: 567–571
76. LeRoux PD, Berger MS, Haglund MM, Pilcher WH, Ojemann GA (1991) Resection of intrinsic tumors from nondominant face motor cortex using stimulation mapping: report of two cases. Surg Neurol 36: 44–48
77. Liepert J, Bauder H, Wolfgang HR, Miltner WH, Taub E, Weiller C (2000) Treatment-induced cortical reorganization after stroke in humans. Stroke 31: 1210–1216
78. Liu Y, Rouiller EM (1999) Mechanisms of recovery of dexterity following unilateral lesion of the sensorimotor cortex in adult monkeys. Exp Brain Res 128: 149–159
79. Magavi SS, Macklis JD (2002) Induction of neuronal type-specific neurogenesis in the cerebral cortex of adult mice: manipulation of neual precursors in situ. Dev Brain Res 134: 57–76
80. Maguire EA, Gadian DG, Johnsrude IS, Good CD, Ashburner J, Frackowiak RS, Frith CD (2000) Navigation-related structural change in the hippocampi of taxi drivers. Proc Natl Acad Sci USA 97: 4398–4403
81. Malenka RC, Nicoll RA (1997) Silent synapses speak up. Neuron 19: 473–476

82. Mandonnet E, Delattre JY, Tanguy ML, Swanson KR, Carpentier AF, Duffau H, Cornu P, van Effenterre R, Alvord EC Jr, Capelle L (2003) Continuous growth of mean tumor diameter in a subset of grade II gliomas. Ann Neurol 53: 524–528
83. Mandonnet E, Capelle L, Duffau H (2006) Extension of paralimbic low-grade gliomas: toward an anatomical classification based on white matter invasion pattern. J Neurooncol 78: 179–185
84. Marque P, Felez A, Puel M, Démonet JF, Guiraud-Chaumeil B, Roques CF, Chollet F (1997) Impairment and recovery of left motor function in patients with right hemiplegia. J Neurol Neurosurg Psychiatry 62: 77–81
85. Marrelec G, Krainik A, Duffau H, Pelegrini-Issac M, Lehericy S, Doyon J, Benali H (2006) Partial correlation for functional brain interactivity investigation in functional MRI. Neuroimage 32: 228–237
86. Marshall RS, Perera GM, Lazar RM, Krakauer JW, Constantine RC, DeLaPaz RL (2000) Evolution of cortical activation during recovery from corticospinal tract infarction. Stroke 31: 656–661
87. Martin SJ, Grimwood PD, Morris RG (2000) Synaptic plasticity and memory: an evaluation of the hypothesis. Annu Rev Neurosci 23: 649–711
88. Meunier S, Duffau H, Garnero L, Capelle L, Ducorps A (2000) Comparison of the somatosensory cortical mapping of the fingers using a whole head magnetoencephalography (MEG) and direct electrical stimulations during surgery in awake patients. Neuroimage 15: S868
89. Meyer D, Isaac W, Maher B (1958) The role of stimulation in spontaneous reorganization of visual habits. J Comp Physiol Psychol 51: 546–548
90. Meyer PT, Sturz L, Schreckenberger M, Spetzger U, Meyer GF, Setani KS, Sabri O, Buell U (2003) Preoperative mapping of cortical language areas in adult brain tumour patients using PET and individual non-normalised SPM analyses. Eur J Nucl Med Mol Imaging 30: 951–960
91. Muller RA, Rothermel RD, Behen ME, Muzik O, Chakraborty PK, Chugani HT (1999) Language organization in patients with early and late left-hemisphere lesion: a PET study. Neuropsychologia 37: 545–557
92. Munte TF, Altenmuller E, Jancke L (2002) The musician's brain as a model of neuroplasticity. Nat Rev Neurosci 3: 473–478
93. Noppeney U, Friston KJ, Price CJ (2003) Effects of visual deprivation on the organization of the semantic system. Brain 126: 1620–1627
94. Nudo RJ, Wise BM, SiFuentes F, Milliken GW (1996) Neural substrates for the effects of rehabilitative training on motor recovery after ischemic infarct. Science 272: 1791–1794
95. Ojemann G, Ojemann G, Lettich E, Berger M (1989) Cortical language localization in left, dominant hemisphere. An electrical stimulation mapping investigation in 117 patients. J Neurosurg 71: 316–326
96. Patrissi G, Stein DG (1975) Temporal factors in recovery of function after brain damage. Exp Neurol 47: 470–480
97. Paus T, Zijdenbos A, Worsley K, Collins DL, Blumenthal J, Giedd JN, Rapoport JL, Evans AC (1999) Structural maturation of neural pathways in children and adolescents: in vivo study. Science 283: 1908–1911
98. Payne R, Lomber S (2001) Reconstructing functional systems after lesions of cerebral cortex. Nat Rev Neurosci 2: 911–919

99. Peck KK, Moore AB, Crosson BA, Gaiefsky M, Gopinath KS, White K, Briggs RW (2004) Functional magnetic resonance imaging before and after aphasia therapy. Shifs in hemodynamic time peak during an overt language task. Stroke 35: 554–559
100. Penfield W, Bolchey E (1937) Somatic motor and sensory representation in the cerebral cortex of the man as studied by electrical stimulation. Brain 60: 389–443
101. Petrovich NM, Holodny AI, Brennan CW, Gutin PH (2004) Isolated translocation of Wernicke's area to the right hemisphere in a 62-year-man with a temporo-parietal glioma. Am J Neuroradiol 25: 130–133
102. Poo MM (2001) Neurotrophins as synaptic modulators. Nat Rev Neurosci 2: 24–32
103. Pulvermuller F, Neininger B, Elbert T, Mohr B, Rockstroh B, Koebbel P, Taub E (2001) Constraint-induced therapy of chronic aphasia after stroke. Stroke 32: 1621–1626
104. Rijntjes M, Weiller C (2002) Recovery of motor and language abilities after stroke: the contribution of functional imaging. Prog Neurobiol 66: 109–122
105. Rosen J, Stein D, Butters N (1971) Recovery of function after serial ablation of prefrontal cortex in the rhesus monkey. Science 173: 353–356
106. Rosen HJ, Petersen SE, Linenweber MR, Snyder AZ, White DA, Chapman L, Dromerick AW, Fiez JA, Corbetta MD (2000) Neural correlates of recovery from aphasia after damage to left inferior frontal cortex. Neurology 55: 1883–1894
107. Rossini PM, Dal Forno G (2004) Integrated technology for evaluation of brain function and neural plasticity. Phys Med Rehabil Clin N Am 15: 263–306
108. Rouiller EM, Yu XH, Moret V, Tempini A, Wiesendanger M, Liang F (1998) Dexterity in adult monkeys following early lesion of the motor cortical hand area: the role of cortex adjacent to the lesion. Eur J Neurosci 10: 729–740
109. Roux FE, Boulanouar K, Ibarrola D, Tremoulet M, Chollet F, Berry I (2000) Functional MRI and intraoperative brain mapping to evaluate brain plasticity in patients with brain tumours and hemiparesis. J Neurol Neurosurg Psychiatry 69: 453–463
110. Roux FE, Boulanouar K, Lotterie JA, Mejdoubi M, LeSage JP, Berry I (2003) Language functional magnetic resonance imaging in preoperative assessment of language areas: correlation with direct cortical stimulation. Neurosurgery 52: 1335–1345
111. Salenius S, Hari R (2003) Synchronous cortical oscillatory activity during motor action. Curr Opin Neurobiol 13: 678–684
112. Sanai N, Tramontin A, Quinones-Hinojosa A, Barbaro NM, Gupta N, Kunwar S, Lawton MT, McDermott MW, Parsa AT, Manuel-Garcia Verdugo J, Berger MS, Alvarez-Buylla A (2004) Unique astrocyte ribbon in adult human brain contains neural stem cells but lacks chain migration. Nature 427: 740–744
113. Sanai N, Alvarez-Buylla A, Berger MS (2005) Neural stem cells and the origin of gliomas. N Engl J Med 353: 811–822
114. Sanai N, Alvarez-Buylla A, Berger MS (2006) Neural stem cells and the origin of gliomas. N Engl J Med 353: 811–822
115. Sanes JN, Donoghue JP, Thangaraj V, Edelman RR, Warach S (1995) Shared neural substrates controlling hand movements in human motor cortex. Science 268: 1775–1777
116. Sanes JN, Donoghue JP (1997) Static and dynamic organization of motor cortex. Adv Neurol 73: 277–296
117. Sanes JN, Donoghue JP (2000) Plasticity and primary motor cortex. Ann Rev Neurosci 23: 393–415

118. Sanes JN, Schieber MH (2001) Orderly somatotopy in primary motor cortex: does it exist? Neuroimage 13: 968–974
119. Sawaya R, Hammoud M, Schoppa D, Hess KR, Wu SZ, Shi WM, Wildrick DM (1998) Neurological outcomes in a modern series of 400 craniotomies for treatment of parenchymal tumors. Neurosurgery 42: 1044–1056
120. Schiffbauer H, Ferrari P, Rowley HA, Berger MS, Roberts TPL (2001) Functional activity within brain tumors: a magnetic source imaging study. Neurosurgery 49: 1313–1321
121. Seitz RJ, Azari NP, Knorr U, Binkofski F, Herzog H, Freund HJ (1999) The role of diaschisis in stroke recovery. Stroke 30: 1844–1850
122. Selnes OA (1999) Recovery from aphasia: activating the "right" hemisphere. Ann Neurol 45: 419–420
123. Shimizu T, Hosaki A, Hino T, Sato M, Komori T, Hirai S, Rossini PM (2002) Motor cortical disinhibition in the unaffected hemisphere after unilateral cortical stroke. Brain 125: 1896–1907
124. Spena G, Gatignol P, Capelle L, Duffau H (2006) Superior longitudinal fasciculus subserves vestibular network in humans. Neuroreport 17: 1403–1406
125. Stein DG, Butters N, Rosen J (1977) A comparison of two- and four-stage ablations of sulcus principals on recovery of spatial performance in the rhesus monkey. Neuropsychologia 15: 179–182
126. Sterr A, Elbert T, Berthold I, Kolbel S, Rockstroh B, Taub E (2002) Longer versus shorter daily constraint-induced movement therapy of chronic hemiparesis: an exploratory study. Arch Phys Med Rehabil 83: 1374–1377
127. Taphoorn MJ, Klein M (2004) Cognitive deficits in adult patients with brain tumours. Lancet Neurol 3: 159–168
128. Taub E, Uswatte G, Elbert T (2002) New treatments in neurorehabilitation founded on basis research. Nat Rev Neurosci 3: 228–236
129. Teixidor P, Gatignol P, Leroy M, Masuet-Aumatell C, Capelle L, Duffau H (2007) Assessment of verbal working memory before and after surgery for low-grade glioma. J Neurooncol 81: 305–313
130. Thiebaut de Schotten M, Urbanski M, Duffau H, Volle E, Levy R, Dubois B, Bartolomeo P (2005) Direct evidence for a parietal-frontal pathway subserving spatial awareness in humans. Science 309: 2226–2228
131. Thiel A, Herholz K, Koyuncu A, Ghaemi M, Kracht LW, Habedank B, Heiss WD (2001) Plasticity of language networks in patients with brain tumors: a positron emission tomography activation study. Ann Neurol 50: 620–629
132. Thiel A, Habedank B, Winhuisen L, Herholz K, Kessler J, Haupt WF, Heiss WD (2005) Essential language function of the right hemisphere in brain tumor patients. Ann Neurol 57: 128–131
133. Turrigiano GG, Nelson SB (2004) Homeostatic plasticity in the developping nervous system. Nat Neurosci Rev 5: 97–107
134. Ullian EM, Sapperstein SK, Christopherson KS, Barres BA (2001) Control of synapse number by glia. Science 291: 657–661
135. Ulmer JL, Hacein-Bey L, Mathews VP, Mueller WM, DeYoe EA, Prost RW, Meyer GA, Krouwer HG, Schmainda KM (2004) Lesion-induced pseudo-dominance at functional magnetic resonance imaging: implications for preoperative assessments. Neurosurgery 55: 569–579

136. Vigneau M, Beaucousin V, Herve PY, Duffau H, Crivello F, Houde O, Mazoyer B, Tzourio-Mazoyer N (2006) Meta-analyzing left hemisphere language areas: phonology, semantics, and sentence processing. Neuroimage 30: 1414–1432
137. Vives KP, Piepmeir JM (1999) Complications and expected outcome of glioma surgery. J Neurooncol 42: 289–302
138. von Monakow C (1914) Die lokalisation im groshirn un der abbau der funktion durch kortikale herde. Bergman JF, Wiesbaden, Germany, pp 26–34
139. Walbran BB (1976) Age and serial ablations of somatosensory cortex in the rat. Physiol Behav 17: 13–17
140. Walker DG, Kaye AH (2003) Low grade glial neoplasms. J Clin Neurosci 10: 1–13
141. Weiller C, Ramsay SC, Wise RJ, Friston KJ, Frackowiak RS (1993) Individual patterns of functional reorganization in the human cerebral cortex after capsular infarction. Ann Neurol 33: 181–189
142. Weiller C (1998) Imaging recovery from stroke. Exp Brain Res 123: 13–17
143. Wessels PH, Weber WE, Raven G, Ramaekers FC, Hopman AH, Twijnstra A (2003) Supratentorial grade II astrocytoma: biological features and clinical course. Lancet Neurol 2: 395–403
144. Xerri C (1998) Post-lesional plasticity of somatosensory cortex maps: a review. C R Acad Sci III 321: 135–151
145. Xerri C, Merzenich MM, Peterson BE, Jenkins W (1998) Plasticity of primary somatosensory cortex paralleling sensorimotor skill recovery from stroke in adult monkeys. J Neurophysiol 79: 2119–2148
146. Xerri C, Zennou-Azogui Y (2003) Influence of the postlesion environment and chronic piracetam treatment on the organization of the somatotopic map in the rat primary somatosensory cortex after focal cortical injury. Neuroscience 118: 161–177
147. Yasargil MG, van Ammon K, Cavazos E, Doczi T, Reeves JD, Roth P (1992) Tumours of the limbic and paralimbic systems. Acta Neurochir (Wien) 118: 40–52
148. Zentner J, Hufnagel A, Pechstein U, Wolf HK, Schramm J (1996) Functional results after resective procedures involving the supplementary motor area. J Neurosurg 85: 542–549

Offprint from
**Advances and Technical Standards in Neurosurgery, Vol. 33**
Edited by J.D. Pickard


# Tumor-biology and current treatment of skull-base chordomas

M. N. Pamir and K. Özduman

Marmara University Faculty of Medicine, Department of Neurosurgery,
Marmara University Institute of Neurological Sciences, Istanbul, Turkey

With 9 Figures

## Contents

## Abstract

Chordomas are rare, slow growing tumors of the axial skeleton, which derive from the remnants of the fetal notochord. They can be encountered anywhere along the axial skeleton, most commonly in the sacral area, skull base and less commonly in the spine. Chordomas have a benign histopathology but exhibit malignant clinical behavior with invasive, destructive and metastatic potential. Genetic and molecular pathology studies on oncogenesis of chordomas are very limited and there is little known on mechanisms governing the disease. Chordomas most commonly present with headaches and diplopia and can be readily diagnosed by current neuroradiological methods. There are 3 pathological subtypes of chordomas: classic, chondroid and dedifferentiated chordomas. Differential diagnosis from chondrosarcomas by radiology or pathology may at times be difficult.

Skull base chordomas are very challenging to treat. Clinically there are at least two subsets of chordoma patients with distinct behaviors: some with a benign course and another group with an aggressive and rapidly progressive disease. There is no standard treatment for chordomas. Surgical resection and high dose radiation treatment are the mainstays of current treatment. Nevertheless, a significant percentage of skull base chordomas recur despite treatment. The outcome is dictated primarily by the intrinsic biology of the tumor and treatment seems only to have a secondary impact. To date we only have a limited understanding this biology; however better understanding is likely to improve treatment outcome.

Hereby we present a review of the current knowledge and experience on the tumor biology, diagnosis and treatment of chordomas.

*Keywords:* Chordoma; chondrosarcoma; skull base; operative technique; Gamma-Knife; radiation therapy.

## Definition

Chordomas are rare, slow growing bone tumors of the axial skeleton. Due to their invasive, destructive growth characteristics and metastatic potential they are considered malignant tumors. Since their first description chordomas have been and continue to be a treatment challenge. As a tumor, that frequent arises in the central skull base, and is widely invasive in this delicate and intricate anatomy, the surgical resection of chordomas is very challenging even for the experienced skull base surgeon. Some chordomas do well even after simple limited resection, while others continue their relentless growth despite aggressive surgery and multimodal adjuvant treatment protocols, finally to result in the patient's demise. Determinants of this difference in behavior is not known, however is assumed to depend on the intrinsic biology of chordomas.

Chordomas derive from remnants of the notochord and arise along the axial skeleton anywhere from the visceral cranium to the sacrococcygeal bone, where these remnants are present. The outcome after diagnosis of skull base chordomas varies considerably. There are at least two subsets of patients with distinct clinical behavior: some with a benign course and another group with an aggressive and rapidly progressive course over 3–5 years. As the suffix "oma" denotes, chordomas have a differentiated morphological phenotype and appear "benign" under the microscope. However, in many cases this phenotype obscures the malignant tumor biology. Progressive chordomas have an indolent but relentlessly progressive course and are very challenging to treat. The outcome is clearly dictated primarily by the intrinsic biology of the tumor and treatment seems only to have a secondary impact. However, determinants of this biology are still unknown to us and this excludes the possibility of a rational or patient based treatment.

Today there is no single best treatment option, or combination, for chordomas and the current favor is a wide resection followed by high dose radiotherapy. Existing literature can only provide level-4 and very limited level-3 evidence. This is mostly a consequence of the rarity of this disease. Since its first description in 1856 there have been only 24 studies of skull-base chordomas that reported cohorts larger than 30 patients. Skull base chordomas grow widely invasive in the skull base and the patients usually succumb to progressive tumor growth despite multimodal treatment. This is because of their widely invasive nature, which makes them difficult surgical targets and because of their poor response to any available adjuvant therapy.

Hereby we will provide a comprehensive review of the existing knowledge on tumor biology and treatment options for chordomas.

## History

We owe the description of chordoma to the important work done in the second half of the 19$^{th}$ century [296]. The famous German pathologist Rudolph Virchow in 1846 found gelatoinous nest like formations in the spheno-occipital synchondrosis and gave the first description of the "physaliferous cells", the large vesicular cells characteristic of chordomas [356]. Speculating a possible relationship to other cartilaginous tumors he called the lesion "ecchondrosis (originating from cartilage) physillaphora (vacuole containing) spheno-occipitalis" and described them as: " growth and mucoid metamorphosis of remains of the sphenooccipital cartilage" [356]. Hubert von Luschka in his article in 1857 [208] and Virchow in his book [356] were the first to report their findings on this pathology in 1857. Hasse [139] and Zenker [376] in the same year confirmed the findings and with reference to Virchow, referred to them as the "mucous or gelatinous tumors of the clivus Blumenbachi". In the following years Kölliker [177] came up with the concept that the mammalian nucleus pulposus was derived from notochord. Subsequently, Heinrich Müller [237] in 1858, rejected the theory that these lesions are cartilagenous tumors and suggested a possible origin from the primitive notochord and induced a nomenclature change to ecchordosis (originiating from Chorda dorsalis) physaliphora. These ideas caused much controversy in morphological sciences and caused a division among the pathologists with some calling these "jelly tumors" a neoplasia while others considering them developmental abnormalities. Klebs [172] gave the first description of pontine compression from a skull base chordoma in 1864. The term "chordoma" was first used by Ribbert [279, 281] in 1894. Ribbert punctured the anterior intervertebral ligament in rabbits and successfully produced experimental chordomas, essentially classifying them as developmental tumors. In 1904 he published his opinion on the origin of chordomas [280]. In his laboratory Fischer and Steiner [325] confirmed Müller's theory by creating a malignant chordoma in rabbits. In 1909 Linck [205] for the first time established criteria for histopathological diagnosis of chordoma and defined formation of mucus, presence of physaliphorous cells, lobular arrangement, nuclear vacuolation and resemblance of notochordal tissue as characteristic findings. The first succesful resection of a skull base chordoma was reported by Harvey Cushing in his 1912 monograph on pituitary adenomas [72]. The operation, performed in 1909, provided symptomatic improvement for motnths and the tumor was initially misdiagnosed as teratoma. With advancements in surgical technique a more radical approach to skull base has been proposed by several authors. In 1914, Alezais and Peyron [6, 7] gave a detailed description of histogenesis and evolution of chordomas. Stewart and Morin [328] were the first to suggest that chordomas may be derived from ecchordosis physaliphora. The experiments of Ribbert were replicated by Congdon [61] in 1952 in a similar rabbit model. Zülch [379] in 1956 noted variable clinical behavior among chordomas and differentiated between slowly growing benign chordomas and rapidly growing malignant chordomas. In the same book, Zülch also proposed that chordomas arise at anatomical locations where the notochord tissue is not surrounded by cartilage [379]. Heffelfinger, analyzing 155 cases of chordoma and all other cartilaginous tumors treated at Mayo clinic from 1910 to 1973, described a "chondroid" subtype in 1973 [141]. Despite major progress in microneurosurgery in the 1960's, a hundred years after the first description of chordomas, the treatment was still very disappointing. In 1975 Krayenbühl and Yaşargil [182] reported an analysis of 221 cases of skull base chordomas collected from the literature until 1970 and 4 cases of theirs. The results of this analysis were discouraging with 17.5% operative- and another 27% late postoperative mortality [182, 375]. The advent of sophisticated neuroimaging techniques in the 1980's brought better preoperative planning and the development skull base surgery in the early 1990's made total resection possible with acceptable morbidity and mortality. Together with advances in radiotherapy the treatment of chordomas has improved significantly in the last 25 years.

Accumulating experience and sophisticated molecular biology techniques brought a better understanding of the tumor biology. Today we know that the major determinant of the disease course of a chordoma is the tumor biology. The treatment, how aggressive or powerful it may be, does only modulate but does not change this behavior.

## Pathogenesis

Etiology of chordomas is not known, nor there any predisposing conditions. Current scientific knowledge supports the theory that chordomas originate from the remnants of notochord (from the Greek notos: "back", chorde: "string"). The notochord is a rod shaped body that defines the primitive axis of the embryo. In higher vertebrates, the notochord exists transiently during embryogenesis provides structural support and secretes signaling molecules to provide position and fate information to the surrounding structures [326]. The human notochord originates from ectoderm during the third week of embryogenesis [269, 369]. It influences the development of peri-notochordial mesenchymal elements, however, being a primitive relative of cartilage, also serves as the axial skeleton of the embryo until the formation of other elements, such as the vertebral bodies. Without a fully developed notochord embryos fail to elongate [326]. Ultimately the notochord that runs through the middle of each vertebra, which is identified by type X collagen expression, is dismantled and replaced by bone, similar to the enchondral bone formation, in which Collagen II rich extracellular matrix (ECM) is deposited by type X collagen and finally replaced by bone [206]. However, between the vertebrae the notochord does not express collagen-X and eventually expands forming the nucleus pulposus [13]. The cranial extension of this embryonic structure extends as far as the sella turcica. In the skull base the notochord is incorporated into the caudal part of the sphenoid and the basilar part of the occipital bone [296, 297]. It is possible for the notochord to bend towards the pharyngeal wall, forming secondary unions with the pharyngeal epithelium [264].

The notochord most likely is a primitive relative of cartilage and shares many characteristics with it such as expression of type II and type IX collagens, aggrecan, Sox9 and chondromodulin [126]. Chondrocytes normally secrete a highly hyrdrated extracellular matrix, which gives cartilage its main structural properties [326]. Notochordal cells, on the contrary, retain hydrated materials in large cellular vacuoles [326].

Benign chordal ectopias (ecchordosis physaliphora) are commonly encountered in the skull base in asymptomatic adults. It is widely believed that these benign chordal ectopias are also precursors of chordomas. Some authors have proposed a progressive tumorigenesis from benign notochordal tumors while others advocated a de-novo origin from notochordal remnants [372, 373]. The hypothesis on the origin of chordomas from pre-malignant lesions (ecchordosis physillaphora) is supported by similar morphology (light microscopy and electron microscopy [148]), similar immunophenotype [126, 295] and similar localization [370, 371]. Ecchordosis physillaphora are reported with an incidence of 0.5 to 2% in autopsy studies [3, 221]. Similar incidences are reported in radiological studies [221]. Alhough most common in the skull base, ecchordosis physillaphora (EP) may also be seen in other locations along the axial skeleton [245, 277, 348]. The supposed origin of ecchordosis physillaphora from the notochord is supported by similar electron microscopy findings and immunohistochemical profile [143, 148, 368].

## Genetics and molecular biology

### Familial chordomas

Familial chordomas are exceptionally rare. However, the presence of several cases in two or more close relatives suggested that the disease may be caused by possible genetic alterations. In 1958, Foote *et al.* [105] reported the familial occurrence of chordoma for the first time in a brother and sister, who presented with metastatic sacrococygeal chordomas. This was flowed by a report of two young brothers with nasopharyngeal chordoma [93], a man, his mother and daughter with nasopharyngeal chordomas [167], a man with sacrococygeal chordoma whose sister and niece developed clival chordomas and whose first cousin had a nasopharyngeal chordoma [327], and a father and daughter with clival chordomas [73, 231]. Stepanek *et al.* [327] reported an autosomal dominant inheritance pattern. This was followed by a genome-wide linkage analysis in an extended pedigree of 10 affected individuals of the same family and the defect was localized to 7q33 [166]. In a recent study the authors reconfirmed this disease region in the same 3 families by linkage analysis, however were unable to detect the same changes in a fourth family [374]. Dalpra *et al.* [73] reported a father and a daughter with recurrent chordoma. Another daughter also had a cerebellar astrocytoma. Cytogenetic analysis revealed pronounced heterogeneity of the karyotypes, with a number of unbalanced translocations leading to 1p losses [73, 231]. An analysis of this family and several other sporadic cases mapped the genetic defect to a 25cM segment between 1p36.31 and 1P36.13 and possibly involving a tumor suppressor gene [231]. A list of reported disease loci in chordomas is presented in Table 1.

### Telomere maintenance

Telomere length is an important regulator of cell life span and is deregulated in virtually all types of cancer to provide limitless replicative potential [19]. Reactivation of the cellular enzyme telomerase is the most common way utilized by tumor cells to maintain telomere length. This reactivation is strongly associated with genomic instability [19]. Butler *et al.* [42] showed increased telomere length in 4 of 4 chordomas they studied and telomerase activity in half of these cases. Pallini *et al.* [258] in their study of 26 skull base chordoma cases concluded that expression of hTERT correlated significantly with shorter recurrence-free survival. Interestingly the majority of the hTERT positive tumors in this study were also positive for p53 mutations, an association that results in increased incidence in human-like carcinomas in mice [54].

### Genome wide studies and genomic integrity

There are only few genome-wide studies on chromosomal abnormalities in chordomas. The NCBI Cancer Chromosomes database, as accessed on

**Table 1.** *Reported disease loci in chordomas*

| Ref. | Reported locus | Mode of analysis | Comments |
|---|---|---|---|
| Foote *et al.* [105] | – | Case report | Chordomas may be inherited. Brother and sister presenting with recurrent and metastatic chordomas |
| Stepanek *et al.* [327] | – | Genetic analysis | Autosomal dominant inheritance in a family |
| Dalpra *et al.* [73] | 1p33 | Linkage analysis | Deletion in familial recurrent chordoma |
| Miozzo *et al.* [231] | 1p36 | Linkage analysis | Tumor suppressor gene suggested at the locus |
| Kelley *et al.* [166] | 7q33 | Linkage analysis | Linkage analysis performed on the same family as Stepanek |
| Colli *et al.* [59] | – | Karyotype analysis | Abnormal karyotype is not correlated with recurrence. It is not different in chondroid chordomas or chondrosarcomas. |
| Scheil *et al.* [304] | 3p, 1p, 7q, 20q, 5q and 12q | Comparative genomic hybridization | Analysis of 16 chordomas in 13 patients Frequent loss at 3p and 1p Frequent gain at 7q, 20q, 5q and 12q |
| Riva *et al.* [284] | 1p36.13 | Linkage analysis | LOH analysis in 27 sporadic chordomas. |
| Bayrakli *et al.* [20] | 1p36, 1q25, 2p13, 7q33 6p12 | iFish | Analysis of 7 primary tumors and 11 recurrences in 7 patients. Gains at 1q25 (66.6%), 1p36 (60%), and 7q33 (37.5%) 4q26-q27 (12.5%), 3p12-p14 (10%), 3p12-p14 (16.6%) in recurrent, 7q33 (33.3%), 3p12-p14 (16.6%), 1q25 (14.2%), and 1p36 (14.2%) in primary tumors. Losses at 1q25 (66.6%), 2p13 (55.5%), 1p36 (30%) in recurrent and 2p13 (83.3%), 6p12 (50%), 1q25 (32.7%), 17p13.1 (20%), 6p12 (12.5%), and 3p12-p14 (10%) and 1p36 (28.5%) 3p12-p14 (16.6%), 7q33 (16.6%), and 17p13.1 (14.2%) in primary tumor samples. |

October 2006, reports chromosome aberrations of 34 chordomas [176]. In our literature analysis we came across 82 karyotypes reported in chordomas as presented in Table 2 [40, 51, 73, 75, 118, 119, 188, 226, 267, 303, 304, 334]. Fifty-one (62.2%) of these karyotypes were abnormal and a majority of those were hypo-diploid or near-diploid. Very diverse chromosome aberrations were detected in the rest and no single characteristic karyotypic abnormality was described in primary or recurrent chordomas [303].

The incidecence of an aneuploid karyotype is comparable in classic and chondroid chordomas and ranges between 27% and 45% [40, 119, 124, 232, 303, 334]. Findings were similar for skull base and sacral chordomas [299]. Three studies reported complex, aneuploid/multiploid karyotypes in dedifferentiated chordomas [119, 150]. Genetic instability may be a late event in chordoma oncogenesis.

Other tumors such as meningiomas or gliomas contain areas with chordoid phenotype [173]. Interestingly, in chordoid meningiomas an unbalanced translocation t(1;3) was shown to be associated with this chordoid phenotype. Chordoid gliomas, in the other hand, have no chromosomal imbalances [276].

Some studies explored a correlation between ploidy and survival. Mitchell *et al.* [232] found polyploidy with similar incidences in chondroid and classic chordomas. In their study none of the tumors containing chondroid areas had aneuploidy and the diploid and aneuploid tumors had comparable survival. Colli *et al.* [59] conducted a ploidy analysis in 2 classic and 5 chondroid chordomas and a karyotype analysis in 11 classic-, 3 chondroid chordomas and 4 chondrosarcomas and confirmed the findings of Mitchell *et al.* [60]. Additionally they have found that patients with an abnormal karyotype had higher recurrence rates.

The largest series of genome wide analysis in chordomas was reported by Scheil *et al.* [304]. In their study the most commonly encountered losses were on 1p (50%) and 3p (44%). Most frequent gains were 7q in 69%, chromosome 20 in 50%, 5q in 38% and 12q in 38% of the cases in this series. Brandal *et al.* also reported similar findings: In their study the most frequently observed changes were 1q23 gain in 50%, 7p gain in 50%, 7q gain in 75%, 19p gain in 50% and loss of 9p in 50% of cases. So far, 4 cases of chordoma with single cytogenetic defects have been described, three with different translocations, 2 with involvement of 6q and 1 case with 1p [40, 50, 226, 267] Sawyer *et al.* [303] found cytogenetic abnormalities in 11 of their 22 skull base and cervical chordoma samples. All of these positive tumors were recurrent lesions and isochromosome1q was a recurrent abnormality in a number of tumor samples, however not the sole abnormality [303]. Bayrakli *et al.* [20] using interphase FISH, have studied 1p36, 1q25, 3p13-p14, 7q33, 17p13.1 (p53 gene locus), 2p13 (TGF-$\alpha$), 6p12 (VEGF), and 4q26-q27 (bFGF/FGF2) loci in 18 primary and recurrent tumor samples from 7 patients. Common gains were found at 1q25 (66.6%), 1p36 (60%), and 7q33 (37.5%) and losses at 2p13 (83.3%), 6p12 (50%), 1q25 (32.7%), and 1p36 (28.5%) loci. In conclusion two loci, 1p36 and 7q33, were found to be associated with chordoma progression and recurrence. Two other newly reported loci, 1q25 and 2p13, displayed abnormalities both in primary chordomas and recurrences. The chromosome 6p12 aberration was only observed in primary chordomas.

**Table 2.** *Abnormal karyotypes reported in chordomas*

| Case # | Study | Main study cohort | Abnormal karyotypes | | | | | |
|---|---|---|---|---|---|---|---|---|
| | | | Age/gender | Tumor site | Tumor status | Histo-pathology | Radio-therapy | Karyotype |
| 1 | Chadduck *et al.* [51] | 1 chordoma | ?F | N/A | N/A | N/A | N/A | 46,XX,t(1;16)(p34;p11) |
| 2 | Persons *et al.* [267] | 2 SAC chrodomas | 56M | SAC | R | N/A | N/A | 44,XY,t(1;3)(q42;q11),−2, der(7)t(2;7)(q23;q32),−21/46, X,t(Y;6)(q12;q22), t(1;14)(q34;q32)t(5;10)(q13;p11) |
| 3 | | | 77F | SAC | R | N/A | N/A | 45,XX,−21 |
| 4 | Gibas *et al.* [118] | 2 SAC chrodomas | 71F | SAC | P | N/A | N/A | 36,X,−X,−1,−3,−4,−11,−13,−14, −18,−21,−22,+der(21)t(1;21)(q21;q22) |
| 5 | | | 75F | SAC | P | N/A | N/A | 72,XX,−X,−1,+del(1)(p22)×2,−2, −3,add(3)(p25),−4,del(5)(p13), add(5)(p15),add(5)(p13),−7, inv(7)(q11.2q22),der(9)t(9;?)(p24;?)×2, −10, −10,−10,+12,−13,−13, der(15)t(15;?)(p11;?),−17, der(18)t(18;?)(p11;?), der(19)t(19;?)(q13;?),der(20)t(20;?)(q13;?), +der(20)t(20;?)(q13;?),−21, +der(21)t(2;21)(q11;q22)×2,+9mar [cp] |
| 6 | DeBoer *et al.* [75] | 1 SAC chordoma | 69M | SAC | P | N/A | N/A | 43,XY,−2,−3,del(4)(q32),−6,+7,−11, der(12)t(9;12)(q12;p11),add(16)(q23), −20,add(22) (q13),+mar |

| | | | | | | | | |
|---|---|---|---|---|---|---|---|---|
| 7 | Mertens *et al.* [226] (also reported by Mandahl *et al.* [214]) | 8 SAC chordomas | 51M | SAC | R | N/A | N/A | 42,XY;add(1)(q31),del(2)(p21),−3, add(3)(p11),−4,t(5;7)(q33;q36), add(8) (q24),del(9)(p13),−10, add(11)(q11),dup(12)(q13q24),−16, −18,ins(18;t)(q21;?),add(19)(p13), der(22)t(4;22)(q11;p11),+mar [3]/46,Y,del(X)(q24),t(1;5)(p36;q33), del(2),der(3)t(3;14)(p21;q24), t(X;3)(q24;q11),der(6)t(3;6)(p21;p21), del(9),10,add(11),del(12)(q13q15), +add(12)(q24),der(14)t(3;14) (q21;q24),der(15)t(6;15)(p21;p13), −16,?add(17)(p11),add(19), +mar [4]/48,XY,del(2), der(2)t(2;?;12)(p14;?;q13), inv(4)(p16q31),add(5)(p15),+7,+8, del(9), 10,del(11)p12),del(12), add(16)(p13),add(17)(q21),add(19), +mar [4] |
| 8 | | | 61M | SAC | R | N/A | N/A | 46,XY(1;6)(q44;q11) [5]/46,XY [20] on recurrence: 46,XY [12] |
| 9 | | | 62M | SAC | P | N/A | N/A | 40,XY,del(1)t(1;21)(p11;q11),−3,−4, −8,der(8)t(1;8)(q21;q23),add(9)(q22), −13,−14, der(20)t(2;20)(q21;q13), del(2)(q35),−21 [13]/77–84,idem×2, +3,+8,+2mar [3]/46,XY [3] |

(*continued*)

**Table 2** (*continued*)

| Case # | study | Main study cohort | Abnormal karyotypes | | | | | |
|---|---|---|---|---|---|---|---|---|
| | | | Age/gender | Tumor site | Tumor status | Histo-pathology | Radio-therapy | Karyotype |
| 10 | Bridge et al. [35] | 1 SAC chordoma | 70M | SAC | P | N/A | N/A | 42,XY,add(1)(p11),−3, der(4)t(4;?;?18;?)(q12;?;?;?),−6,−9, −14,der(16)t(4;?;16)(q12;?;q11), der(17)add(17)(p12) t(17;18)(q11;p11), der(18)del(18)(p11)add(18)(q?) [6]/42, idem,der(9)t(6;9)(q11;p11) [4]/46,XY [10] |
| 11 | Butler *et al.* [41] | 5 SAC chordomas | 34F | SAC | P | N/A | N/A | 46,X,−X,t(5;12)(q13;p13), t(6;7)(q25;q22),+14 |
| 12 | Buonamici *et al.* [40] | 3 SB, 1SPl chordomas | 47M | SP | P | classic | N/A | 46,XY,(6;11)(q12;q23) |
| 13 | Dalpra *et al.* [73] | 1 SB chordoma | 39M | SB | R | Classic | No | 39,XY,dic(1;9)(p36.1;p21),add(1)(p12), del(3)(p13),−4,−4,der(6)t(1;6;14) (6pter →6q2:1p36 →1p13:14pter →14qter), −7,−8,−8,−11,−17, −17,−18,−18, −19,−20,−20,−22,−22,+8mar on recurrence 46,XY [18]/40,XY, del(2)(p12pter),del(3)(q21qter), del(3)(q21qter),−3,−6,−9, del(12)(q21qter),−13,−13,−15, −19,−19,−20,+mar1,+mar2, +mar3/45,X,−Y,add(6)(p25)/46,XY, del(7)(q32qter)/47,XY,+mar1/48, XY,+r1, +r2,(ace and dmin)/44,X, |

| |
|---|
| −Y,−2,del(2)(q31qter), t(2;Y)(p25;q11.2),add(10) (q26),−13, −14,−15,del(15)(q15ter),+20,+22, +mar1/45,XY,−4,add(10) (q26)/46, XY,del(6)(q21qter),add(D)(q?)/46,XY, add(6)(q27),add(10)(q26)/44,XY,-D, −16,−17,−18,+21,+mar1/45,XY, inv(1)(p21;q32-44),−4,−20,+mar/46, XY,add(1)(q21),add(10)(q26)/48,XY, del(3)(q21qter),−7,add (9)(q34), t(9;10)(q11;p15)+add(20)(q13.3)/43, XY,del(2)(p12pter),−6, add(10)(p15), −11,−13,−16,+mar1/46,XY, del(2)(p12pter),add(11)(q14 o q22)/ 46,XY,−2,−7,t(15;15)(p?;p?),−19, +mar1,+mar2,+mar3/46,XY,−4, +add(10)(q26),del(12)(q22qter)/45, Y,−X,add(1)(p12),−20,+mar/45,XY, del(6)(q25qter),del(10)(q23-24qter), −12,der(16)t(q12-13;q23-24)/46,XY, del(3)(q21qter),add(9)(q34)/44,XY, add(1)(p?),del(2)(p12pter),−6,−8,−11, −18,+mar1,+mar2/46,XY,−2, add(11)(p?),−12,+iso(12p), +mar1/43,XY, −2,add(3)(p23),−4, −21/46,XY,−6,+mar1/45,XY, del(3)(p21),−16,+mar1/43,XY, del(1)(q11qter),add(1)(p12-p13) [2], |

(*continued*)

**Table 2** *(continued)*

| Case # | study | Main study cohort | Abnormal karyotypes | | | | | |
|---|---|---|---|---|---|---|---|---|
| | | | Age/ gender | Tumor site | Tumor status | Histo- pathology | Radio- therapy | Karyotype |
| | | | | | | | | −15,−17,−20/46,XY,add(6) (q27), del(4)(q21.3qter) or t(4;6)(q21.3;q27)/44,XY,del(4)(p12), −5,t(5;11) (q12;p15),−7,−8, +10/46,XY,add(10)(q26) [2]/46,XY, +mar1/46,XY,del(2) (p12pter), add(16)(p12-p13)/47,XY,t(1;10)(p36;q24) |
| 14 | Scheil *et al.* [304] | 7 SAC,5 SB, 1 SP chordomas | 46M | SAC | R | N/A | Yes | gains: 7; 8p;9q34; 12q34; 15q; 17, 20 q Losses: 1p34-p21; 3; 10; 11; 14q; 18; 22 |
| 15 | | | 77F | SAC | R | N/A | Yes | gains: 7q36, 20 Losses: 1p31.3-p22; 3p21-p12; 13q21-q32; 18q22-q23 |
| 16 | | | 70F | SAC | R | N/A | Before 2nd surgery | gains: 1p34.2-p36; 7p21-qter; 12p; 15q; 22qLosses: 1p31-p21; 3p; 6q11-q21; 9p; Xp On recurrence(1 year later) gains: amp1p34.2-p36; 7; 12p; 15q; 22qLosses: 1p31-p21; 2q33-q36; 3p; 6q11-q21; 9p-q31; Xp |
| 17 | | | 69F | SAC | R | N/A | Before 2nd surgery | gains: 7q22-qter; 12pLosses: On recurrence gains: 7q22-qter Losses: 3; 4; 5; 9p; 10 |
| 18 | | | 61F | SAC | R | N/A | Yes | gains: 17; 20q Losses: 1p31; 4p; 9p21-p24; 13q21 |

| | | | | | | | | |
|---|---|---|---|---|---|---|---|---|
| 19 | | | 46F | SAC | R | N/A | Before 2nd surgery | gains: 5q23-qter; 7; 12q24; 20 Losses: 3; 4q35 On recurrence 6 years later gains: 5q31-qter; 7q34-qter; 12q24; 20; 22q; Xq23-qter |
| 20 | | | 74F | SAC | P | N/A | No | gains: 1q, 3p, 4q12-q27, 5q, 7, 8pter-q21.1, 8q24, Losses: 9q22-qter, 11pter-q22, 12, 13q22-qter, 15q, 17q, 21, 22 |
| 21 | | | 26M | SB | P | N/A | No | gains: 20; 21q22; 22q; Xp, Xq26-q28 Losses:- |
| 22 | | | 66F | SB | R | N/A | Yes | gains: 11q24-q25; 12q24; 14q21-qter; 17q; 20q; 21q21-q22 losses: 6q; 12p; 13q |
| 23 | | | 51F | SB | R | N/A | Yes | gains: 7q34-qter; 20q Losses: 1p31-p21; X |
| 24 | | | 37M | SB | P | N/A | No | gains: 12q24Losses: 13q21-q31; Xq25-Xqter |
| 25 | | | 58F | SB | P | N/A | No | gains: 1q; 11q24-q25Losses: 1p; 3; 4; 9p; 10; 13q; 14q; X |
| 26 | | | 80F | SP | P | N/A | No | gains: 5p15; 7q34-qter; 9q34; 22qLosses: 3p12-p14; 13q; 18q |
| 27 | Sawyer *et al.* [303] | 22 SB chordomas | 57F | SB | R | Chondroid | Yes | 46,XX,inv(1)(q23q42),t(1;10)(q32;p11), t(3;14)(p21;q13),inv(4)(p14q31), add(12)(q22),del(14)(q32) [5] 46–48,XX,add(1)(q?32),del(3)(p25), del(5)(q31),del(6)(q15),add(11)(p13), +del(12)(q22),−13, |

(*continued*)

**Table 2** *(continued)*

| Case # | study | Main study cohort | Abnormal karyotypes | | | | | |
|---|---|---|---|---|---|---|---|---|
| | | | Age/ gender | Tumor site | Tumor status | Histo-pathology | Radio-therapy | Karyotype |
| | | | | | | | | add(16)(p11),add(16)(q24),+17,<br>der(18)t(1;18)(q12;q23)x2,<br>add(19)(q13) [cp3]46,X,del(X)(p22.1),<br>t(1;9)(p36.1;p13),t(4;9)(p12;q34),<br>t(6;16)(p11;q24) [2]<br>45,X,del(X)(p11.2p11.4),<br>der(5)t(5;14)(p13;q11),?add(11)(q22),<br>del(12)(q22),−13,<br>der(17)t(13;17)(q14;p13),add(21)(q22) [3] |
| 28 | | | 25M | SB | R | Chondroid | No | 48,XY,+5,+7,+12,−13,<br>add(13)(q34),−18,+20 [2]49,idem,<br>+19 [16] |
| 29 | | | 34M | SB | R | Classic | No | 44–45,XY,t(2;14)(p23;q11),<br>?t(3;12)(p21;p13),del(4)(q?23),−5,<br>−6,der(11)t(6;11)(q11;p12) [cp2] |
| 30 | | | 58F | SB | R | Classic | Yes | 46,XX,t(4;17)(q23;q21),<br>t(8;9)(q11;q11) [3]<br>46,XX,t(2;20)(p31;p11.2),<br>t(3;22;16)(p21;q11.2;q22),del(6)(p23) [2] |
| 31 | | | 41M | SB | R | Classic | Yes | 52–66,−X,−X,−Y,add(1)(q22)x2,i(1)(q10),<br>+2,−3,der(3)t(3;4)(p?24;q?13)t(1;3)(q21;q21)X2,<br>4,der(4)del(4)(p12)add(4)(q13)x2,add(6)(q?21)+7, |

| | | | | | | |
|---|---|---|---|---|---|---|
| | | | | | | −9,−10,add(11)(q13)x2,add(11)(q25),+add(11)(q25), −12,13,add(13)(?q13),?del(15)(q11.1q13)×2, ?dup(15)(q11.1q13),add(17)(q24),−18,+19, −20,+21,+22 [cp9] |
| | | | | | | 46,XY,1,der(1)?t(1;4)(p13;q?27), +der(3)t(3;11)(q29;q11)add(3)(p13),del(4)(p12), der(4)add(4)(p16)t(1;4),inv(7)(p?21q?34),add(8)(p22), del(9)(q21),del(10)(q22),der(11)add(11)(p15)?del(11) (q13q22),?inv(14)(q11.2q32),+add(15)(q22), der(15;16)(q10;q10),?t(17;20)(q?23;q?13.3) [cp4] |
| 32 | 33M | SB | R | classic | Yes | 38,X,−X,i(1)(q10),−3,−4,add(6)(q27),+7,−9, −10,−13,−14,−18,−22 [cp5] |
| 33 | 65M | SP | R | Classic | Yes | 43–45,−Y,del(X)(q?26),t(2;17)(q21;p13),del(6)(q?25), add(9)(p24),inv(14)(q13q24) [cp10] |
| | | | | | | 46–47,XY,t(1;2)(q44;q13),inv(3)(p?24.2q29), t(4;9)(q33;q22),t(8;16)(q24.1;q24),t(10;13) (p13;q12) [cp5] |
| 34 | 15F | SB | R | Classic | Yes | 44–46,XX,t(1;22)(p32;q11.2),?t(2;20)(q33;q11.2), der(3)t(3;4)(p21;q?31;1)t(3;22)(q21;q13),der(4)t(3;4), ?t(9;15)(p22;q22),t(17;18)(q21;q23) [cp15] |
| 35 | 52M | SB | R | Classic | Yes | 45–47,Y,del(X)(p22.1),del(1)(q24),?t(8;18)(q24.1;q23), add(9)(q34),?inv(9)(p11q22),del(16)(q?22),add(17)(p11), add(19)(q13),del(20)(q11.2) [cp20] |
| 36 | 69M | SB | R | Classic | Yes | 45–46,XY,der(1)t(1;1)(q42;p34.1), der(1)t(1;1)t(1;14)(q24;q11.2),t(3;5)(p23;p11), t(3;10)(q21;q24),t(4;6)(q31.1;p11.2), t(4;16)(q25;p11.2),der(?6)del(6)(p12p21.2)t(6;12) (q?27;?21.2),t(13;16)(q12;q22),der(14)t(1;14) [cp10] |

(*continued*)

**Table 2** *(continued)*

| Case # | study | Main study cohort | Abnormal karyotypes | | | | | |
|---|---|---|---|---|---|---|---|---|
| | | | Age/ gender | Tumor site | Tumor status | Histo-pathology | Radio-therapy | Karyotype |
| 37 | | | 47F | SB | R | Classic | Yes | 46,X,?del(X)(q26q26),inv(3)(p23q?25),inv(7)(p22q22), add(8)(p23),der(8)t(8;9)(p11.2;q22)t(8;13)(q13;q11), der(9)t(8;9),t(10;15)(q26;q12),der(13)t(8;13), del(17)(p11.2p11.2),t(21;22)(q11.2;q13) [cp11]46, XX,inv(20(p13q11.2),del(7)(q11.1q11.2), t(14;19)(q11.2;p13.3),del(16)(q23)46, der(X)del(X)(p11.4)del(X)(q21),der(X)t(X;X)(q26;p11.4) der(5)t(5;9)(q11.2;q32),inv(6)(p23q?13), der(7)t(7;9)(p15;p24),t(7;15)(p12;q15), t(8;12)(q24.1;q22),?t(8;19)(p22;p11), der(9)t(7;9)(p15;p24)t(5;9)(q11.2;q?32), t(10;20)(p13;q11.2),del(22)(q13) [3] 37–40,XX,i(1)(q10),−3,?t(3;13)(p26;q11), −4,?t(4;5)(p14;q33),der(5)t(?4;5)(q?21;q?33),−6, +7,der(9)add(9)(p24)del(9)(q22),−10,−13,−14, del(15)(q21),−18,add(20)(p11.2),−22,+mar [cp3] |
| 38 | Tallini *et al.* [334] | SAC chordomas | 80 M | SAC | N/A | N/A | N/A | add(1)(p11),−3,−4,−10,−11,−14, der(14;15)(q10;q10),−22,−mar |
| 39 | | | 60 F | SAC | N/A | N/A | N/A | 43,t(X;1)(q28;p31),der(X;7)(q10;p10),add(1)(p11), add(3)(p13),add(3)(p25),add(5)(p15), _der(7)t(1;7)(p21;p22),add(8)(q24),−10,add(11)(p11), der(12)t(7;12)(q11;p11),ins(12;?)(q13;?),−13, del(14)(q32),−17,−18,−mar |

| | | | | | | | | |
|---|---|---|---|---|---|---|---|---|
| 40 | | | 55 M | SAC | N/A | N/A | N/A | 44,X −3, −9,−Y, -mar |
| 41 | | | 60 M | SAC | N/A | N/A | N/A | 47,XY,+X/46,XY |
| 42 | | | 61 M | SAC | N/A | N/A | N/A | 46,XY,t(1;16)(q44;q11)/46,XY |
| 43 | Gil *et al.* [119] | 3 SB chordomas | 66 F | SB | R | Classic | N/A | 45–46,X,del(X)(q23) [3],t(2;9)(p23;p24) [5],t(3;19)(q26;q13) [4],t(5;15)(p13;q26) [5],+der(8) [3] [cp7] |
| 44 | | | 47 M | SB | P | Dedifferentiated | N/A | 71,XY,+X,+1,+1,+2,+2,+5,+6,+6,+7,+7,+8,+9,−11,add(11)(p15),+12,+14,+14,+16,+7mar,3dmin |
| 45 | Kuzniacka *et al.* [188] | 7 SP and SAC chordomas | 74M | SAC | P | N/A | N/A | 40–42,XY,−3,der(6)t(6;9)(q?25–27;q11-12),−8,−9, der(9)t(9;10)(p24;?) or der (9)t(9;16)(p24;?),−10, dic(12;?16)(?p1?3;?)?inv(12)(p11p13), der(21)t(8;21) (q11;p13),−22 |
| 46 | | | 60F | SAC | P | N/A | N/A | 43,−X,der(X;1)(q22-24;p13),der(1)t(1;11)(p1?3;p1?3), der(1;22)(q10;q10),add (3)(p1213), der(3)t(3;12)(p25;?p11),der(5)ins(5;19)(p15;p11p12) or der (5)ins(5;19)(p15;q11q12), der(7)t(2;7)(p15-16;q21-22) or der(7)t(2;7)(q31-32;q2122),+der(7)t(7;13)(p15;?q14)t(1;13)(p22;q22),der(8)t(7;8)(?q32;q24), ?der(10)del(10)(p11)del(10)(q22), der(11)t(11;16)(p11;q11),der (12)t(7;12)(q11;p11), ?inv(12)(q13q15),−13,del(14)(q32),−16,−17,−18 |
| 47 | | | 51M | SAC | R | N/A | N/A | 42,X,−Y,der(1)t(1;3)(p31;p11-12),der(2)t(2;3)(p21;?), −3,der(3)t(2;3)(?;p12), −4,der(5)t(5;16)(q33;?p?), der(7)t(5;7)(q33;q36),+der(8)t(1;8)(?;q24),del(9)(p13),−10,del(11)(q13),dup(12)(q13q24), +del(12)(q13),−16,−18,dup(18)(q?), ?add(19)(q13), der(22)t(4;22)(q11;p11)/40,X,−Y,der(1)t(1;3), der(2)t(2;3),der (2)t(2;7)(p?;?),−3,der(3)t(2;3), |

(*continued*)

**Table 2** *(continued)*

| Case # | study | Main study cohort | Abnormal karyotypes | | | | | |
|---|---|---|---|---|---|---|---|---|
| | | | Age/ gender | Tumor site | Tumor status | Histo- pathology | Radio- therapy | Karyotype |
| | | | | | | | | der(4)t(4;7)(p?;?),der(5)t(5;16),der(6)t (6;7)(q?;?),der(7) t(5;7),del(9),−10,del(11),dup(12),+del(12),der(13)t(8;13) (q?;q?),−16,der(17)t(6;17)(?;q?),der(19)t(3;19),der(22) t(4;22)/46,del(X) (q24),−Y,der(1)t(1;9)(p36;?),der(2) t(2;16)(p21;?),der(3)t(3;14)(p21;q24)t (3;16)(q11;?)t(2;16) (?;?),der(4)t(4;13)(q3?;?),der(5)t(5;16),der(6)t(6;8) (p23;?p21),?del(7)(q?),der(8)t(6;8)(?;p?),del(9),del(11), der(12)t(7;12) (q?;q24)t(5;7)(q33;?),+del(12)(q13q15), der(14)t(3;14)(q21;q24),−16,der(16)t (Y;16)(q11;p13), der(17)t(9;17)(q?;p?),?add(17)(p11),der(19)t(X;19) (?q24;p13) |
| 48 | | | 71M | SP | P | N/A | N/A | 47–48,XY,+2,inv(9)(p11q12)c,+13,−14,−16, −16,+2mar |
| 49 | | | 71M | SP | R | N/A | N/A | 40–44,XY,−1,der(3)t(1;3)(q11;q11),?−4, der(9)t(9;14)(p11;p13),−22 |
| 50 | | | 59M | SP | P | N/A | N/A | 47,X,−Y,+6,+7 |
| 51 | | | 50M | SAC | MET | N/A | N/A | 33–40,X,−Y,−1,add(1)(p11)x1-2,+2, der(2;14)(q10;q10),−3,add(4)(p15),−5,−6, ins(6;?1)(q24;q25q44),−8,−9,−10,add(11)(p15), −12,der(12)t(8;12)(q13;q24), −13,−13,−15, add(16)(q22),−17,−18,−20,−21,−21,−22, +der(?)t(?;13)(?;q13), +1−4r,+4mar |

P: primary, R: recurrent, SAC: Sacral, SB: skull base, SP: spinal, MET: metastatic.

Several solid tumors are known to have microsatellite instability (MIN), a term used for allelic size alterations in microsatellites, oligonucleotide tandem repeats dispersed throughout the genome. This is a signal of defective DNA mismatch repair and resultant genomic instability. Klingler *et al.* [174] found MIN in 6 of their tumor samples. In contrast Pallini *et al.* [258] found no MIN in the 9 tumor tissues they studied.

## Cell cycle control

The retinoblastoma (Rb) gene is a well characterized tumor suppressor gene which is shown to have several important roles in oncogenesis. Eisenberg *et al.* [90] demonstrated LOH at intron 17 of the retinoblastoma gene in 2 of 7 chordomas they studied but in none of the 2 chondrosarcomas.

Naka *et al.* [244] found alterations in cyclin D1, and pRb proteins, all of which take roles in the G1-S checkpoint of the cell cycle in 10–45% of primary chordomas.

## Tumor suppressor genes

Riva *et al.* [284] performed a linkage analysis in 27 sporadic chordoma cases and mapped a defect to 1p36.13, common to 85% of the cases [231, 284]. By performing RT-PCR analysis on candidate genes in this region the authors suggested that Caspase 9, Ephrin-2A and DVL1 (which is also a candidate for neuroblastoma transformation) genes may play a role in chordoma tumor-suppression [284]. Defects at 1p may be an early change in chordoma oncogenesis.

P53 plays an important role in the response to genetic damage and metabolic disturbance and modulates, cell cycle arrest, repair and apoptosis. Deregulation of this tumor suppressor gene is found in majority of human cancers. Bergh [26], Kilgore and Prayson [168], Naka *et al.* [244], Pallini *et al.* [258] found p53 overexpression in 0, 27%, 30%, 40% of the chordoma cases in their cohorts respectively. In a comprehensive analysis, Naka *et al.* [244] showed that high p53 levels in this 30% of their cases correlated well with increased mitotic index and decreased patient survival. In a significant proportion of human cancers increased p53 levels result from mutations in the p53 gene. However, the authors found no mutations in the p53 gene in cases with increased p53 levels, possibly indicating an alternative mechanism for p53 protein accumulation. Mdm2 overexpression is a common mechanism of p53 inactivation in sarcomas, but not in chordomas [244].

There are numerous case reports on occurrence of chordomas in patients with the tuberous sclerosis complex [32, 43, 178, 201]. Lee-Jones *et al.* [201] showed somatic mutation of corresponding alleles in patients with TSC-1 or TSC-2 tumor suppressor gene germ line mutations. A causal relationship is not proven.

### *Oncogene activation*

Most studies on oncogene activation in chordomas were motivated by the availability of small molecule receptor tyrosine kinase (RTK) inhibitors and the prospect of the use in recurrent/refractory chordomas [364]. No studies on the significance or downstream signaling of these or RTK's is available. Weinberger *et al.* [364] in their study 10 chordomas (30% skull base, 50% sacral, 20% sacral) found consistent immunoreactivity for EGFR and c-Met receptors, robust expression in 50% and 70%, respectively. HER2/neu receptor expression was present in 70% of the tumors [364].

### *Experimental models of chordoma*

Spontaneous chordomas are documented in several animals including rats rats, ferrets, cats, dogs and minks, however currently there are no animal models with spontaneous chordomas. Explant cultures of chordoma cells have been performed by Horten and collegues [147] who also have generated several commonly used human glioma cell lines. Another cell line, U-CH1, was generated from a recurrent sacral chordoma by Scheil *et al.* [304], who also described its chromosomal abnormalities in detail.

## Pathology

Chordomas are slow growing, unencapsulated, extraaxial tumors that are locally invasive within bone of the skull base (Table 3). They have an extradural origin; however, few completely intradural cases have also been reported [261].

**Table 3.** *Definitions*

| | |
|---|---|
| Chordoma | A rare neoplasm of skeletal tissue mostly in adults, derived from persistent portions of the notochord; composed of cells arranged in lobules, with abundant myxoid stroma with some clear vacuolated cells |
| Chondrosarcoma | A sarcoma derived from cartilage cells which produce cartilage matrix<br>May develop de-novo or secondarily from a preexisting benign cartilaginous neoplasia such as such as enchondroma or osteochondroma. This is the third most common primary malignant tumor of the bone but only 2% arises in the skull base |
| Chondroma | A benign neoplasm derived from mesodermal cells that form cartilage |
| Parachordoma | A neoplasm that develops outside the axial skeleton in muscle, adjacent to tendons, synovium and bone and has morphological features identical to chordoma |

On gross examination they have a smooth or lobulated surface, gelatinous. The cut surface is usually homogenous, and inside the tumor is often soft with occasional semi-translucent gray and blue areas, focal hemorrhages, cyst formations cartilage and calcifications. The high mucin content is responsible for the semi-fluid consistency. Chordomas are unencapsulated and grow infiltrative along the lines of least resistance in the bone [141]. However a pseudocapsule may be seen, especially in skull base cases that grow into soft tissues or the dura mater.

Skull base chordomas are not primary tumors of the nervous system and classified among tumors that involve the nervous system by local extension. Three histopathological variants are recognized: Classic (International classification for disease-oncology [ICD]: M-9370/3), chondroid (ICD: M-9371/3) and dedifferentiated chordomas (ICD: M-9372/3). Light microscopy of chordomas shows a differentiated morphological phenotype, despite the malignant biology in most cases. Light microscopy of the **classic chordoma** reveals cells with a clear but granular appearance (Fig. 1). The cytoplasm is eosinophilic and stains positive with the periodic-acid Schiff (PAS) stain [283]. Distinct, larger cells with eccentric nuclei abundant vacuolated and reticulated cytoplasms due to intracellular accumulation of glycoseaminoglycans are called physaliferous cells and are typical of chordomas [283]. The nuclei are eccentric, hyperchromatic, have prominent nucleoli and rarely demonstrate atypia. These cells rarely present the majority [283]. The biological nature of physaliphorous cells is still not clear. It is widely accepted that the vacuoles are droplets of mucoid material in the cytoplasm. An ultrastructural and histochemical study showed intracellular enrichment in the enzymes leading to synthesis of stromal glycosamino-

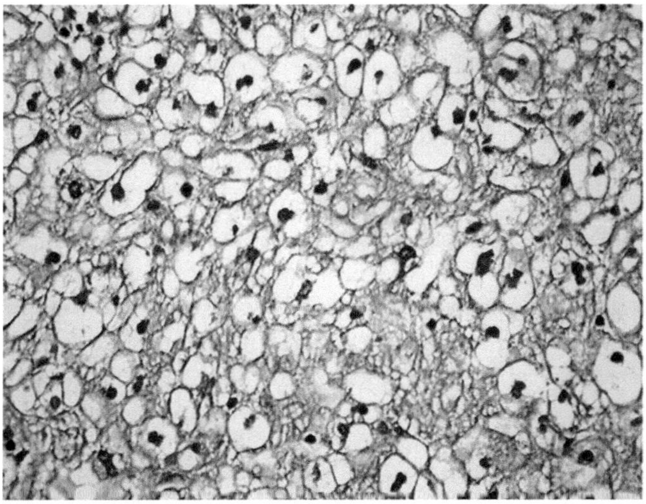

**Fig. 1.** Light microscopy of chordoma. Cells with vacuolated cytoplasm and small, uniform hyperchromatic nuclei are seen (Hematoxylin-eosin stain)

glycans and the excessive synthesis and storage of sulfated glycosaminoglycans, which suggests that the vacuoles result from the breakdown and utilization of membrane-bound glycogen in sulfated glycosaminoglycans biosynthesis [191]. Signet-ring appearance may be seen in cells containing an intermediate quantity of mucin [141]. Electron microscopy also reveals parallel bundles of criss-crossing microtubules within the rough endoplasmic reticulum, but the significance of these structures is not known [156].

A lobular configuration may be marked with cell clusters divided by thin fibrous septa in the myxoid extracellular matrix. The fibrous septa may be thin or thick and hyalinized Naka *et al.* [243] found fibrous septa in 79 (64.8%) of the 122 chordoma samples they studied. Forty-two per cent of the tumors with septa had also a lobular growth pattern and a more favorable prognosis when compared to those without a lobular pattern. The lobules either contain a sheet of cells or a pool of mucin [141]. The mucoid matrix stains strongly with Alcian blue.

Mitoses, necrosis, hypervascularity or spindle cells are typically absent or rare in the classic chordoma. Pools of mucin containing cords of eosinophilic syncytial cells can be found. These cords often attach peripherally to the septa and are projected toward the center, giving an impression of a continuum from polyhedral cells containing little mucin. **Cellular chordomas** have very little extracellular matrix while others contain numerous cells resembling adipocytes and are called **lipoid chordomas** [291] None of these pathological subtypes are associated with distinct tumor biology and likely represent individual variations of the classic chordoma.

Low grade chondrosarcomas and chordomas can have similar localization, imaging characteristics and pathological appearance and have traditionally been analyzed together to create sufficiently large artificial cohorts to enable conclusive analyses. Accumulating evidence has shown, however, that chondrosarcomas have a more benign and predictable tumor biology and therapeutic response when compared to chordomas [290]. Low-grade chondrosarcomas respond much better to surgical resection, to conventional, stereotactic, charged particle therapies and recur less frequently. In selected cohorts more than 99% of patients with chondrosarcomas were still alive 10 years after diagnosis [290]. Chondrosarcoma patients also fare much better than patients with chordoma in terms of median and long-term survival. Therefore, to come up with realistic conclusions, chordomas and chondrosarcomas should be considered separately.

The distinction of chordoma, pleomorphic adenoma, mucinous adenocarcinoma, and chondrosarcoma may pose difficulties to the neuropathologist but immunohistochemical techniques are usually adequate to establish the diagnosis [273]. Chordomas exhibit an epithelial phenotype [232, 289]. Morphologically they possess atypical epithelial markers in conventional microscopy and desmosomes and simple cell junctions in electron microscopy. Immunohistochemical analysis also presents an epithelial phenotype with staining for EMA [33, 223,

**Table 4.** *Immunohistopathological findings in chordomas*

| | Classic chordoma | Chondroid chordoma | Chondro-sarcoma | Ref. |
|---|---|---|---|---|
| EMA | 88–94 | 24–33 | 0 | [223, 232, 289] |
| Cytokeratin | 94–100 | 32–33 | 0 | [223, 232, 289] |
| S100 | 44–94 | 85–100 | 20–100 | [2, 223, 232, 289] |
| Vimentin | 94 | 92 | 100 | [2, 223, 232, 289] |

232], low molecular weight cytokeratins 7, 8, 18, and 19 (simple epithelial), as well as high molecular weight 4, 5, and 6 (mucosal epithelial). In contrast chondrosarcomas do not express epithelial markers. Despite this clear distinction there were no survival difference between cytokeratin positive and negative tumors [232]. There are very conflicting reports on the incidence of S-100 or CEA positivity in chordomas, so we presented the results of large studies in Table 4.

In 1973 Heffelfinger *et al.* [141] described a variant of chordomas that contained islands of chondroid differentiation, resembling chondrosarcomas. The authors called this **chondroid chordoma** and also documented lower rates of recurrence and longer survival when compared to classic chordomas. Since this observation there has been an ongoing debate about existence and the prognostic significance of this phenotype. Chondroid chordomas contain areas of typical chordoma intermixed with islands of stellate cells in lacunar spaces, resembling chondrocytes. The chondroid component may be in the form of small scattered foci or even dominate the picture [141]. As in classic chordoma, anaplastic features are lacking. Electron microscopical studies supported the dual nature (epithelial-mesenchymal) of these neoplasms by showing that the chondrocyte-like cells have mesenchymal features while other cells have epithelial features [353].

Some authors speculated that chondroid chordoma may be in fact a low grade myxoid chondrosarcoma with good prognosis [157]. As the conclusion of an analysis of 7 chondroid chordomas, 18 classic chordomas, 2 peripheral chondromas, 8 peripheral chondrosarcomas, fetal notochord and fetal cartilage of 9-week and 12-week gestational age, Brooks *et al.* [36] even questioned the existence of any cartilaginous differentiation in chordomas. In the contrary later studies from Mayo clinic did not replicate the prognostic findings of the previous study by Heffelfinger *et al.* and it was suggested that this difference in survival might be related to the younger age of the chondroid chordoma patients in that study [106, 232]. The immunopositivity of classic and chondroid chordomas for epithelial markers was demonstrated by Mitchell *et al.* [232], who analyzed 16 classic chordomas, 25 chondroid chordomas and 12 condrosarcomas at the Mayo clinic. In this study the authors found immunopositivity for EMA in 88%, 24%, 0, for cytokeratins in 100%, 32%, 0, for S100

**Table 5.** *Comparison of chondroid tissues, tumor and chordomas*

| | Fetal chorda dorsalis | Pediatric nucleus pulposus | Adult nucleus pulposus (cartilage) | Classic chordoma and Chordoid areas in chondroid chordoma | Chondroid areas in chondroid chordoma | Chondrosarcosma |
|---|---|---|---|---|---|---|
| Primary cell type | Physalipherous cells | Chondrocyte like rounded cells | Chondrocytes | Physalipherous neoplastic cells | Chondrocyte like rounded neoplastic cells | Chondrocyte like rounded neoplastic cells |
| Typical ECM molecules expressed | Collagen VI, (focal Collagen I and III) Chondroitin Sulphate and Keratan Sulphate rich Proteoglycan | Collagen II | Collagen IIB | Collagen VI (focal Collagen I, II and III) Chondroitin Sulphate and Keratan Sulphate rich Proteoglycan | Collagen II Aggrecan | Collagen II, Collagen X Aggrecan |
| Typical immuno-histochemical markers | EMA pan-cytokeratin cytokeratin 19 vimentin S-100 | EMA pan-cytokeratin cytokeratin 19 vimentin S-100 | Vimentin S-100 | EMA pan-cytokeratin cytokeratin 19 vimentin S-100 | Vimentin S-100 | Vimentin S-100 |

44%, 88% and 100 and for vimentin in 94%, 92% and 0% for classic chordomas, chondroid chordomas and chondrosarcomas respectively. Rosenberg *et al.* [289] reported a comparative analysis of 38 classic chordomas, 12 chondroid chordomas, 28 chondrosarcomas, fetal notochord, ecchordosis physaliphora, and fetal hyaline cartilage. All classic and chondroid chordomas in this study were positive for cytokeratin, and the majority was also positive for EMA and CEA. In contrast, none of the chondrosarcomas stained for cytokeratin, EMA, or CEA. Vimentin and S-100 were positive in more than 95% of both classic chordomas and chondroid chordomas, and chondrosarcomas. Histopathological findings and immunoistochemical profiles of the tumors correlated well with their proposed physiological counterparts (Table 5). The authors concluded that chondroid chordoma is a subtype of chordoma and not chondrosarcoma. In another study on chondrosarcomas by Rosenberg *et al.* [290] the authors found S100 positivity in 96 of 97 (98.9%), cytokeratin expression in 0 of 97 (0%) and a faint staining for epithelial membrane antigen in 7 of 88 tumors (7.95%). Chordomas have chondrogenic potential as demonstrated by the expression of Collagen II protein expression in the tumors, even in the absence of chondroid areas [336, 365]. It has also been shown that chondroid areas in chondroid chordomas mimic nucleus pulposus development. In an elegant immunohitochemical study, Gottschalk *et al.* [126] showed that the physalipherous cells in the fetal chorda dorsalis expressed collagen VI (focally I and III), Chondroitin- and keratin-sulphate rich proteoglycan and was positive for EMA, epithelial cytokeratin, vimentin and S100. The pediatric nucleus pulposus had chondrocyte like rounded cells and was positive for Collagen II expressed EMA, Epithelial Cytokeratin, Vimentin and S100 while the adult nucleus pulposus had round chondrocytes, Collagen II, vimentin and S-100. Classical chordomas, chordoid areas of chondroid chordomas, fetal chorda dorsalis have similar cellular features and matrix composition while chondrosarcomas have a different pattern. Additionally the expression of intercellular adhesion molecule (NCAM, VCAM-1, CD44, N-Cadherin, B-Catenin) expression in chordomas also mimics fetal notochord. Neural cell adhesion molecule (NCAM) expression is associated with the formation and maintenance of chordoma tissue architecture. NCAM is not expressed by chondrosarcomas and therefore of important value in the differential diagnosis of chordoma versus CS. In their tissue comparison with microarray Fujita *et al.* [111] found CD24 overexpression in the nucleus pulposus. The same study also reported CD24 immunoreactivity in 6 of 7 studied chordomas, however in none of the chondrosarcomas. CD 24 is a P-Selectin (CD62P) ligand, however its role in chordomas is not known. Valderrama *et al.* [353] studied ultrastructural characteristics of chordomas and found that the presence of well-formed tonofilament desmosome complexes as well as complexes composed of alternating profiles of rough endoplasmic reticulum and mitochondria were seen only in chordoma and chondroid chordoma, but not in cartilaginous tumors. Deniz *et al.* [79] studied the expression of several extracellular matrix proteins and growth factors (basic fibroblast growth factor, transforming growth factor $\alpha$, vascular endothelial growth factor, fibronectin, collagen III, and collagen IV) that take part in oncogenesis in chordomas with aggressive and benign courses. This descriptive data from immunohistochemical analyses of chordomas suggested that high levels of transforming growth factor $\alpha$ and basic fibroblast growth factor expression, ligands of two important cellular kinase pathways that are shown to be important in a wide variety of cancers, were linked to higher rates of recurrence and an aggressive behavior [79].

Taken together, these clinical, immunohistochemical and ultrastructural findings quite strongly support the hypothesis that chordoid chordomas are a subtype of chordomas and not of chondrosarcomas. However, it remains unproven still if chondroid chordomas, in fact, have a better outcome than classic chordomas.

In a minority of patients chordomas exhibit atypical histopathological features of a round cell tumor or spindle cell sarcoma. Such tumors are usually composed of sheets of relatively small epitheloid cells with oval to irregular nuclei with a minimal amount of eosinophilic to clear cytoplasm and commonly exhibit tumor necrosis. Atypical chordomas usually have higher mitotic activity (1–3/10 hpf) and more commonly demonstrate cellular atypia than conventional chordoma, chondroid chordoma or cellular chordoma. This histology is commonly observed in the pediatric population and is almost exclusively associated with aggressive behavior [31, 58, 144]. Chordomas with such a sarcomatous component are called **dedifferentiated chordomas** [104, 207, 222]. Only very few cases have been reported in the literature, mostly in sacrococcygeal location and in pediatric population. Dedifferentiated chordomas constitute less than 4% of chordomas at initial presentation and are documented through the course of a chordoma in 4–9% of the cases [341].

There is scant information on the evolutionary process of a dedifferentiated chordoma in comparison with classic chordomas. The clonality of the two tumor components has not been analyzed. Some authors suggested that dedifferentiated chordomas might arise secondary to sarcomatous transformation after radiotherapy, or even be a collision tumor. However roughly ¼ of the dedifferentiated chordomas arise in patients who did not receive any radiation and this speaks against the exclusive role of radiation in causality [119]. Other authors postulated that a sarcomatous progression could be regarded as a failure of differentiation rather than a reversal of differentiated cell to an embryonic undifferentiated cell. Sarcomatous areas of dedifferentiated chordomas are negative for the epithelial markers such as cytokeratin and EMA [119]. The usual finding in dedifferentiated chordomas is such that the high-grade malignant spindle cells stain strongly for vimentin and weakly for cytokeratin, S-100 protein, and epithelial membrane antigen (EMA), whereas the areas of conventional chordoma in these same neoplasms stain moderately for vimentin and S-100 protein, and strongly for cytokeratin and EMA [150]. Immunohistochemistry studies in dedifferentiated chordomas report that the transitional areas between conventional and dedifferentiated chordoma exhibited EMA and CK positivity, despite an absence of the same markers in the center of the sarcomatous areas [150, 294]. Vimentin and alpha1-antichymotrypsin are also reported positive in these areas and this supports the pathogenesis of sarcomatous transformation from chordoma [294].

## Local invasion

Chordoma is a locally aggressive tumor and almost exceptionally invades the surrounding bone. The process of bone invasion requires active proteolytic activity, and Heackel *et al.* [130] showed that chordomas were positive for Cathepsin K, an osteoclast protease. In their study of 44 chordomas, 10 chondrosarcomas and 10 fetal specimens the authors showed that Cathepsin K and its mRNA were present in the advancing tumor front in chordomas [130]. This protease was not present in fetal notochord or in skull base chondrosarcomas, except for in entrapped osteoclasts. Naka *et al.* [242] studied the expression of extracellular matrix proteases MMP-1, MMP2, MMP9, Cathepsin B and urokinase plasminogen activator in non-skull base chordomas and found that patients with high MMP2 activity has a significantly worse prognosis.

Although they are widely invasive in the bone, skull base chordomas do not invade, but simply displace surrounding soft tissues [253]. This is especially noteworthy from the surgical standpoint, because adjacent vessels, nerves and dura are not invaded [101]. In 6 cases involving the cavernous sinus Goel *et al.* [122] did not find any vessel wall invasion.

## Metastasis

Metastases occur in 3–48% of adult patients with chordomas and sacrococcygeal and vertebral chordomas are more likely to metastasize than intracranial cases [26, 52, 252, 320]. One study reporting post mortem results in 27 skull base chordomas found a 37% incidence of metastases [209]. Borba *et al.* [31], in their extensive review of pediatric chordoma cases in the literature found the incidence to be 57.9% in patients younger than 5 years. Interestingly 87.5% of these cases had atypical histopathology. Metastases usually are encountered late in the disease course, usually years after the initial presentation and most commonly become manifest in the bone and skin [52]. However lesions in lungs and lymph nodes are also frequently seen. Most common sites of involvement in the pediatric population were lungs followed by lymph nodes, bone, liver, dura mater, kidney, adrenal glands, cerebrospinal fluid, and heart (7.1%). Seeding through the cerebrospinal fluid has been reported [329, 347]. Surgical seeding of chordoma is reported in 7.3% of the cases along the operative route or even at distal sites such as fat tissue graft harvest site [11].

### *Intraopertative diagnosis and cytology*

Smear preparations from chordomas are generally satisfactory. Usually chords or clusters of discohesive cells set in an abundant mucinous background is observed. Tumor cells are uniform and have rounded nuclei. Physaliphorous cells can be seen but these must be differentiated from freezing artifacts. The ECM stains metachromatically with toluidine blue.

Fine needle aspiration biopsies (FNAB) are seldom possible in skull base chordomas but are of significant diagnostic importance especially when retropharyngeal extension is present [34, 140]. Studies on the cytology of chordomas most consistently report moderate to hypercellular smears of typical physaliphorous cells in a myxoid background [64, 140, 181, 234, 355]. However hypocellular smears have also been reported [246]. In addition to the physilaphorous cells, a second population of non-vacuolated epitheloid cells is also commonly reported [64]. Tumor cells are usually clustered in groups and have indistinct cytoplasmic borders [64, 360]. Occasionally well demarcated cells surrounded by the myxoid background are seen [64, 360]. Cytoplasmic vacuolization in pysaliphorous cells in a minority of cases leads to nuclear indentation or even "signet ring-like" cells [64]. Layfieled *et al.* [200] reported the cytological diagnosis of a dedifferentiated chordoma in a patient with radiographic appearance of a conventional chordoma, emphasizing the importance of cytological diagnosis.

### Incidence

Chordoma is a rare bone tumor of the axial skeleton. The incidence varies considerably among studies and is dependent on the methods used for analysis. Clinical studies report incidences between 0.2% and 6.15%. However, most studies are affected by selection bias associated with referral and treatment patterns. Population-based studies avoid these type of bias and report incidences ranging from 0.18 to 0.8 per million (Table 6). A detailed list of population based studies on chordomas is presented in Table 6. The prevalence of chordoma has been stable in the last 3 decades [220] The incidence increases with advancing age [141, 349]. The peak incidence is reported to be in the 4$^{th}$ to 7$^{th}$ decades [220] decades. Mean age at diagnosis ranged 48 to 55 years among studies [96, 141, 251, 256, 349]. Median age reports vary between 58.5 and 62 years (range 3–95 years) [85, 89, 220, 270]. Although chordomas may be encountered in virtually any age group congenital or infant cases are exceptional and pediatric cases are rare [88, 217]. Patients younger than 20 years only

**Table 6.** *Population based studies on chordoma*

| Study | Origin of registry or study cohort | Study period | Total number of cases | incidence | F/M ratio | Age at diagnosis (years) | Peak Incidence (decades) | Anatomical localization | | | Follow-up (years) | Median survival (years) | 5 and 10 year survival (%) |
|---|---|---|---|---|---|---|---|---|---|---|---|---|---|
| | | | | | | | | Sacral | Spinal | Skull-base | | | |
| Paavolainen and Teppo [256] | Finland | 1953–1971 | 20 | $0.3/10^6$ in males $0.18/10^6$ in females | 1:1.5 | Mean 55.5 | 6–7 | 75 | 15 | 10 | Complete* | N/A | 35/18 |
| Eriksson [96] | Sweden | 1958–1970 | 51 | $0.51/10^6$ | 1:1 | Mean 57 | 6–7 | 57 | 16 | 27 | 8–20 | 4.6 for sacral 3.3 for S/B 3.5 for spinal | N/A |
| O'Neil [251] | Scotland | 1953–1971 | 34 | N/A | 1:1 in S/B 2.6:1 in sacral | Mean 49.6 | N/A | 52.9 | 11.8 | 35.3 | N/A | 7.2 for sacral 7.7 for S/B | N/A |
| Price and Jeffree [270] | England | 1946–1974 | 11 | N/A | N/A | Median 59 | N/A | 45 | 37 | 18 | N/A | N/A | N/A |
| Dreghorn [89] | England | 1958–1989 | 13 | N/A | N/A | Median 62 | N/A | 70 | 30 | Not included | Mean 6.2 | 3.75 | N/A |
| Dorfman and Czerniak [85] | USA | 1973–1987 | 221 | $0.3/10^5$ for 75–79 years age group | 1:1.6 | Median 59 | 6–7 | N/A | N/A | N/A | N/A | N/A | 63.8/– |
| McMaster *et al.* [220] | USA | 1973–1995 | 400 | $0.08/10^5$ | 1:1.7 | Median 58.5 | 7–8 | 29.2 | 32.8 | 32 | N/A | 6.29 | 67.6/39.9 |

* Patients were followed until all were deceased. S/B: Skull base.

make up 5% of the cases [31, 144, 217, 261, 320]. Pediatric cases constituted 5.5% of our cohort and only 35.71% of the patients were younger than 40 years at presentation [261]. Female to male ratio ranged from 1:1 to 1:2 [85, 89, 96, 141, 204, 220, 251, 256, 270, 349, 358]. Chordomas were very rarely reported in the black race [85, 220]. In a study of 221 chordomas Dorfman and Czerniak [85] found only 4 cases (1.8%) in blacks.

Chordomas represent 3–8.4% of all primary bone tumors, 17.5% of the primary bone tumors of the axial skeleton, 0.2% of all intracranial tumors and 6% of all skull base tumors [141, 209, 220, 357]. Among primary bone cancers chordomas are the fourth most common pathology [85, 209, 220]. In their analysis of 2627 histologically verified primary malignant bone tumors, Dorfman and Czerniak reported that chordomas comprised 8.4% of the cases [85]. Unni [349] analyzed 11087 cases of malignant bone tumors seen at the Mayo clinic from 1901 to 1994 and reported that chordomas comprised 4%. There is no gender predilection for skull-base cases.

Although chordomas can be seen anywhere along the axial skeleton, where remnants of the notochord are present, they are more commonly localized at the two craniocaudal extremes (Table 7). Most studies report a higher incidence for sacral chordomas but comparable incidences for sacral and skull base cases have also been reported by other authors both population based and clinical studies [220]. Young age (<26 years; $p = 0.0001$) and female sex ($p = 0.037$) were associated with greater likelihood of cranial presentation [220]. McMaster *et al.* [220] reported a higher incidence of skull base cases in the youngest age quartile and a higher incidence of sacral cases in the oldest group. Heffelfinger *et al.* [141] and Unni [349] both reporting Mayo clinic experience found that the average age at presentation was a decade earlier in skull base chordomas when compared to spinal or sacral cases. This may be related to the late presentation for treatment in nonskull base chordomas, which tend to be symptomatic

**Table 7.** *Anatomical localization of chordomas along the axial skeleton*

| Study | *n* | Mean age at diagnosis | Skull base (%) | Sacral (%) | Spinal (%) |
|---|---|---|---|---|---|
| Harvey and Dawson [138] | 240 | | 37 | 12 | 51 |
| Heffelfinger *et al.* [141] | 155 | 48 | 36 | 49 | 15 |
| Paavolainen and Teppo [256] | 20 | 55 | 10 | 75 | 10 |
| Price and Jeffree [370] | 11 | 59 | 18 | 45 | 37 |
| Eriksson *et al.* [96] | 51 | 57 | 27 | 57 | 16 |
| O'Neil *et al.* [251] | 34 | 49.6 | 35.3 | 52.9 | 11.8 |
| Unni [349] | 356 | 48 | 38.2 | 47.5 | 14.3 |
| McMaster *et al.* [220] | 400 | 55.8 | 32 | 29.2 | 3 |
| Total | 1124 | | 39 | 41 | 20 |

much longer and considerably larger in size at the time of presentation [141, 241, 349]. Alternatively the difference may be explained by different biological nature and behavior of chordomas in two different localizations.

Analyzing 128 skull base cases that have been diagnosed in the USA 1973 through 1995, McMaster *et al.* [220] reported that 51.8% of the patients were treated surgically alone, 44.6 with a combination of surgery and radiotherapy, 1.8% with radiotherapy alone. Another 1.8% did not receive any treatment. Median survival reported in this analysis was 6.29 years; 5- and 10-year relative survival rates were 67.6% and 39.9%, respectively. Dorfman and Czerniak reported a five year relative survival rate of 63.8% [85]. The 5 year survival numbers have not changed in the last 3 decades [220]. There was no overall increased risk for second primary cancers after the diagnosis of chordoma [220].

## Clinical manifestations and natural course of disease

There are no exclusive signs or symptoms of skull base chordomas and the presentation depends on the localization, extent and direction of expansion of the tumor [225]. The usual presentation is of vague complaints of headache and/or neck pain, followed by rapid progression of one or more of the symptoms [225]. The average time between the onset of symptoms and clinical presentation reported for all chordomas is 3.44 years. However there is much variation in this and presentations as quick as 1 week and as late as 16 years have been reported. Acute presentations are however rare and related to unusual complications such as intratumoral hemorrhage [110]. Skull base chordomas present to clinical attention in average one decade earlier than sacral chordomas [349]. Diplopia and headache are the most common symptoms in patients with skull base chordomas [114, 282]. Diplopia is present in the majority of patients. Symptoms may be persistent or intermittent [16]. On examination CN-VI is the most commonly involved nerve followed by CN-III and CN-IV. Ptosis may be seen in up to 50% of the patients.

Headaches are of aching character and are most commonly poorly localized. Retroorbital pain or pressure sensation is also frequently reported. Bone destruction and neuralgia are the most common causes of pain. Trigeminal nerve is the most frequently affected. Visual loss is reported in only a minority of patients. Facial numbness may also be reported in up to 30% of the patients. Facial paresis may also be encountered. Lower cranial nerve involvement most commonly presents as hoarseness and dysphagia. Dizziness, hearing loss and vertigo may be encountered due to CN VII and CN VIII traction, compression or cervicomedullar junction compression. Neural axis impingement by lower clival tumors may result in spastic paresis in the extremities. Compression at the craniovertebral junction can cause hydrocephalus, syringobulbia and syringomyelia and resultant symptomatology.

Natural course of chordomas after they become symptomatic is dismal. Kamrin *et al.* [162], estimated that the average survival of an untreated chordoma would be between 6 and 24 months. Eriksson and colleagues reported a less than 1 year survival without treatment [96]. Menezes *et al.* [225] reported an average survival of 28 months after the onset of symptoms.

## Diagnosis

### *Neuroradiology of chordomas*

Preoperative diagnosis of chordoma mainly relies on neuroradiology. Computerized tomography (CT) and magnetic resonance imaging (MRI) are the backbone of modern neuroradiological imaging of chordoma. Sensitivity of CT and MRI for chordomas are similar and the information provided is complementary [332]. MRI is superior in delineating the extent of the tumor, its relation to surrounding structures including neural parenchyma, cranial nerves, vessels and the CT is superior in imaging bone involovement [332, 362]. Current neuroradiological technology can reliably diagnose chordomas and chondrosarcomas, however differential diagnosis between chordomas and chondrosarcomas or between classic and chondroid chordomas is not reliable [87, 229, 255, 261, 317, 362].

The classic appearance of intracranial chordoma on CT is that of a centrally located, well-circumscribed but invasive, lytic soft tissue lesion within the clival bone [87]. Bone margins are not sclerotic. The mass usually contains large calcifications and bone sequestra [87, 261, 332, 362]. The lesion is usually slightly hypodense to brain parenchyma and usually enhances well after injection of iodinated contrast agents [95]. Single or multiple small hypodense areas may be seen [95]. CT is of great importance in evaluating erosion of cranial foramina.

MRI is the single best imaging modality for chordomas of the skull base [38, 87, 195, 203, 229, 255, 261, 332]. The typical small chordoma will arise within the clivus, cause expansion of the bone, will have a homogenous hypointense T1 and bright hyperintense T2 signal, enhance moderately and heterogeneously after contrast injection [38, 87, 95, 195, 203, 229, 255, 332].

#### MRI and CT correlates of pathological findings

Physaliphorous cells contain intracytoplasmic mucopolysaccharide accumulations and have a high water content [141]. Most chordomas and chondrosarcomas appear iso- to hypointense to adjacent brain parenchyma on conventional spin echo T1w images [38, 87, 95, 195, 203, 229, 255, 261, 332]. In our analysis only 4.8% of cases had a hyperintense signal on T1w images [261]. Such hyperintense signal on T1W images in a minority of patients has also been demonstrated by other authors, however the pathological correlate is not known [87, 299]. On T2w images most chordomas exhibit high to very-high signal intensity [229, 261].

Chordomas are the second most common mass lesion within the clivus after metastases [170]. Normal clivus has a uniformly low signal on T1w images which changes to uniformly high signal intensity in the third to fourth decades [170, 254]. This incidence of a T1 bright clivus increases with advancing age. Especially in the elderly the chordoma will thus appear as a clear cut hypointense focus within the hyperintense signal of the fatty bone marrow of clivus [95]. In larger lesions the clear demarcation from the surrounding tissue may be lost [170]. Doucet *et al.* [87] suggested that the incomplete delineation of chordomas on MRI may indicate microscopic distal extension of tumor cells. Meyers *et al.* [229] indicated that indistinct and irregular borders are found at sites of marrow invasion. Enhancement of the normal clivus is mild, howeve the contrast enhancement of the hypoientese tumor tends to be intense [170].

Majority if chordomas have a homogenous cut surface and in our experience 64.3% of cases had also homogenous signal on T1w images. Lobule formation is also a hallmark of chordomas, and this feature is more readily appreciated on T2w images, where hypointense fibrous septae will separate highly hyperintense lobules [195, 229, 261, 332]. Lobulation is seen in approximately half of the cases and with the same incidence both in chordomas and chondrosarcomas [261]. In less than half of the cases areas of recent and old hemorrhage, collections of mucin, necrotic regions, dystrophic calcification, and/or entrapped bone trabeculae will result in a heterogenous signal intensity on MRI [87, 225, 229]. Some chordomas show focal areas of low attenuation, and these are thought to represent myxoid and gelatinous material found in pathology specimens [227]. This feature is more commonly observed in spinal chordoma variants [227]. Small hemorrhagic foci, which are common in chordomas, appear as hyperintense in T1w images will appear hypointense in spin echo sequences [95]. Bone sequestrae, hemorrhages or mucus pools with high protein content will appear as hypointense foci on T2w images.

Major vascular structures in the region such as the ICA and the basilar artery are easily appreciated as flow-voids on T2W MRI [229, 261]. Meyers *et al.* [229] indicated that 79% of skull base chordomas displaced or encased major vascular structures. Vascular flow voids must be differentiated from a speckled pattern of low signal, which most likely represent calcifications. The absence of the flow voids of major vessels should prompt for angiography as this might indicate vascular narrowing, however this is very rare [229, 261]. Abnormal vascularity or tumor staining is generally absent on angiography.

Chordomas and chondrosarcomas show varying degrees of contrast enhancement [87, 332]. Enhancement is usually moderate and only a very small proportion of chordomas do not enhance [229, 261]. Strong enhancement is seen only in a small minority of cases [261]. Heterogenous contrast enhancement

, the known "honeycomb" pattern [87, 95, 362]. Intravenous contrast can ectively demonstrate meningeal, cavernous sinus or sellar involvement, intracranial or retropharyngeal extension as well as invasion of cranial foramina. Strong enhancement of the dura may also help aid in indirect demonstration of the tumor extent and will strongly facilitate diferential diagnosis [229]. Fat suppression can aid in differentiating between enhancing tumor mass and the surrounding fatty marrow or fat grafts from previous surgery, however susceptibility artifacts, especially around the paranasal sinuses can be a limiting factor. Several studies reported similar contrast enhancement patterns in CT and MRI. In our analysis contrast enhancement was less frequently observed on CT [261].

## Osseous invasion

Bone destruction is demonstrated in 95% of chordomas and chondrosarcomas and this is almost always accompanied by expansion of involved bone and no reactive bony changes surrounding the area of destruction [182, 261]. This finding is lost with further enlargement of the tumor [87].

We detected advanced erosion of the occipital condyle on CT in roughly 26% of our cases that involved the inferior clivus and 60% of these cases required postoperative occipitocervical fusion [261].

Chordomas and chondrosarcomas may feature bone sequestra as well as dystrophic calcification or mineralization of the chondroid matrix (ring-and-arc pattern). CT is reported to demonstrate calcification in 41% to 88.1% of chordomas [87, 114, 229, 261, 332]. It is not always possible to differentiate bone sequestrae from calcification on CT. Weber *et al.* [362] suggested that linear, globular, or arc-like calcifications may help differentiate chordomas from chondrosarcomas. Erdem *et al.* [95] found that dystrophic calcification was more common in chondroid chordomas than in classic chordomas. In our analysis there were no significant differences among the 3 groups (classic chordoma, chondroid chordoma, chondrosarcoma) with respect to proportions of lesions with calcification [261].

## There are no characteristic radiological findings of chordoma subtypes

A differential diagnosis between skull-base chordomas and chondrosarcomas preoperatively using radiological methods would be extremely valuable but currently there are no reliable radiological markers to differentiate chondrosarcomas from chordomas or classic chordomas from chondroid chordomas [255, 261].

All three histopathological types of chordoma have a classic chordoma background or at least have some classic chordoma component to it. Chondorid chordomas have additional chondroid foci and atypical chordomas have sarcomatous foci. Sze *et al.* [332] reported that in their cohort chondroid chordomas had shorter T1- and T2-signal when compared to classic chordomas and speculated that this may be related to the replacement of gelatinous-watery matrix by the chondroid foci. This has been largely cited in the literature despite the lack of any studies confirming this finding. On the contrary many studies, including three studies with large cohorts of 42, 28 and 22 patients, did not find such a difference [87, 228, 229, 255, 261, 317, 362].

Some authors argued that chordomas are midline pathologies whereas chondrosarcomas are more often located off the midline and speculated that this finding may be used for differential diagnosis [229, 362]. We and others did not find any differences concerning location relative to the midline between chordomas and chondrosarcomas [261, 285].

## Tumor size and extent

It is extremely difficult to identify the site of origin of a chordoma or chondrosarcoma because neither of these neoplasms has a radial growth pattern. Both tumors tend to invade surrounding bone in rather unpredictable fashion, and only those that are confined to a specific anatomical compartment (intradural tumor, cavernous sinus, and others) exhibit radial growth. In our series, we observed no significant difference in tumor volume between skull-base chordomas and chondrosarcomas. To specifically define the extent of each mass, we divided the skull base into 18 zones and recorded whether tumoral tissue was present/absent in each. Our detailed analysis of the extent of the 42 tumors revealed no difference between chordomas and chondrosarcomas [261]. This finding is consistent with prior reports [69, 285]. We also observed no significant differences between the 2 chordoma subtypes (classic and chondroid) with respect to lesion volume or tumor extent [261].

Skull base chordomas occur at the spheno-ocipital synchondrosis and grow within the clival bone [305]. In an analysis of 28 chordoma cases, Meyers *et al.* [229] reported extension into the middle fossa in 32.1% of cases and into the posterior fossa in 78.5%. Albeit rare, other localizations outside the central skull base are also encountered and include purely intrasellar [161, 339], purely intracavernous [117, 123, 192, 193, 312, 318], within Meckel's cave [22, 261] and those that are purely intradural [261] chordomas.

Although the sella and parasellar area is very frequently involved, pure intrasellar chordomas are rare [261, 339]. Cavernous sinus is involved in 54 to 75% of the chordoma cases [375]. In addition to cases arising purely within the cavernous sinus larger tumors can involve the cavernous sinus secondarily. There is still no consensus on the nature of cavernous sinus invasion. Cases of chordomas arising within the cavernous sinus or those which secondarily invade the cavernous sinus are known]. Goel *et al.* [123] reported their observation that the cavernous sinus involvement was in the form of displacement rather than invasion while others like El-Kaliny *et al.* [92] concluded that chordomas were invasive in the cavernous sinus. In our experience aggressive surgical resection for cavernous sinus involvement was associated with poor surgical outcome and high morbidity. Surgical results of chondrosarcomas were better than those achieved in chordomas [260].

The relation of the tumor to the petrous and intracavernous internal carotid artery is of clinical significance. Displacement or partial encasement is frequently observed, but complete encasement is exceptional [122, 123]. Chordomas displace the relatively immobile parts of the internal carotid artery in the petrous and precavernous segments along its anterolateral border [122]. In massive tumours, the entire intrapetrous segment of the artery can ne displaced. At the petrous apex, the fifth nerve is displaced superiorly while the carotid artery was displaced anteriorly [122]. Luminal narroving may be due to stretch but not due to invasion [122].

Intradural extension is a frequent feature of chordomas. Of the 38 chordomas in our series, only 47.2% were completely extradural [261]. The pathogenesis of this intradural extension is unknown. As with invasive pituitary adenomas, it is not known whether skull-base chordomas actually invade and penetrate the dura or extend through small dural defects or around cranial nerve sleeves [253]. Some reports have stated that chordomas do not penetrate the dura, and that the exact mechanism of this intradural extension is yet to be proven. Interestingly, several cases of intradural ecchordosis physillaphora have been reported within the pons which were connected with a pedicle to their intraclival part, however no such case has been documented in chordomas [3, 221]. MRI is the modality of choice for assessing intradural extension of chordomas and chondrosarcomas. CT myelography can also be used for this purpose, but this modality is seldom indicated given the extraordinary tissue resolution of MRI [332]. It is very rare for a chordoma to be purely intradural. Dow *et al.* [88] found a total of 19 reported purely intradural chordoma cases in the literature and we have also reported another case [261]. No age or gender predisposition is noted in cases reported so far. Median age of the reported cases is 38 (range 9–57 years). Males constituded 42.11% of the cases and 37.89% were females. Interestingly, it is easier to totally resect chordomas that are completely intradural than it is to totally remove other chordomas [88]. Complete resection is reported to be commonly achieved in intradural chordomas and no recurrence has been reported in any of the intradurally located chordomas with follow up periods ranging from 1 month to 12 years [5, 88, 229, 261, 367]. Our patient who had the strictly intradural chordoma is recurrence-free 10 years after complete surgical removal with no adjuvant therapy. MR spectroscopy may aid in differential diagnosis of purely intradural chordomas [215].

Skull base and cervical chordomas can spread by para- or retro-pharyngeal extension. Pharyngeal extension is seen in 7.1–25% of cases. We only observed retropharyngeal extension in tumors that involved the inferior clivus. Chordomas have been reported within the craniofacial skeleton [125], frontal, ethmoid and maxillary sinuses [142, 319], mandible and scapula. Although extension into sphenoid or ethmoid sinuses is seen in chordomas, subfrontal extension has not been reported [228, 229, 261].

Metastatic chordomas are found in 3 to 48% of the cases but become manifest very rarely [252, 320]. Chordomas may seldom seed through cerebrospinal fluid pathways [329, 347]. Surgical seeding of chordoma is also documented in 7.3% of the cases along the operative route or even at distal sites of fat tissue graft harvest [11].

## Differential diagnosis

Several different pathologies can mimic the radiological appearance of chordomas and chondrosarcomas in the skull base [87, 95, 115, 203, 283], however chordomas and chondrosarcomas of the skull base can be reliably differentiated from other tumors of the skull base with current neuroradiological technology. Meningiomas of the region are differentiated by their homogenously intense contrast enhancement on MRI, presence of a dural tail, and hyperostotic bone reaction on CT and frequent tumor blush on angiography [87]. Chordomas with sellar involvement should be differentiated from an invasive pituitary adenomas [301]. Although sellar encasement is very common in chordomas and chondrosarcomas, pure intra-sellar cases are exceptionally rare [339]. Endocrinological studies may be suggestive of an adenoma, however several endocrinological disturbances may also be seen in sellar chordomas [339]. Chordomas may also contain hemorrhages and mimic pituitary apoplexy [202]. Other pathologies that should be ruled out include malignant lesions such as plasmocytoma, lymphoma, metastasic as well as nasopharyngeal or paranasal carcinomas. Rhabdomyosarcomas should also be suspected in the pediatric population. Benign lesions that should be considered in the differential diagnosis are histiocytosis X, fibrous dysplasia, dermoid and epidermoid cysts as well as giant carotid aneurysms [87, 95, 115, 203].

Ecchordosis physaliphora (EP) are believed to be the precursors of chordoma. These benign lesions are common incidental findings and are found in roughly 2% autopsies or imaging studies for done for other reasons [3, 221]. Exceptionally rare symptomatic cases have been reported [3, 49, 186, 210, 286, 340]. To date there are only 12 reported EP cases with MRI findings [3, 49, 186, 210, 221, 286, 340, 361]. Eleven of the 12 cases were hypointense on T1W images and all were hyperintense on T2w images. In several cases a pedicle connecting the intradural lesion to the clivus was demonstrated [3, 221]. None of the cases showed contrast enhancement. At times an EP may be symptomatic and in these cases it may be difficult to differentiate these notochordal remnants from chordomas and clinical follow up may be needed. Wolfe *et al.*

[367] suggested that all such lesions should be considered intraaxial chordomas. Rodriguez *et al.* [286], in the contrary, stated that all MRI findings suggestive of symptomatic, intradural, extraosseous physaliphorous cell growth should be classified as giant or symptomatic EP as long as the existence of an intradural chordoma is not definitely proven.

## Classification schemes

At present, aggressive surgical resection remains the most effective available treatment for chordomas [100, 199, 259]. Chordomas and chondrosarcomas vary much in their localization and extent in the skull base. Therefore, preoperative neuroradiological workup has an enormous impact on the choice of the optimum surgical approach to maximize resection and minimize morbidity. Through the years, several classification systems have been proposed to aid surgical planning (Table 8). The first scheme was described by Schisano and Tovi [305], who categorized skull-base chordomas as sellar or clival types. Falconer *et al.* [99] classified skull-base chordomas and chondrosarcomas as sellar, parasellar or clival subtypes. Subsequently, Sekhar and Janecka [314] classified chordomas as superior middle and inferior clival subtypes. Each of these classification schemes was very valuable in its time, but became less significant as operative approaches to the skull base evolved. This evolution continues.

With the need for an improved classification method and aware of the weaknesses of the current classification schemes, we devised a new method to quantify and define tumor extent within the skull base structures [261].

**Table 8.** *Surgical-anatomical classification schemes of chordomas reported in the literature*

| | |
|---|---|
| Krayenbühl and Yasargil [182] | 1. Clival<br>2. Parasellar<br>3. Sellar |
| Schisano and Tovi [305] | 1. Basiocciput<br>2. Basicsphenoid |
| Raffel [274] | 1. Basi-occiput<br>2. Basi-sphenoid |
| Falconer *et al.* [99] | 1. Sellar<br>2. Parasellar<br>3. Clival |
| Sekhar and Janecka [314] | 1. Superior clival<br>2. Middle clival<br>3. Inferior clival |
| Goel *et al.* [122] | 1. Petroclival<br>2. Others |

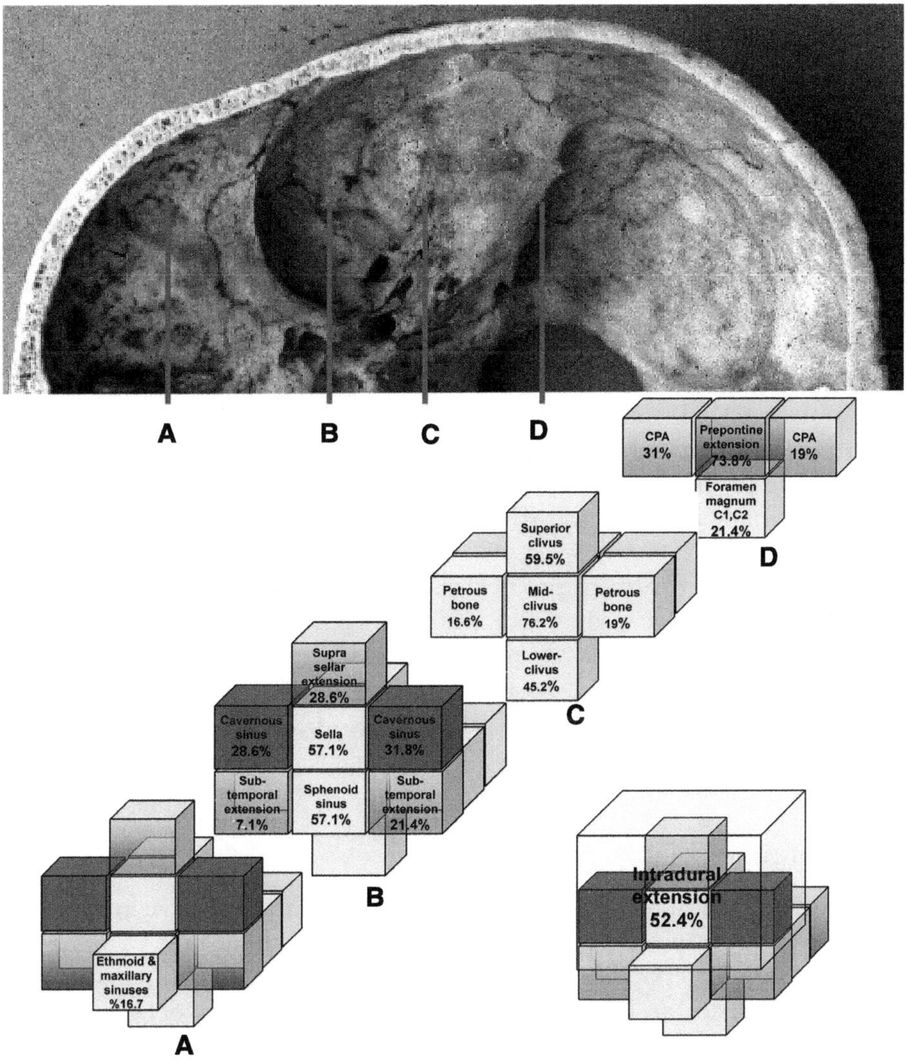


**Fig. 2.** Schematic representation of the 18 zones within the skull base. Red lines (A–D) represent the planes at which the schematic descriptions are made. Such a division of the skull base allows a detailed and objective description of the extent of each skull base chordoma to aid in surgical decision making, postoperative evaluation of resection and follows up. Please refer to the text or reference 273 for further details

For each tumor we analyze the presence/absence of tumor involvement in 18 distinct anatomical zones in the skull base (Fig. 2).This system addresses specifics of tumor location and extent, and thus provides very valuable information both for selecting the optimal surgical approach and systematic comparison. In our analysis of 38 skull base chordomas and 4 chondrosarcomas (42 tumors total) a mean of 6.7 (SD ± 2.9) zones was involved in each tumor [261].

## Early and late postoperative imaging

Aggressive surgical debulking remains the most effective treatment option for chordomas Although total resection is rarely possible, extensive removal is correlated with a longer survival [60, 65, 114, 259, 345]. The extent of surgical removal is of crucial importance for planning of further treatment as recurrence is most commonly observed as persistent growth of a residual tumor mass [316]. Early postoperative MRI within the first 48 hours is performed in all neurooncological operations at our clinic. Its efficiency has been proven for several tumor types including chordomas and thus it has become a part of our current treatment paradigm for chordomas [91, 169, 259]. Early postoperative MRI led to a second attempt of surgical removal in 10.6% of our patients [259]. With increasing availability intraopertive MRI may supplement or substitute early postoperative MRI.

Despite modern treatment protocols a significant percentage of skull base-chordomas recur regardless the mode of therapy [259]. Recurrence is most frequently observed as hyper-intense mass in T2w images [95]. Most recurrences occur at the main tumor mass, most commonly as persistent growth of residual tumor. Recurrence along the surgical path has also been reported in 5% [103]. Distant metastasis is seen in up to 7–14% of patients, more so in children and with the dedifferentiated phenotype [31, 52, 252, 331].

## Intraoperative imaging

Ultasonography, CT and MRI have all been used for intraoperative imaging for skull base tumors. Intraoperative MRI is used in both resective surgery or biopsy sampling of chordomas [29, 86, 219, 233, 262]. Intraoperative MRI caries a high potential to improve surgical result as it can show details, location and extent of known or unexpected residual tumor tissue and feed this information to neuronavigation equipment improving the extent of tumor removal [262]. Short term results of intraoperative MR imaging in different pathologies such as pituitary adenomas, low and high grade glial tumors, epilepsy surgery, suprasellar tumors are very encouraging [29, 39, 57, 98, 247, 248, 262]. Use of intraoperative MRI can be useful for chordoma surgery in several perspectives. First it has a high potential in assuring a safer and more extensive surgical resection, possibly decreasing the need for staged surgeries. In several approaches, and maybe most importantly in the transsphenoidal approach, it can provide dynamic image guidance. Finally the availability of objective feedback on operative success facilitates planning of further treatment.

We have been using an intraoperative 3 tesla MRI system for more than a year and early results have been reported [262]. We are using the Siemens 3T

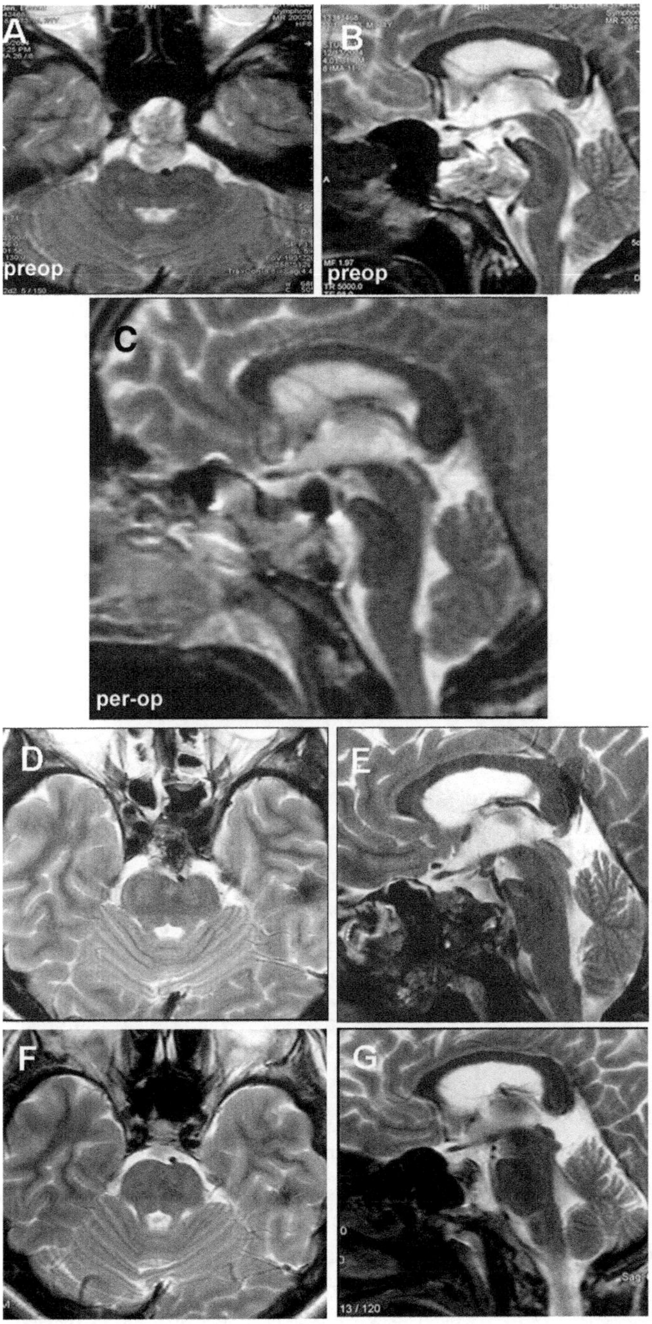


**Fig. 3.** Use of intraoperative MRI. for a clivus chordoma. T2w MRI of a patient showing preoperative (A and B), intraoperative (C), early postoperative (D and E) and postoperative 15$^{th}$ month (F and G) images

Trio (Erlangen-Germany) system which is capable of intraoperative imaging and functions as a clinical scanner as well. Our preliminary experience indicated that, as with many other tumors, the ioMR is very useful in the surgery for chordomas to help decrease complications and to increase the total resection rate. An exemplary figure of gross total chordoma resection without complications is demonstrated in Fig. 3.

### *Other diagnostic tests*

Plain X-ray films may demonstrate an osteolytic lesion, osteosclerosis or may be normal in a minority of cases [351]. Calcifications or bone sequestrae are less readily diagnosed than with CT [229, 261]. Technetium Tc 99m bone scans are seldom performed but may reveal hot areas within the tumor. PET scans can also demonstrate chordomas, however are not routinely utilized.

For accessible lesions fine needle aspiration biopsies, with or without image guidance, may be performed to verify diagnosis. However, it should be kept in mind that such interventions will interfere with imaging findings. Presence of retropharyngeal tumor poses a unique opportunity for transpharyngeal biopsy in exceptional cases when preoperative radiology is not conclusive. However the incidence of retropharyngeal tumor extension is low (8.33–25%) and is only present in cases involving the lower clivus [5, 182, 229].

## Treatment of chordomas

Current treatment options of skull base chordomas rest mostly on level-4 and very limited level-3 evidence. This is mostly a consequence of the rarity of this disease [220]. Since its first description in 1856 there have been only 24 studies of skull-base chordomas that reported cohorts larger than 30 patients [15, 28, 47, 65, 106, 114, 117, 142, 145, 152, 168, 211, 229, 234, 253, 254, 265, 278, 307, 313, 314, 350, 361b, 368].

There are three different philosophies regarding the treatment of chordomas: aggressive surgical resection, with radiotherapygiven only in patients who have remnants, aggressive resection followed by radiotherapy, and partial resection followed by radiotherapy. Sekhar and Crockard have followed the policy of aggressive surgical resection and no radiotherapy unless distinct remnants remain [315, 317, 345]. In contrast, Al-Mefty advocated administering radiotherapy to all patients postoperatively, regardless of extent of resection [5, 30, 60].

In a recent study Tzortzidis *et al.* [345] have presented the clinical outcome and recurrence rates of 74 cranial base chrome patients at long term follow-up after aggressive microsurgical resection. On the basis of the experience gained from this series, they have stated that tumor resections are much easier if the patient is seen initially, before the patient has had a previous resection or radiotherapy and recurrent tumors are not only more difficult to remove, but also carry a higher complication rate. Thus, the surgeon's aim should be to administer the optional treatment during the initial treatment session, which may consist of tumor resection and/or radiotherapy. In this paper the thoughts of the senior author, Sekhar were stated as: "whenever possible, radiotherapy should be reserved for recurrences rather than initial therapy". In this series, better long-term results were obtained in primary tumors than recurrent tumors. However, they have also stated that this may be caused by more aggressive biological behavior (recurrent tumors) rather than complete removal (in primary patients). For the recurrent tumors their policy was summarised as:" when a patient presents with recurrent tumors, the approach should be different and more conservative. If the tumor can be removed completely without causing disability, it should be removed. However, the surgeon (and the patient) should be aware that the chances of long-term survival and the potential for complications (resulting in disability) are higher in reoperation cases. The treatment strategy should be planned appropriately".

It is widely accepted today, based on critical analysis of available data, that surgical resection is the mainstay of chordoma treatment. A more complete resection is correlated with longer survival. And It is possible that younger patients benefit from resection and its extent [259]. The importance of intraoperative or early postoperative MRI cannot be overemphasized in the shaping of adjuvant treatment. The surgeons assessment of the completeness of resection is often unreliable and MRI interpreted by a team consisting at least of the operating surgeon and a competent neuroradiologist is required to assess completeness.

Maybe the most important factor determining how a patient will fare from surgery is the biology of the tumor. Today we know very little on oncogenesis of chordomas, however it is well established that not all chordomas behave the same. There are at least two subsets of patients with distinct clinical behavior: Some with a benign course and another group with an aggressive and rapidly progressive course over 3–5 years. The outcome is clearly dictated primarily by the intrinsic biology of the tumor and treatment seems only to have a secondary impact. However understanding the oncogenesis and intrinsic behavior will enable us to shape our treatment protocols rationally or even tailor it to the needs of the individual. With advancing molecular biology and increasing knowledge of tumor biology such a possibility is not remote.

Most chordomas are not surgically treatable and recurrences create a clinical picture of ever increasing complexity. Surgical resection, even when gross total, cannot exclude the possibility of recurrence and some form of adjuvant therapy is almost always required. Therefore management of chordomas by a multidisciplinary team is of crucial importance. Particle based radiation treatment was shown to be the most effective adjuvant therapy for residual chordomas after maximal surgical resection. However it is a very expensive treatment modality and most institutions do not have the luxury of particle based radiation therapies.

Few authors have reported such prospective management protocols. Protocols differ in the timing of postoperative imaging and the mode of postoperative radiation treatment and its timing. Increased understanding of chordoma biology and development of definitive conclusions on the optimal adjuvant therapy will eventually dictate optimal, patient based treatment protocols.

## Surgical treatment

### *Patients benefit from aggressive but safe surgery*

Accumulating evidence indicates that a simple debulking procedure is not the optimal surgical treatment for chordomas. Just in the contrary, an extensive resection of the tumor is shown to be of benefit to the patient. A subset of patients, if not all, benefits form the extent of surgical resection. This is especially true for the young patient population.

Extensive resection requires the use of more advanced surgical techniques. Chordomas arise in the center of the craniofacial skeleton and invade the surrounding structures with an unpredictable pattern, creating a very large and invasive tumor bulk. This oftentimes necessitates combination of several approaches or staged procedures to address tumor extension into different parts of the skull base [345, 346]. Facing such challenging tumors, Al-Mefty and Borba [5] classified chordomas according to their resectability. Type I chordomas can be resected along with a margin of normal bone and soft tissue. These tumors are small, symptomatic or asymptomatic and separated from critical structures. The most commonly encountered type is the Type II tumor which is larger and involves contiguous anatomic areas. Type II chordomas are still resectable with a single operative approach. Type III chordomas have extensive skull base involvement and require multiple approaches for resection.

It is commonly accepted that an extensive resection is feasible. However, there is no consensus to date regarding how aggressive the surgeon should be. Should a cavernous sinus involvement be addressed aggressively at the cost of cranial nerve morbidity? Does such an aggressive approach increase our chances of assuring local control? Can a similar outcome be obtained by "safe, maximal surgical resection" and adjuvant therapy? Current literature cannot provide definitive answers most of these questions [12, 84, 117, 132, 165, 193, 312]. However some facts have been proven by accumulating experience: Safe maximal resection is of benefit to the patient at initial resection, but is influenced by other factors such as history of prior surgery or radiotherapy, which greatly increase the risk of complications and force us to being more conservative [345, 346].

## *Evolution of the surgical technique*

Surgical techniques used for the treatment of chordomas are in constant evolution. Forsyth *et al.* [106] reported 78% subtotal removal and an 11% biopsy rate in patients treated with conventional techniques between 1960 and 1984. Skull base surgery, as it entered our routine armamentarium in the 1990's has provided major improvements in treatment of chordoma, which grows widely invasive in the skull base. Cumulative experience of the last 20 years has proven the usefulness of several of these approaches. For treatment of lower clival lesions with lateral extension the far lateral transcondylar approach has been a major improvement over transoral approaches with a limited reach and high complication rate. During this evolution limitations have been defined and the degree of success defined for each approach and emergence and popularization of newer technologies have helped define more precise indications. For example the limited midline reach of the traditional transsphenoidal transseptal approach was considerably widened with the popularization of extended transsphenoidal approaches [63, 109, 163, 302]. Couldwell *et al.* [63] reported that the extended transsphenoidal approach can expose the skull base from the cribriform plate of the anterior cranial base to the inferior clivus in the anteroposterior plane, and laterally to expose the cavernous cranial nerves and the optic canal. Similarly Kouri *et al.* [180] described the modifications to the standard trasnsphenoidal approach for accessing to suprasellar tumors. Increased interest in surgical neuroanatomy [236], wider use of endoscopes [159, 160], image guidance, and development of inntraoperative MRI have been major driving factors in the field [29, 86, 219, 233, 262]. Jho *et al.* described routine successful use of endoscopy for transsphenoidal approaches and described endoscopic removal of large posterior fossa chordoma [158–160].

With advanced surgical techniques gross-total tumor removal is achieved in approximately 50–71.6% of these patients, with estimated rates of mortality and major complications at 5% and 10%, respectively [259, 345]. Our analysis showed that the initial tumor volume was also correlated with operative outcome. Tumor progression was almost the rule if initial tumor volume exceeded 20 $cm^3$ [259]. In most studies the extent of resection was inversely related to the risk of recurrence [60, 65, 114, 259, 345]. And in many cases the patients have residual, albeit controlled, disease. To achieve high rates of complete tumor removal, 16 to 50% of patients require multiple skull-base operations [5, 60, 114, 259, 345]. These above-mentioned results represent dramatic improvement over conventional surgeries. The 5-year rate of progression free survival after this aggressive skull-base surgery is approximately 76% [259, 345].

Several different studies on the postoperative functional performance status of patients indicated that there was no improvement postoperatively [60, 114]. It should be noted that there is a small but significant group of patients, who experience functional deterioration due to the operative procedure and never improve [60].

## Principles of tumor resection

When treating chordomas the aim of surgeon is to reach the most extensive resection with the least morbidity. Preoperative evaluation includes, in addition to detailed neurological examination, neuroopthalmological, otolaryngological and endocrinological testing if appropriate and general medical assessment. Electrophysiological testing is also of great value. Comprehensive neuroimaging should also be undertaken to delineate tumor location, extent, invasion and relation to vital structures both using MRI and CT and additional techniques such as CTA, MRA or DSA as needed. Basic concepts of skull base surgery apply in their entire to chordoma surgery. As one of the pioneers of the radical skull base surgery for chordomas, Sen *et al.* [316] indicated that the tumor resection should follow pathways created by the tumor and follow an intracapsular route. Removal of bone is preferred over retraction of neurovascular structures. When dura is opened into communication with nasopharyngeal or oropharyngeal spaces, repair with vascularized large pedicle-flaps is required to prevent cerebrospinal fluid (CSF) fistulas.

## Choice of the surgical approach

With the current surgical techniques there is no single best operative approach to treat chordomas and all approaches have limitations as well as weaknesses. The choice of surgical approach is dictated by the tumor's location, extent, growth pattern, relation to the dura and surrounding vital structures. Other factors that must be taken into consideration are the general health of the patient, previous surgery or radiation treatment and the experience and choice of the surgeon.

We prefer to tailor the approaches according to the extension of each individual tumor. The extent of the tumor is analyzed according to our method, which simply marks the presence/absence of tumor tissue in 18 distinct anatomical zones in the skull base [261]. Details of this method and other previous classification schemes is described in the radiology section. Capabilities of each surgical approach to reach these 18 compartments are outlined in the Table 9. Details of each surgical approach are also presented below. Rough outlines are as follows: Midline central skull base can be reached by anterior or lateral transcranial approaches. Lateral extension of chordomas is best approached by lateral approaches. Tumors at the craniovertbral junction can be approached with midline subfrontal, maxillotomy or transoral approaches. Lateral extension of the tumor at the craniovertebral junction will necessitate

**Table 9.** Common surgical approaches to the skull base and extent of anatomical exposure. A positive sign denotes that the anatomical zone (columns) can be exposed with the corresponding surgical approach (rows).

| Approaches | Intradural extension | Sellar encasement | Suprasellar extension | Subtemporal extension | Cavernoussinus involvement | Sphenoidsinus involvement | Ethmoid–maxillary sinusinvasion | Superiorclivus involvement | Middleclivus involvement | inferiorclivus involvement | Prepontine extension | Petrousbone involvement | Cerebellopontine angleextension | Foramenmagnum/atlas/axisinvasion |
|---|---|---|---|---|---|---|---|---|---|---|---|---|---|---|
| Anterior approaches | | | | | | | | | | | | | | |
| Extended transbasal/subfrontal | + | + | + | – | +/– | + | – | +/– | + | + | + | – | – | +/– |
| Subcranial | – | + | – | – | +/– | + | – | +/– | + | + | + | – | – | +/– |
| Conventional transsphenoidal | – | + | + | – | – | + | – | + | +/– | – | – | – | – | – |
| Extended transsphenoidal | – | + | + | +/– | – | + | + | + | + | + | + | – | – | – |
| Transethmoidal-sphenoidal | – | + | – | – | – | + | + | + | + | – | + | – | – | – |
| Le-Fort maxillotomy | – | + | – | – | – | – | + | + | + | + | + | – | – | + |
| (extended) Transoral | – | – | – | – | – | – | – | – | – | + | – | – | – | + |
| Anterolateral approaches | | | | | | | | | | | | | | |
| Pterional | + | – | + | + | + | – | – | – | – | – | – | – | – | – |
| Fronto-orbitozygomatic | + | – | + | + | + | – | – | +/– | – | – | – | – | – | – |
| Cavernous sinus exploration | + | – | + | + | + | – | – | +/– | – | – | – | – | – | – |
| Lateral and posterolateral approaches | | | | | | | | | | | | | | |
| Subtremporal | + | + | – | + | – | – | – | + | – | – | – | – | – | – |
| Transpetrous apex | + | + | – | + | + | – | – | + | +/– | – | – | – | – | – |
| Presigmoid-Retrolabyrinthine | + | – | – | – | – | – | – | + | + | – | + | + | + | – |
| Presigmoid-Translabyrinthine | + | – | – | – | – | – | – | + | + | – | + | + | + | – |
| Total petrosectomy | + | – | – | – | – | – | – | + | + | + | + | + | + | – |
| Retrosigmoid | + | – | – | – | – | – | – | +/– | – | – | +/– | +/– | + | – |
| Extreme lateral | + | – | – | – | – | – | – | – | + | + | + | + | + | + |

the use of an extreme lateral approach. We have previously shown that use of tailored skull base techniques as opposed to conventional approaches decreased the postoperative residual tumor volume decreased from 20% to 9.2% [259]. Use of 3T intraoperative MRI and neuronavigation further improves surgical results [262].

## *Anterior approaches*

Midline central skull base can be reached by anterior or lateral transcranial approaches. These approaches expose the whole clivus in its entire from different angles. Entry may be performed by a bicoronal or facial incisions or through nasal or oral cavities or the neck. Within the facial skeleton a subfrontal, ethmoidal, transnasal, transseptal, transfacial, transmaxillary or a transoral route may be taken, either alone or in combination. All anterior approaches are in essence midline approaches and are limited in their lateral exposure.

### Midline Subfrontal approaches

Chordomas with significant suprasellar and anterior extension in addition to widespread disease in the clivus can be addressed with the transbasal, extended subfrontal approaches or their modifications [80]. These two approaches combine various degrees of bifrontal craniotomy and orbitonasal osteotomies. As described by Derome [80] in 1972 the transbasal approach is a capable and versatile anterior midline approach. Derome [81] published his experience with the results of 33 skull base chordomas and documented its versatility. This approach has been extended by several authors with the addition of varying orbital, nasal or ethmoidal osteotomies [53, 145, 187, 275, 313, 322, 377]. Sekhar *et al.* [313] described the extended subfrontal approach, and advocated a radical ethmoidectomy to improve exposure of the clivus. Spetzler *et al.* [323] further refined the approach by the addition of an osteotomy of the cribriform plate to preserve olfaction and facilitate the reconstruction of the floor of the anterior fossa. Several similar techniques involving varying slightly in their fronto-orbito nasal osteotomies have been described. Cadaver dissection studies report that the transbasal approach increases the viewing angle twice and the extended subfrontal approach five times when compared to the simple subfrontal approach [145]. The extended subfrontal approach involves a bifrontal craniotomy, followed by orbital, frontal and ethmoidal osteotomies. Planum sphenoidale is removed and both optic nerves are exposed and protected. Laterally the internal carotid arteries are identified and protected. Piecemeal removal of the tumor starts from the core and tumor boundaries within clivus are drilled until normal bone architecture is seen. Possible tumor remnants at blind spots at the dorsum sella or the petrous apices can be addressed using endoscopic assistance. Such an invasive skull base exposure also requires careful reconstruction with closure of

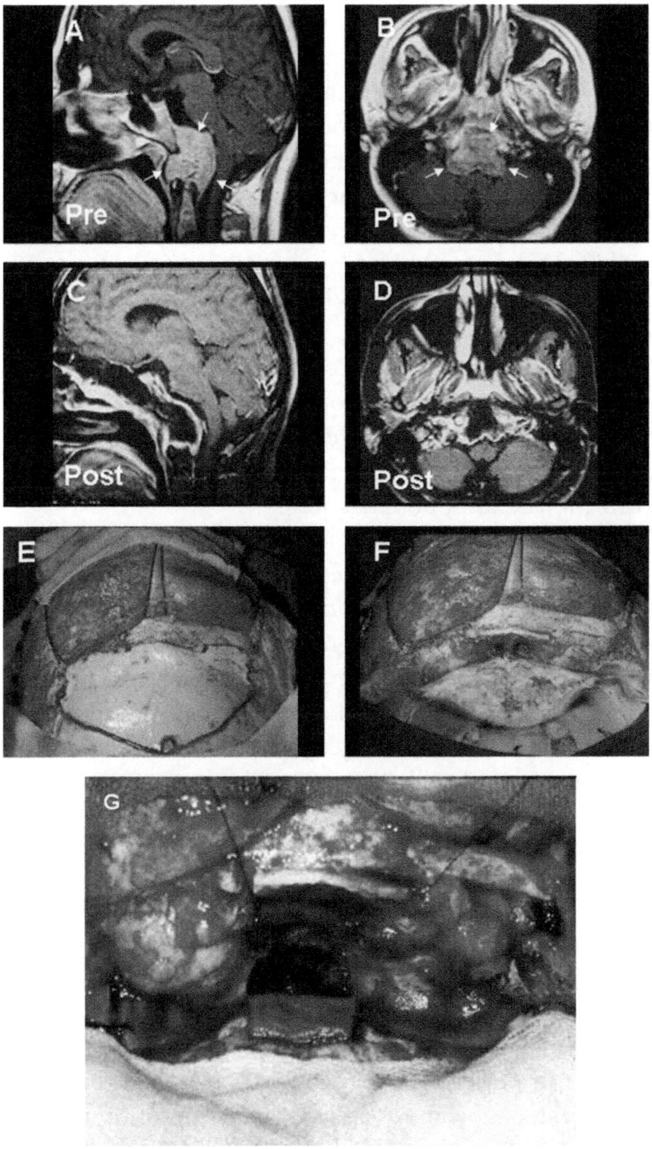


**Fig. 4.** Transbasal approach for the removal of an inferior clival chordoma. This approach is well suited for resection of midline tumors and provides access to as low as the axis. A and B present the preoperative T1w contrast enhanced images and show the inferior clival contrast enhancing chordoma impinging on the pontomedullar junction. C and D represent postoperative T1w contrast enhanced images with fat supression. E shows the monobloc bifrontal osteotomy. F shows the exposure after removal of the bone flap and (G) represents the deep exposure to the inferior clivus

dural defects, lying of a large pedicle-flap of pericranium along the surgical path and generous packing with fat on the cranial side.

Such midline subfrontal approaches provide an exceptionally deep view down to the skull base as low as the odontoid process of C2 (clival dura posteriorly and roof of the nasopharynx anteriorly) with very little brain retraction (Fig. 4) [81]. Superiorly the exposure of the superior clivus and the dorsum sella is limited by the dorsum sella [81]. Lateral boundaries of the approach decrease with the depth of exposure [80, 313]. Lateral boundaries in the ethmoid bone are formed by the orbital apices and the optic nerves. Within the sphenoid the lateral resection can extend into the cavernous sinus [80, 313]. Chordomas involving the medial wall of the cavernous sinus can be resected and venous bleeding which starts after resection of the tumor bulk can be stopped with surgical packing, however the risk of injury to the internal carotid artery and cranial nerves within the cavernous sinus becomes significant. Down at the clivus trigeminal roots and the hypoglossal nerves form the lateral boundaries [80].

These approaches are very versatile but they also have significant limitations. The exposure is deep and at times requires specialized equipment to reach the lesion that lies 8–10 cm away from the opening [53, 145, 187, 275, 313, 377]. These approaches are essentially designed to address lesions in a midline corridor but can be combined with some type of lateral approach to address for lateral extensions of the tumor. Possible complications of transbasal and subfrontal approaches are frontal lobe injury, CSF leak, injury to the optic, abducens and olfactory nerves, carotid rupture and hypopituitarism [70].

## Transsphenoidal approaches

Their extradural origin, their predominantly extradural extension and little hemorrhage make chordomas attractive targets for endonasal approaches (Fig. 5). Traditionally, the conventional transseptal-transsphenoidal approach was considered appropriate only for biopsy or for subtotal removal of small midline lesions of the upper (retrosellar) clivus only [12, 136, 196, 198, 212, 317, 335]. However with the development of newer technologies such as image guidance, intraoperative MRI and neuroendoscopy endonasal and description of alternative techniques these approaches are gaining popularity and with more reports of success its role is being reconsidered. To date, despite all the encouraging preliminary results, only few reports exist on use of microsurgical transsphenoidal [63, 74, 190, 197] or the endoscopic transnasal approach [44, 74, 109, 159, 160] for the treatment of clival chordomas. Apart from its ever increasing use for resective surgery, the transsphenoidal technique also still maintains its valuable role for biopsy [29].

The main limitation of classical-midline approaches was their inability to address lateral extension adequately. Several new techniques have been proposed to overcome these shortcomings both for microsurgical and endoscopic

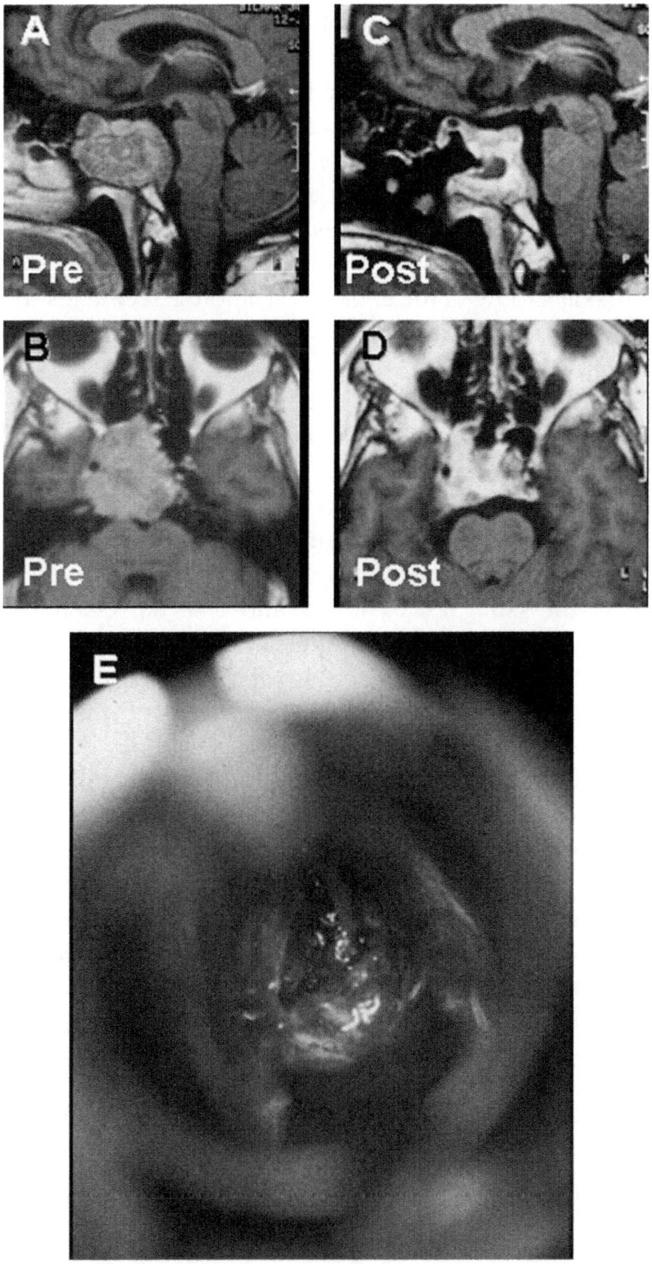


**Fig. 5.** Standard transseptal transsphenoidal approach to the sella for removal of a sellar chordoma. A and B represent sagittal and axial preoperative T1w contrast enhanced MRI's. C and D are the corresponding postsurgical 26$^{th}$ month images. E shows the visualization of the chordoma through the transnasal transseptal exposure

approaches [316]. Laws [63, 197, 198] was one of the pioneers of extended transsphenoidal approaches [197, 198, 366]. Couldwell *et al.* [63] described their experience of extended transsphenoidal approach for 18 chordomas of the inferior clivus and noted that the superior clivus can be accessed posterior to the sphenoid sinus and that the middle or inferior clivus can be reachedafter removal of the sphenoid floor. Kitano and Taneda [171] described the submucosal removal of the posterior ethmoid to gain access to gain a wider access to the suprasellar area or the cavernous sinus. Addition of transmaxillary approaches or addition of a maxillectomy in the endoscopic approach extends the lateral exposure and provides access to the medial compartment of the cavernous sinus [62, 108, 272, 293].

Radical resection of chordomas is possible with the transsphenoidal approach and its modifications in selected cases. In such suitable cases the technique is less invasive and results in fewer complications than craniotomy [63, 109, 197, 212]. Rates of macroscopic total resection for selected clival chordomas with transsphenoidal approaches ranges from 45% to 70% [63, 197]. Intraoperative MRI, neuronavigation and endoscopy can greatly facilitate resection of an invasive tumor in the skull base. The limitations of current transsphenoidal techniques, either endoscopic or microsurgical, are tumors primarily situated in the lower clivus with lateral extension into the occipital condyles. The course of the internal carotid artery and the brainstem narrow the surgical space to the petrous apex.

Complications reported with the transsphenoidal approaches for chordoma include carotid rupture (with resulting hemiparesis), basilar thrombosis, venous cavernous sinus hemorrhage (intra or postoperative), CSF leak, anosmia, CN III and CN VI palsies [63, 198]. Couldwell *et al.* [63] reported a very high incidence (3 of 18 cases) of carotid artery rupture during chordoma resection from the clivus. Laws *et al.* [198] noted that the complication risk in repeat surgery was significantly higher.

## Anterior midface approaches

Anterior midface approaches take advantage of the fact that the clivus lies immediately posterior to the nasal cavity, paranasal sinuses and the nasopharynx. The entire length of the clivus can be accessed through the nose with a substantially shallow operative depth [137, 155]. Transethmoid and sphenoid approaches can expose the area from dorsum sella down to the hard palate [155]. Addition of a maxillotomy or maxillectomy extends the inferior down to the craniovertebral junction [155]. The superior and inferior limits of various transnasal approaches are similar and these approaches differ mainly in the extent of lateral exposure. A wider lateral exposure provides access to lateral extension of the tumor but also widens the surgical field, decreasing the working distance.

Incisions for midface approaches can be rhinal or mucosal [155]. Mucosal incisions include the posterior septal, septal transfixion, sublabial and "midfacial degloving" procedures and provide easy and relatively less invasive approaches to the midfacial skeleton with good cosmetic results. However, except for the "midfacial deglowing" procedure these procedures provide a more limited surgical field, being more suitable for the resection of smaller tumors or tumors that may be removed from a small window. The "midfacial deglowing" procedure was described by Casson *et al.* [46] in 1974 and provides a complete exposure of the visceral cranium without the need for facial skin incisions. Another very important advantage of this approach is that the submucosal dissesction for closure and repair decreasing the risk of a CSF fistula [189]. Facial-rhinal incisions can be limited to the superior, full, extended or bilateral extended [137, 155]. A lateral rhinotomy permits entry into ethmoid and sphenoid sinuses and the superior half of the clivus can be accessed through this approach [155]. Spanning the whole length from Glabella to philtrum, the Weber-Ferguson incision starts from the glabella, extends around the medial canthus deep into the orbicularis muscle, lateral aspect of the nose and down to the philtrum [155]. This incision provides access to the ethmoid, sphenoid and medial maxillary sinuses and makes lateral reflection of the nasal cartilage and bone possible [155]. This can expose the clivus in its entire length [155]. For mobilization of midfacial skeleton this incision may be extended laterally beneath the eye and the lower eyelid and from the lateral canthus to the preauricular area.

Exposure to the clivus can be gained with various facial osteotomies. Maxillary osteotomies, especially Le Fort-I or hemi-Le Fort-I osteotomy procedures have frequently been reported to approach clival lesions [10, 155, 189, 235, 352, 354] These procedures have in common a horizontal maxillary osteotomy. The drop-down maxillotomy procedure exposes the sphenoid bone, the superior and the middle clivus. The translocated maxilla, however, limits the visualization of the inferior clivus and the craniovertebral junction [155, 189]. On the axial plane the approach is limited by the carotid arteries. One of the important advantages of midline transfacial approaches is due to its embryological development the facial skeleton is quite symmetrical and each half has its own neurovascular supply. This creates a unique opportunity to "hinge" any part of the facial skeleton from the orbit down to the maxilla and mandible to create a midline surgical corridor [235]. The so called "swing approaches" were first described on the mandible by Spiro in 1981 [324]. A maxillary swing procedure involves an extended Weber fergusson incision followed by a hemi Le fort III osteotomy and mobilization of the nasal septum [324]. Alternatively the extended "open door maxillotomy" procedure consists of midfacial deglowing exposure, a Le-Fort I osteotomy and a midline division of the hard and soft palate. Each flap of the palate is supplied by its own palatal artery and nerve. This approach provides a more extensive caudal exposure than the drop down maxillotomy and can visualize as low as the body of C2. Superior limits are formed by the sella superiorly, the optic canals superolaterally and the cavernous sinuses laterally. Lateral boundaries are the carotid arteries and the occipital condyles. Using a maxillotomy approach the carotid artery can be visualized from its bifurcation to the petrous canal, however proximal control is not possible.

Major disadvantages of anterior midface approaches are the contaminated surgical field, cosmetical concerns and functional problems (nasal crusting and chronic sinusitis) in the upper airway [155]. Maxillotomy approaches are of significant complexity and complications include carotid artery injury, cranial nerve injuries, CSF fistula, oral malocclusion, palatal and dental numbness, maxillar osteonecrosis and loss of tooth viability [10, 155, 189, 235, 352, 354].

## Transoral approaches

The transoral transpharyngeal approach provides an easy and direct access to the extradural structures in the ventral aspect of the craniovertebral junction without the risk of manipulation of brainstem, spinal cord or the vertebral arteries [69, 94, 224, 343]. With the standard approach a midline corridor spanning from the inferior one third of the clivus down to the C3 can be exposed [224]. However exposure can be extended to as high as the middle clivus by splitting the soft and hard palate [224]. As for the lateral exposure, it can extend to the jugular foramina [224]. For tumors with larger lateral extension a posterolateral exposure is indicated, which also makes occipitocervical fusion possible in the same setting [224]. Alternatively a combination with transethmoidal, transmaxillary or maxillectomy procedures may be performed to increase superior and lateral exposure [224]. In case of limited oral exposure, in patients with small interdental space (<2.5 cm) or less commonly in those with micrognathia or macroglossia, addition of a glossotomy may be required [9, 78, 224, 240]. A glossotomy is more commonly required in children than in adults [134, 343]. A midline mandibular splitting procedure may also be used to increase inferior exposure. The removal of occipital condyles to resect tumor may necessitate an occipitocervical fusion, which must be done as a separate procedure. Tuite *et al.* reported several cases with acute neurological deterioration after the transoral procedure with possible injury occurring during repositioning for the posterior fusion procedure. Crockard *et al.* [67] described a one-stage procedure for transoral approach and fusion in cases with rheumatoid atlantoaxial subluxation.

This is an old and established approach with much accumulated experience. However despite initial optimism, transoral transpharyngeal-transpalatal approaches fell of favor for the treatment of chordomas at the craniovertebral junction, mostly due to their high infectious complication rate and limited exposure [8, 70, 213, 224, 311, 343, 359]. The contaminated surgical field also precludes its use for chordomas with intradural extension. Such an approach is best suited for partial resection of purely extradural tumors located at the midline on the craniovertebral junction with no or very little lateral extension.

The overall complication rate for transoral approach is 18 to 26% and there is also a high mortality rate (6%). Surgical wound infection is of great concern with transoral approaches. Pulmonary infectious complications are also commonly seen. Other complications include CSF fistula, vertebral artery rupture, velopharyngeal insufficiency (with resultant hypernasal voice, nasal regurgitation, and dysphagia) and occipitocervical instability.

## Anterolateral approaches

Parasellar structures are very commonly involved by chordomas. Fifty-four to 75% of chordomas involve the cavernous sinus. Pterional approach alone or in combination with orbital or orbitozygomatic osteotomies or frontotemporal interdural approaches (cavernous sinus exploration as described by Dolenc, Hakuba and Kawase) with or without addition of orbitozygomatic osteotomies are frequently utilized for resection of parasellar, suprasellar cavernous sinus extension of chordomas [12, 82, 84, 117, 123, 192, 193, 312, 318]. However, exposure of the clivus with these approaches is limited [82].

Tumor within the cavernous sinus are approached with frontotemporal interdural approaches [12, 84, 117, 132, 165, 193, 312]. These are collectively known as cavernous sinus explorations. The Dolenc approach involves an extradural anterior clinoid resection and stripping of the two layers of the lateral wall of cavernous sinus after an incision along the occulomotor nerve (Fig. 6) [82, 84]. The similar Hakuba approach exposes the cavernous sinus purely extradurally [164, 165]. The Kawase approach involves a frontotemporal-orbitozygomatic craniotomy (or alternatively a simple subtemporal craniotomy) [132]. Anterolateral approaches such as the transcavernous or Kawase approaches can only provide a very limited and narrow exposure of the dorsum sella and the petrous apex, far less than what is required for the average chordoma [82, 164, 165]. The approaches are well suited for lesions arising in the superior clivus and the petrous apex invading the posterior cavernous sinus and can be extended into the petrous apex or the posterior fossa [164, 165].

## Lateral approaches

Lateral approaches use floor of the middle cranial fossa to approach the central skull base. They include the subtemporal approach, the standard middle fossa approach to the internal auditory canal and its extensions. The middle fossa approach was first described by House as an extradural, infratemporal approach to the internal acoustic canal for resection (with hearing preservation)

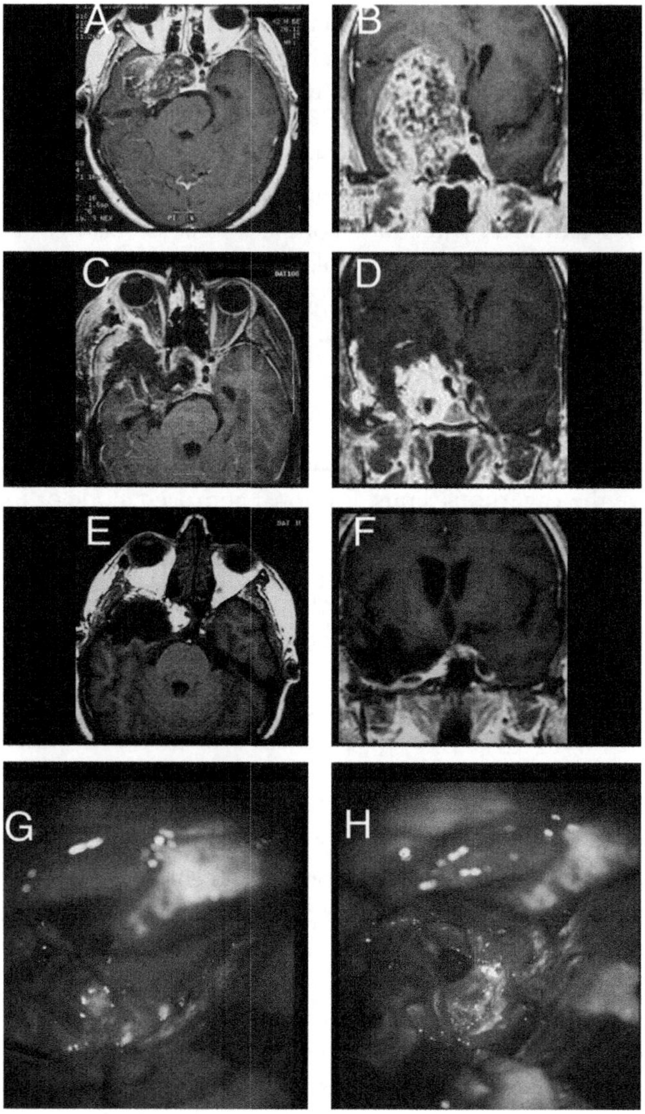


**Fig. 6.** Cavernous sinus exploration with the Dolenc procedure. A and B present the preoperative T1w contrast enhanced images and show the tumor within the left cavernous sinus. Early postoperative images show the tumor cavity. C and D which has collapsed at late postoperative imaging. G shows intraoperative exposure of the characteristic greenish looking chrodoma. H shows the resection cavity after piecemeal removal of the tumor

of small vestibular schwannomas with limited posterior fossa extension [149]. This approach because of its very limited exposure it is used in its extended form. The extension involves an anterior petrosectomy through a subtemporal approach and exposes posterior cavernous sinus, anterolateral mesencephalon, pons and the upper half of the clivus [121]. Lateral inferior approaches divide the temporomandibular joint and reach the central skull base through the infratemporal fossa [23, 102].

### *Posterolateral and inferolateral approaches*

Posterolateral and inferolateral approaches are mainly indicated for chordomas with marked lateral extension. Various presigmoid approaches can be used for chordomas invading the petroclival area [141, 315, 317, 344a, 345]. Lateral extension at the craniovertebral junction are best addressed with an extreme lateral approach, which involves mobilization of the vertebral artery, partial or complete resection of the occipital condyle and provides a lateral viewing angle to the caudal brain stem.

#### Presigmoid approaches

The transpetrosal approach was first described in the neurosurgical literature in 1985 by Hakuba *et al.* [131]. In this report they described the surgical technique and results of the transpetrosal transtentorial route used in 8 patients with a retrochiasmatic craniopharyngioma. In 1988 Al-Mefty *et al.* [4] and Samii and Ammirati [298] independently described their experience with the technique and the results of the transpetrosal approach. Al-Mefty reported on 13 patients with a petro-clival meningioma treated using, what he called the "petrosal" approach [4]. Al-Mefty's original work was a key literature in popularizing this approach.

Presigmoid approaches combine a simple mastodidectomy with various degrees of petrosectomy (Fig. 7). The extent of petrosectomy depends on both the desired exposure and the preoperative symptoms of the patient and includes partial labyrinthectomy, total labyrinthectomy (translabyrinthine approach) and petrosectomy (transcochlear approach). The translabyrinthine exposure exposes the anterolatral brainstem and the cerebellopontine angle and the transcochlear approach further exposes the anterior brainstem, however at the expense of hearing and transient facial nerve palsy. All levels of petrosectomy can be combined with middle fossa or far lateral approaches for resection of extensive tumors.

We are currently using small petrosal approach to petroclival region [344a]. The small petrosal approach allows safe access to this region without the need for brain resection or retraction [344a].

#### Extreme lateral approach

Extreme lateral approach is of great value for resection of chordomas of the lower clivus with lateral extension into the craniovertebral junction. The approach allows the surgeon to view the craniovertebral junction (CVJ) from a

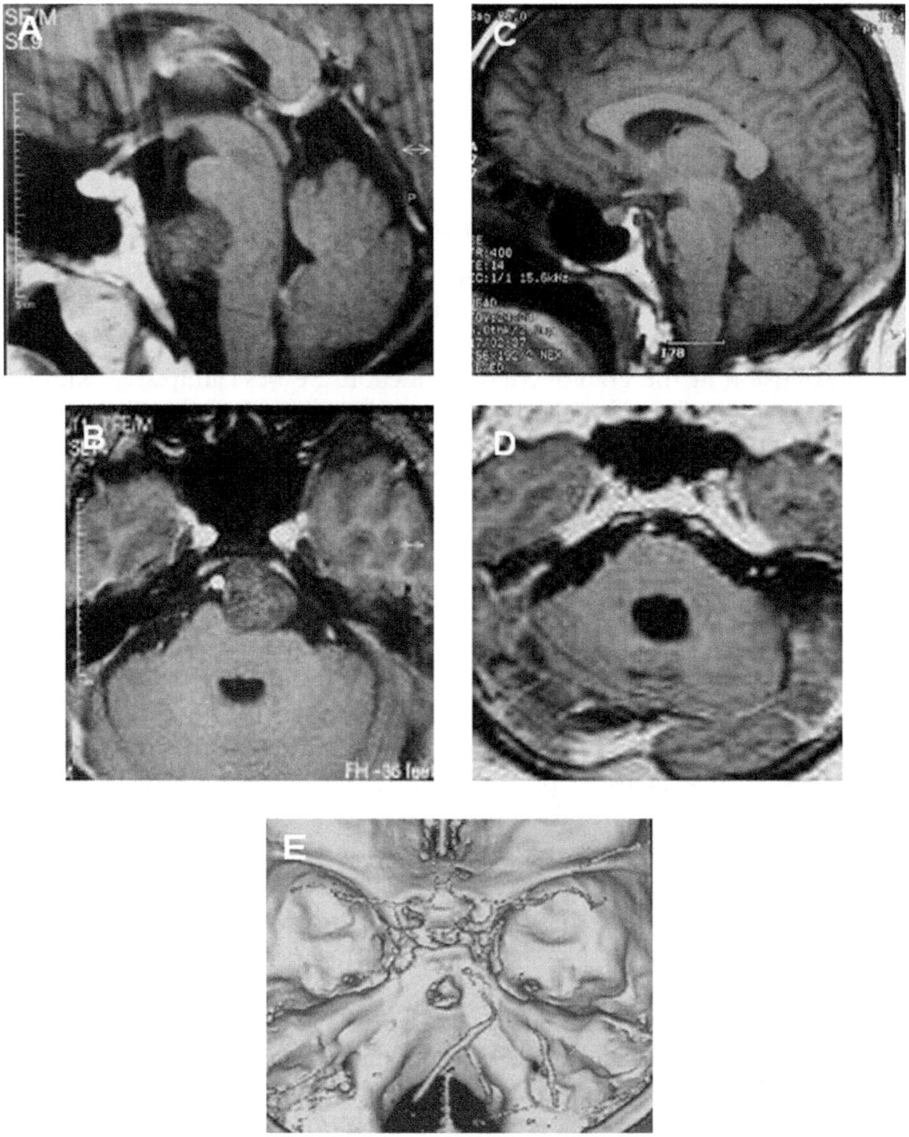


**Fig. 7.** Presigmoid approach for resection of a predominantly extraosseus prepontine chordoma. A and B represent sagittal and axial preoperative T1w contrast enhanced MRI's withsignificant impingement on pons. C and D are the corresponding postsurgical images. E presents a preoperative CT reconstruction of skull base showwing localized bone destrucion at the level of mid-clivus

lateral perspective and this is of great importance as most chordomas arise either anterior or anterolateral to the neuraxis [18]. The extreme lateral approach can be used alone or in combination with presigmoid or subtemporal approaches [18].

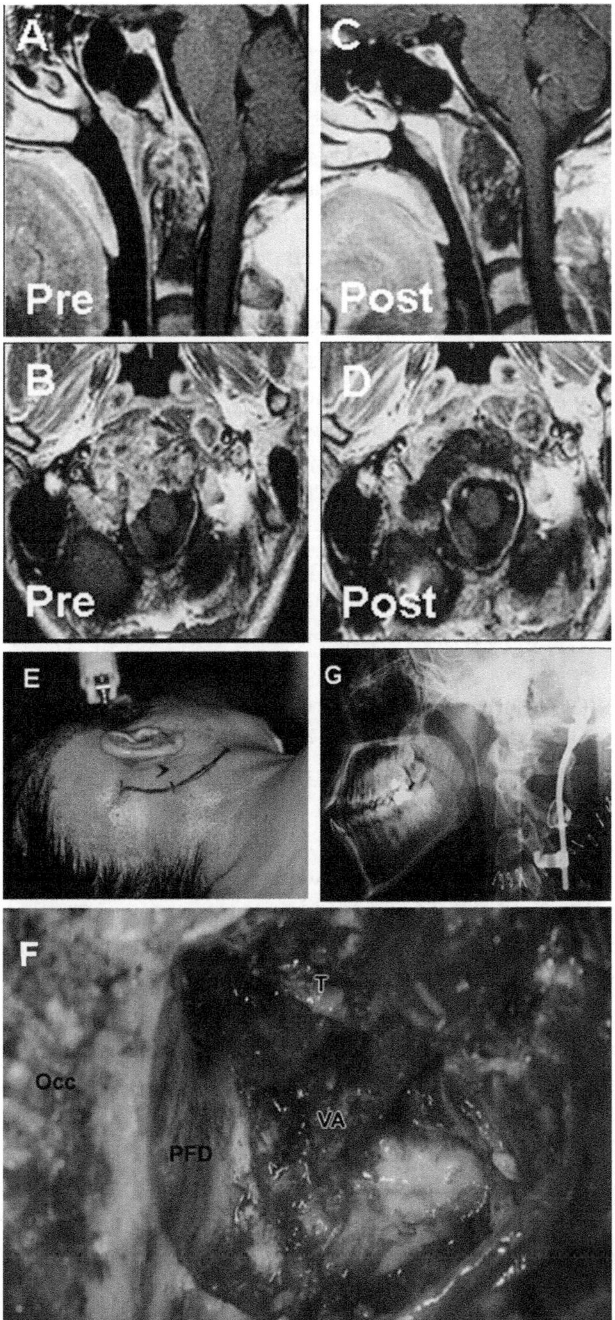


**Fig. 8.** Extreme lateral transcondylar approach for the removal of an inferior clival chordoma with significant lateral extension. A and B represent sagittal and axial preoperative T1w contrast enhanced MRI's with involvement of the craniovertebral junction. C and D are the corresponding postsurgical images. Through a retroauricular incission the craniovertebral junction is exposed (E). A demonstration of the surgical field is given in F. Extensive condylar resection necessitated a fusion procedure (G). *Occ* occipital bone, *PFD* Posterior fossa dura, *T* tumor, *LC VA* vertebral artery

The extreme lateral approach involves a vertical retromastoid incision extending down to the neck to expose the vertebral artery within the foramen transversarium of axis (Fig. 8).

Occipital bone, arch and lateral mass of atlas and the lamina of axis are exposed. The vertebral artery is identified within the suboccipital triangle and unroofed at the foramen transversarium of atlas. Exposure and subsequent mobilization of the vertebral artery for protection was first described by George *et al.* [116]. The V3 segment is identified using bony landmarks. Between atlas and axis the ventral ramus of the C2 nerve root passes lateral to the artery and at this portion (between the atlantooccipital membrane and the posterior fossa dura) the vertebral artery courses within a venous plexus. Parkinson [263] compared this venous plexus to the lateral sellar compartment and Arnavutovic *et al.* [11] called it "the occipital cavernous sinus". The exposure of the venous plexus greatly facilitates protection of the vertebral artery and minor bleeding form the plexus is easily controlled by packing with surgicell and gentle compression. A gentle posteromedial translocation of the artery exposes the lateral mass of C1 and subsequently a durotomy to explore intradural tumor extension may be performed. It is of extreme importance to avoid kinking of the vertebral artery as it may cause brainstem infarction. Calcification of the periosteal sheath and tunneling of the vertebral artery groove should be considered during mobilization of the artery, especially if the artery is the dominant one. The muscular branch of the VA above the posterior arch of the atlas is usually coagulated during exposure, and care must be taken not to confuse the muscular branch with the posterior inferior cerebellar artery which, although rarely, may originate from the extradural VA [344]. A retrosigmoid craniotomy is performed, followed by unroofing of the sigmoid sinus and the jugular bulb and a posterior fossa craniectomy involving the foramen magnum. Transcondylar approach caries a risk of injury to the hypoglossal nerve or the jugular bulb during drilling of the condyle. Extradural tumor removal is removed and invaded bone is drilled until healthy tissue is recognized. Intradural tumor extension can also be accessed after posteromedial mobilization of the vertebral artery.

A wide condylar resection (more than the posterior 2/3 of the condyle) either to resect involved bone or the gain exposure causes craniocervical instability. In our experience 60% of inferior clival cases with condylar involvement required craniocervical stabilization. Bejjani *et al.* [24] reported a need for fusion in 5 of 6 chordoma cases, all of which needed more than 70% resection of the condyle. The most devastating complications in this approach, however, are vertebral artery injury and lower cranial nerve palsies. The risk of lower cranial nerve injury is especially high in the case of tumor removal from the jugular and hypoglossal foramina and this may be very debilitating to the patient. Other complications include hemiparesis or quadriparesis, CSF fistula and pseudomeningocele [18].

*Author's experience:* We presented our experience with 26 pathologically confirmed skull-base chordomas which were managed by conventional or specialized skull-base surgery initially, and subsequent radiosurgery in selected cases [259]. The results of this study indicate that skull-base techniques should be used instead of conventional surgical approaches for first-line treatment of skull-base chordomas. According to data in this study, the residual tumor volume after specialized skull-base techniques is approximately half that associated with conventional surgical approaches. The second comment in this study is that the critical initial tumor volume at the time of diagnosis is $20\,cm^3$ and all patients with initial tumors which exceed this tumor volume developed recurrence or progression after the resection regardless of whether a conventional or specialized skull-base approach was used. We have also concluded that performing Gamma-knife surgery immediately after the initial operation yields better control of tumor growth than if this modality is used to treat tumor progression at a later date. Since this report our patient cohort grew and within 20 years (between September 1986 and December 2006) 44 patients with skull-base chordomas were treated at the Marmara University, Department of Neurosurgery; Institute of Neurological Sciences and Acibadem Medical center. The cohort included 27 females and 17 males and the median age was 39 years (range 3–82 years). Presenting symptoms were headache in 32 (72%), diplopia in 18 (41%), difficulty swallowing in 16 (36%), nausea-vomiting

**Table 10.** *Surgical approaches in 69 tumor excision procedures*

| Surgical approaches | No. of patients | (%) |
|---|---|---|
| Conventional approaches (before 1992) | | |
| Transoral | 5 | 7 |
| Transsphenoidal | 4 | 6 |
| Subtemporal | 1 | 1 |
| Suboccipital aramedian | 4 | 6 |
| Skull Base approaches (after 1992) | | |
| Subfrontal | 12 | 17 |
| Transsphenoidal | 10 | 15 |
| Transfacial approach | 2 | 3 |
| Cavernous sinus exploration | 12 | 17 |
| Presigmoid (petrosal) approaches | 13 | 20 |
| Mastoidectomy | 7 | |
| Mastoidectomy + labirynthectomy | 1 | |
| Total petrosectomy | 1 | |
| Partial petrosectomy | 4 | |
| Transcondylar | 6 | 9 |
| Total | 69 tumor excisions | |

in 15 (33%), ataxia in 13 (29%), motor deficit in 10 (23%), slurred speech in 4 (8%). During the course of treatment a total of 78 operations (excluding Gamma-Knife procedures) were performed, and 69 of those were for tumor resection and 9 were for other purposes (4 occipitocervical fusions, 4 ventriculoperitoneal shunt placements, and 1 hematoma evacuation) (Table 10). In addition to these 78 operations, 16 of the patients underwent 19 stereotactic radiosurgery procedures with the Leksell Gamma-Knife system. All patients underwent T1-weighted (with and without gadolinium enhancement) and T2-weighted magnetic resonance imaging (MRI), as well as computerized tomography (CT) with bone density studies which included three-dimension skull-base constructions. Tumor volume was measured on an Image Analyzer (Image Inc., Canada). All tumors were pathologically diagnosed as chordoma. Conventional approaches were used in 14 of the 69 operations for tumor resection (20.3%) and skull-base approaches were used in the rest (Table 10). Complete tumor resection rate, as judged by early postoperative or intraoperative MRI, was 70% with conventional approaches and 84.8% with skull-base approaches. Surgical mortality is 2.6% and the morbidity rate was 28.2% (Table 13). Mean follow-up period is 67.6 months (range 6–88 months). A total of 25 patients (56.8%) experienced recurrence during this follow-up period. In subtotally resected cases recurrent was defined as persistent tumor growth after surgery. Nine of 44 patients (20.5%) died in the follow-up period. Eight of these 9 patients died due to tumor relate reasons (2 due to surgical complications, 6 due to related clinical deterioration) and 1 died of myocardial infarction. Complications seen are presented in Table 11. The data on our growing patient cohort still supports our conclusions we have drawn in our published study [259].

**Table 11.** *Surgical complications in 44 surgically treated chordoma cases*

| Complications | No. of patients | (%) |
|---|---|---|
| Hydrocephalus (requiring VP shunt) | 4 | 5.1 |
| Lower cranial nerve palsy (transient in 2 cases, gastrostomy required in 2) | 4 | 5.1 |
| Craniocervical instability (requiring OC fusion) | 3 | 3.8 |
| CN-III palsy (2 transient, 1 permenant) | 3 | 3.8 |
| CSF fistula (treated with lumbar drainage) | 2 | 2.6 |
| Facial paresis | 1 | 1.3 |
| Hearing loss | 1 | 1.3 |
| Postoperative hematoma at resection bed | 1 | 1.3 |
| Vertebral artery rupture | 1 | 1.3 |
| Hemihypoesthesia (1 case) | 1 | 1.3 |
| Hemiparesis (1 case) | 1 | 1.3 |
| Total | 22 | 28.2 |

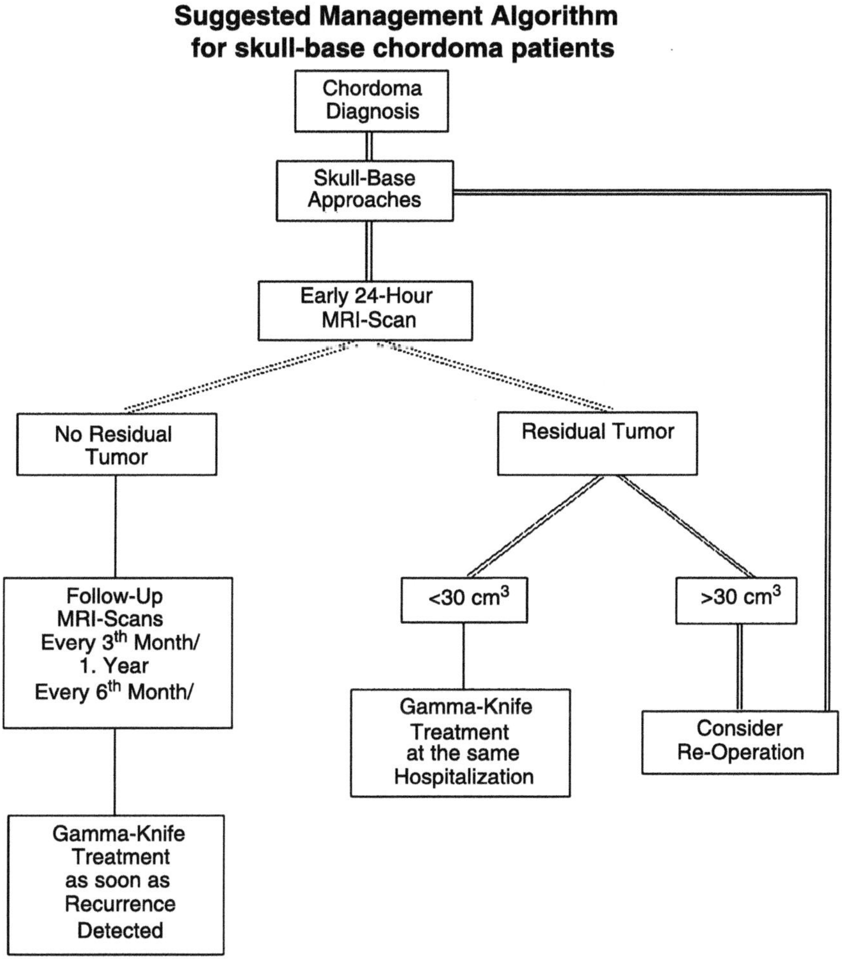


**Fig. 9.** An algorithm was formulated based on our institution's experience with skull-base chordomas

We have adopted a prospective algorithm for treatment of skull base chordomas which relies on maximal safe surgical resection followed by Gamma-Knife radiosurgery of residual lesions smaller than 30 $cm^3$ (Fig. 9). When the residual tumor volume exceeds 30 $cm^3$, immediate reoperation should be considered. The use of intraoperative MRI enabled us to decrease the residual tumor volume after maximal safe resection during the first operation [262].

## Radiotherapy

Most chordomas recur after surgical resection and some form of adjuvant therapy is almost always needed. Radiation therapy is therefore used in an

**Table 12.** *Studies on radiation therapy of chordomas*

| Study | Treatment method | n | Total dose (Gy/CGE) | Follow-up (months) | Overall survival rate % | Local control rate % | | |
|---|---|---|---|---|---|---|---|---|
| | | | | | | 3y | 5y | 10y |
| Magrini *et al.* [211] | photon | 12 | Median 58 (48–60) | Median 72 (12–300) | 58 at 5 years, 35 at 10 years | N/A | 25 | 25 |
| Forsyth *et al.* [106] | photon | 39 | Median 50 (22.93–67.42) | Median 99.6 (67.2–356.4) | 51 for biopsy and 64 for resection at 5 years | N/A | 39 | 31 |
| Romero *et al.* [287] | photon | 18 | Median 50.1 (29.9–64.8) | Median 37.2 (4–240) | N/A | N/A | 17 | N/A |
| Catton *et al.* [48] | photon | 24 | Median 50 (25–60) | Median 62.4 (4–240) | N/A | N/A | 23 | 15 |
| Zorlu *et al.* [378] | photon | 18 | Median 60 (50–64) | Median 43.2 (12–96) | 35 at 5 years | N/A | 23 | N/A |
| Austin Seymour *et al.* [15] | Particle (Proton beam) and photon combined | 68 | Median 69 (56.9–75.6) | Median 34 (17–152) | N/A | N/A | 82 | 58 |
| Benk *et al.* [25] | Particle (Proton beam) and photon combined | 18 | Median 69 (55.8–75.6) | Median 72 (19–120) | 68% | N/A | 78 | N/A |
| Berson *et al.* [28] | Particle (Proton beam) and photon combined | 45 | 59.4–80 | 33 patients longer than 12 months | 62% at 5 years | N/A | 59 | N/A |

| | | | | | | | | |
|---|---|---|---|---|---|---|---|---|
| Hug *et al.* [152] | Particle (Proton beam) | 58 | Mean 70.7 (66.6–79.2) | Mean 33 (7–75) | 97 at 3 years, 79 at 5 years | 67 | 59 | N/A |
| Munzenrider and Liebsch [238] | Particle (Proton beam) and photon combined | 621 | 66–83 | Median 41 (1–254) | 80 at 5 years and 54 at 10 years | N/A | 73 | 54 |
| Igaki *et al.* [154] | Particle (Proton beam) and photon combined | 13 | Median 72 (63–95) | Median 69.3 (14.6–123.4) | 66.7 at 5 years | 67.1 | 46 | N/A |
| Noel *et al.* [250] | Particle (Proton beam) and photon combined | 100 | Median 67 (60–71) | Median 31 (0–87) | 94.3 at 2 years, 80.5 at 5 years | 86.3 at 2 years | 53.8 at 4 years | N/A |
| Castro *et al.* [47] | Particle (Helium ion) | 80* | Mean 65 (60–80) | Median 51 (4–191) | N/A | N/A | 63 | N/A |
| Shultz-Ertner *et al.* [308] | Particle (Carbon ion) | 44 | Mean 60 | Median 16 (4–38.3) | 89.4 at 3 years | 87.1 | N/A | N/A |
| Weber *et al.* [363] | Particle (Carbon ion) | 29 (11 cases CS) | Mean 74 (67–74) | Median 26 (8–70) | 93.8 at 3 years* | 87.5 | N/A | N/A |
| Muthukumar *et al.* [239] | Gamma-Knife | 15* (6 cases CS) | Mean 20 Gy to margin | Median 40 (6–84) | N/A | N/A | N/A | N/A |
| Pamir *et al.* [259] | Gamma-Knife | 7 | Mean 16.2 Gy to margin | Mean 23.3 mo | N/A | N/A | N/A | N/A |
| Feigl *et al.* [100] | Gamma-Knife | 13* (10 cases CS) | Mean 17 Gy to margin | Mean 17mo | N/A | N/A | N/A | N/A |
| Krishnan *et al.* [183] | Gamma-Knife | 29* (4 cases CS) | Median 15 Gy to margin | Median 57.6mo | N/A | 70 | 32 | N/A |

* Marked studies do not indicate results selectively for chordomas but report cumulative outcome data for chordomas, chondrosarcomas and (in one study) other tumors.

attempt to gain local control. However, failure of initial attempts at conventional radiation therapy to control chordomas resulted in the notion that chordomas are radioresistant. This concept was challenged by more recent series showing modest benefit with conventional radiotherapy and improved results with higher dose regimens and stereotactic methods (Table 12) [31, 106, 141, 333].

## *Conventional radiotherapy*

Early studies showed that conventional radiotherapy after subtotal resection of chordomas was associated with a high rate of treatment failure and recurrence (Table 14). Progression free survival rates in these studies ranged form 17 to 39% at 5 years [48, 106, 112, 287, 378]. Some studies from the 1970's however, indicated better response rates with the use of escalated radiation doses [142, 265, 338]. Pearlman and Friedman [265] concluded that doses lower than 40 Gy were not effective and doses >80 Gy were more likely be of benefit. Despite reports of improved results with escalated doses, other studies failed to reconfirm this increase in efficacy [48, 333]. Cummings *et al.* [71] showed a survival benefit even with a low dose (40–55 Gy) radiotherapy compared to surgery alone. Currently it is fairly well established that conventional postoperative radiotherapy can result in approximately 50% 5-year survival and effective palliation [1]. However long-term local control and cure are not possible in most instances [1]. Salvage therapy is effective in alleviating symptoms, but is associated with a grim survival [97].

Conventional radiotherapy has frequently been combined with particle beam radiotherapies or radiosurgery and some authors claim that there may be an advantage to this as chordomas and chondrosarcomas have intermediate proliferative indices and presumably intermediate $\alpha/\beta$ ratios for linear quadratic modeling purposes [107]. Results from a recent Gamma-Knife study from Mayo clinic however reported complications only in patients who received a combination of radiosurgery and fractionated radiotherapy and not those who received their adjuvant therapy with radiosurgery alone [183].

Rhomberg *et al.* [278] showed promising results with the addition of the radiosensitizing agent razoxane to conventional radiotherapy. The authors presented 5 patients with chordoma who were alive with local control 5 years after this combination treatment.

## *LINAC based stereotactic radiotherapies*

The need for higher doses and concern with complications associated with such high doses resulted in the adoption of advanced technologies such as particle irradiation and stereotactic radiosurgery with more conformal dose distributions [333]. Stereotactic techniques and radiosurgery allow for precise, image guided, highly conformal and high dose radiation treatment of chordomas. Current radiosurgical modalities include Gamma-Knife radiosurgery; LINAC based fractionated stereotactic radiotherapy technologies and particle beam irradiation technologies such as proton beam, helium ion and carbon ion. Better results in treatment of skull base chordomas have been reported using radiosurgical technologies, when compared to conventional radiation treatment [175].

Use of stereotactic techniques, multileaf collimators and sophisticated inverse three-dimensional dose planning for sparing of critical structures in the delivery of intensity modulated radiotherapy is increasing the efficacy of LINAC based radiation treatments [175]. Debus *et al.* [76] reported the results of fractionated stereotactic therapy on 45 skull base chordomas and chondrosarcomas. After delivery of 66.6 Gy for chordomas and 64.9 Gy for chondrosarcomas, the authors reported complete local tumor control at 5 years in chondrosarcomas and 82% 2 year and 50% 5 year local control rates in chordomas. Gwak *et al.* [128] reported the results of hypofractionated Cyberknife stereotactic radiotherapy for skull base and upper cervical chordomas. A tumor dose of 21 to 43.6 Gy was delivered in 3 to 5 fractions and after a median follow up of 24 months only one asymptomatic recurrence was noted. The authors, however, also reported radiation induced myelopathy in 2 of 9 cases.

## Gamma-Knife radiosurgery

Gamma-Knife radiosurgery is reported to be a safe and effective treatment for small chordomas [179]. However there are only a handful of studies using the Gamma-Knife and most of the studies lack long follow-up periods, which prevents us from drawing definitive conclusions. Kondziolka and coworkers [239] showed no progression after Gamma-Knife treatment with a dose of 20 Gy to the tumor margin in chordomas less than 30 $cm^3$, however with only a very short follow up period (mean, 22 months; range, 8–36 months). A newer study by the same group reported a cohort of 9 chordomas and 6 chondrosarcomas with a median follow-up of 40 months (range 6–84) [100]. In this study 73% of patients either improved clinically or remained stable following treatment, and two thirds showed either a reduction or stabilization of tumor size on follow-up imaging with no patients having any complications related to the treatment. We have reported the treatment of 7 patients with adjuvant Gamma-Knife therapy after maximal surgical resection [259]. This treatment for residual lesion is administered in the same hospital admission after maximal radical surgical excision if the residual tumor volume does not exceed 30 $cm^3$. Feigl *et al.* [100] used adjuvant Gamma-Knife radiosurgery 2 to 10 months after radical surgery for skull base chordomas and chondrosarcomas and reported a 93.3% tumor control rate at a mean of 17 months after the treatment. Krishnan *et al.* [183] reported 25 chordomas and 4 chondrosarcomas with a 15 Gy marginal dose. Nineteen patients had prior conventional radiation therapies. Actuarial tumor control rates were 89 and 32% at 2 and 5 years.

Previously we reported the results of 7 patients with adjuvant Gamma-Knife therapy after maximal surgical resection [268]. A total of 30 patients underwent 38 Gamma-Knife radiosurgery at our clinic from January 1997 through December 2006. Of these 30 patients 22 were male, 8 patients were female and the median age was 50 years (range 25–82). All patients had pathologically confirmed diagnosis of chordoma. A mean dose of 15.8 Gy was delivered to 50% isodose line. The patients were followed for 36 ± 41 months and 7 of 30 patients showed progression after the first Gamma-Knife radiosurgery session and a second Gamma-Knife procedure was performed. Only one of these continued to progress after the second radiosurgery and a third Gamma-Knife procedure was performed. We should stress the unlucky localization of skull-base chordomas here. Because these tumors are very close to eloquent areas, such as brain stem, very limited dose can be delivered to tumors for protecting the brain stem from radiation related complications. Two patients (6.6%) died during the follow-up. We did not experience any adverse reactions related to the Gamma-Knife treatment such as brain necrosis, vascular damage, or cognitive dysfunction.

In conclusion Gamma-Knife radiosurgery is potentially useful in the treatment of small sized residuel chordomas, but it is not so effective in treatment of recurrence. However, the definitive role needs to be addressed in larger studies with adequate follow-up durations.

### Brachytherapy

There are only few anectodal reports on the use of brachytherapy for skull base chordomas [27, 127, 184, 185]. Orecchia *et al.* reported combination of brachytherapy with external beam radiotherapy. Although it is an appealing technology due to very high local dose delivery and sparing of surrounding structures it is invasive, does not have any superiority to existing noninvasive stereotactic radiation treatment modalities and therefore used only by very few centers.

### Charged particle radiation therapies

Charged particle irradiation technologies are capable of a sharp cut-off outside the target volume and therefore deliver higher doses to the lesion with relative sparing of the surrounding normal tissue when compared to conventional radiotherapy. This sharp dose escalation curve is both due to a finite range in tissue and a sharply defined lateral beam edge. Charged particles deposit a dose along their path, however much more so at the end of their range. This is due to the "Bragg peak" effect which denotes that the maximum dose delivery to the tissue occurs shortly before the particle lost all its energy and stops [268] and because of their heavy mass the particles.

The largest experience with charged particle irradiation is with proton radiotherapy (Table 14). Proton-beam radiotherapy does not produce resolution of chordomas but provides local tumor control and the results are considerably improved over conventional radiotherapy. Radiotherapy schedules involving a mixed treatment with protons and photons have achieved an approximately 60% local control rate at 5 years [28, 152]. This rate ranged from 46% to 73% in different studies. The most recent study on 100 patients with skull base and upper cervical chordomas from Centre de Protontherapie d'Orsay in France reported 2 and 4 year local tumor control rates of 86.3% and 53.8% with a combination of photon and proton therapy [250]. Using spot scanning proton beam radiation therapy, Paul Scherrer Institute team in Switzerland reported a actuarial local control rate of 87.5% for skull base chordomas. Despite its superior results the proton beam radiotherapy is an expensive technology and the experience is limited to very few centers around the globe.

The results reported by the Carbon ion therapy team in Darmstadt-Germany were significantly better than with LINAC based methods [308, 363]. The authors reported 87.1% 3 year survival in 44 chordomas using a dose of 60 Cobald-Gray equivalent (CGE). This study.

These results are encouraging, however longer follow up is required to draw final conclusions.

## *Predictive factors on outcome after radiation treatment*

Several prognostic factors for local control and overall survival have been reported. Few of these studies indicated better results with smaller tumors and the use of higher radiation doses [15]. Local control rates are correlated with homogeneity of the dose delivered to the tumor and inadequate dose delivery is associated with a high local failure rate [97]. The limit to the total prescribed dose is dictated by the proximity to surrounding radiation sensitive structures such as optic apparatus and brain stem. Frequently this is also the cause of local innadequate dose delivery. Austin-Seymour *et al.* [15] indicated that over 75% of the treatment failures were due to dose limitations. Only 25% of the failures were in areas that received the planned dose. Fagundes *et al.* [97] reported that one third of the patients had treatment failures after proton beam treatment. Ninety-five percent of these patients had a local recurrence, and in 78%, this was the only site of failure. The use of a dermal fat graft as a spacer to maintain a separation between the brain stem and the tumor bed during resective surgery has been described as a means to protect radiation injury to the surrounding parenchyma [66]. Tumor histology is also a very important indicator of treatment response. Low grade chondrosarcomas seem to have a better treatment response but are commonly analyzed as a single group together with chordomas, which complicates the interpretation of the current results [194]. In several studies female sex was associated with a poorer prognosis, and a study analyzing several hypotheses concluded that it was most likely due to a statistical artefact [133]. Age was also commonly reported as a prognostic factor [25, 31, 129, 134, 153, 342, 366]. Forsyth *et al.* [106] reported a 5 and 10 year overall survival of 75% and 63% in patients under 40 years of age; these rated were 30% and 11% for older patients. This may be a reflection of poor tolerance of surgery by the elderly and choice of more conservative treatment options. Children are reported to have chordomas with more aggressive histopathology and also metastasize more frequently. Borba *et al.* [31] reported a poor prognosis for children under 5 years of age, but another study by Benk *et al.* [25] failed to replicate this finding.

### Complications of radiation therapy

Present literature suggests that low to moderate doses of conventional radiotherapy are well tolerated. Serious complications are rarely encountered. Charged particle therapies, which delivery considerably higher doses to the brain also have higher complication rates. Most commonly reported complications are endocrine dysfunction, temporal lobe, brain stem or cord injury, visual loss, hearing loss and memory impairment. In the most recent clinical series on proton therapy of skull base chordomas, Noël *et al.* [249] reported hypopituitarism in 25%, occulomotor impairment in 3%, memory impairment in 2%, hearing loss in 2% and bilateral visual loss in 2% of the patients.

Temporal lobe or brain stem radiation injury are the most serious complications but are seldom encountered after proton beam therapy despite despite very high doses delivered to these structures. In a study of 96 patients, Santoni *et al.* [300] reported 8% and 13% temporal lobe complication rates 2 and 5 years after treatment, respectively. Complications were more common in males. Debus *et al.* [76] reported 12% 10 year incidence of brain stem complications. Ninety per cent of these complications occurred within the first 3 years after treatment. Wenkel *et al.* reported a 2.2% incidence of brainstem complications after proton beam therapy for skull base meningioma. Noël *et al.* [249] reported only 1 incidence (1%) of transient myelopathy after a dose of 55CGE to the spinal cord.

Harbrand *et al.* reported a 20% incidence of visual complications after a dose of 60 Gy to the optic apparatus. Noël *et al.* [249] reported a 8% visual complication rate, which was most commonly a decrease in visual acuity. Radiation injury to other cranial nerves is also commonly encountered. Radiation induced hearing loss is also reported in several series [238, 250, 257, 321].

Cognitive side effects are uncommon. Glosser *et al.* [120], in their study of 17 patients who were treated for skull base tumors with doses up to 66CGE, did not report any early or late cognitive side effects.

The incidence of endocrine dysfunction after proton beam therapy ranged between 26 and 84% among studies in the present literature and included hyperprolactinemia, hypothyroidism, hypogonadism and hypoadrenalism [257, 321]. Complications are reported to be most common 14 to 45 months after therapy, increase with time [257]. Doses of >50CGE to the pituitary axis and >70CGE to the pituitary gland are reported as risk factors [183].

There is only one study that reports complications related to Gamma-Knife radiosurgery for skull base chordoma [183]. This series from Mayo clinic reported a 34% incidence of radiation related complications which included cranial nerve deficits, radiation necrosis and pituitary dysfunction, all of which occurred only in patients who had previous radiation treatment [183].

## Chemotherapy

The role of chemotherapy in the treatment of chordoma remains limited. There is no evidence at this stage that chemotherapy has any beneficial role in the treatment of patients with intracranial chordomas. It is mainly used as a salvage therapy in patients with widespread or recurrent disease not amenable to further surgery or radiotherapy.

As there was no obvious therapeutic target to guide a rational treatment, chordomas mostly have been treated with chemotherapy regimens intended for sarcomas and several of those reported either a lack of response or only a modest therapeutic response [17]. Sundaresan [330] reported treatment of 8 recurrent or disseminated chordomas with different chemotherapy regimens containing 5-fluorouracil, vinblastine, actinomycin-D, cyclophosphamide, methotrexate, epoxy-piperazine, and chlorambucil without any treatment response. Azzarelli *et al.* [17] reported treatment of 33 cases of chordoma with only limited success. Horton *et al.* described a pediatric patient without any response to chemotherapy. Chetty *et al.* [55] also described a pediatric case who responded to a combination of surgery, radiotherapy and chemotherapy, however the role of chemotherapy in this treatment response is not known. Fleming *et al.* [104] also reported two patients with sacral dedifferentiated chordoma and lung metastases. One of the patients was responsive to treatment with a regimen consisting of vincristine, dacarbazine, doxorubicin, etoposide, and cisplatin. The second patient did not respond to the combination treatment but only had a brief response to ifosfamide. Schönegger *et al.* [306] reported one patient treated with repeated surgery, radiotherapy and a subsequent short (2) course of chemotherapy with EVAIA protocol (Etoposide-Ifosfamide-doxorubicin-vinchristine) before he developed toxicity. Reportedly the patient received isoretinoin and IFN-$\alpha$ for 12 months, thaliodomide and finally liposomal doxorubicin for systemic metastases and local progressive disease and was stable with a Karnofsky score of 80 at last follow up 8 years after first diagnosis. Casali *et al.* [45], after demonstrating the presence of PDGF receptors on a chordoma biopsy, reported the use of imatinib mesylate, a small molecule inhibitor of several receptor tyrosine kinases including PDGF receptors, BCR-ABL and KIT and described clinical benefit in treating patients with advanced sacral chordoma. The authors have taken this treatment to a phase II clinical trial. In the only prospective phase II trial of systemic chemotherapy in chordoma a Topoisomerase I inhibitor 9-Nitro-Camptothecin was tried in recurrent inoperable chordoma to show moderate benefit with moderate toxicity [51].

## Chordomas in the pediatric age group

Most chordoma cases are seen in the adult population and patients younger than 20 years only make up 5% of the cases [31, 144, 153, 220]. So far, at least 159 cases of skull base chordomas have been reported in the pediatric population [31, 37, 51, 75, 87, 113, 144, 153, 217, 259, 271, 292, 320, 342, 343]. The youngest case is the congenital chordoma reported by Probst *et al.* [271]. Among those cases there is no gender predilection reported. In this age group skull base cases are more commonly seen than sacral chordomas [31]. Matsumoto *et al.* [217] analyzed 56 pediatric cases younger than 16 years. 63.3% were in the skull base, 21% were sacrococygeal and 16% were spinal. Common cranial localizations are orbital, maxillary, nasopharyngeal, clival and upper cervical regions and here they constitute 15% of pediatric brain tumors. Tumors usually become manifest with pain, headache, neurological dysfunction nasopharyngeal obstruction and/or failure to thrive and are reported to have more aggressive behavior than those observed in adult patients [31, 58]. In a large series of skull base chordomas reported neurological symptoms were intracranial hypertension, CN VI palsy, quadriparesis, dysphagia, dysarthria, torticollis, hydrocephalus, diplopia, nystagmus, palatal weakness, pneuomonia, CN III palsy, lower cranial nerve palsies, pathological laughter, deafness and ataxia [31].

There are 159 reported cases of pediatric chordomas in the literature. Several authors have indicated that the histopathological findings in pediatric chordomas, especially those in patients younger than 5 years are much different from those of the adult population [31]. In dedifferentiated chordomas of the pediatric population, commonly a very aggressive clinical behavior accompanies a tumor with abundant mitotic activity, hypercellularity, and pleomorphism [31]. Symptomatic metastases are also more commonly reported in the pediatric population and this is associated with the atypical phenotype in 85.7% of the cases [14, 31]. One study reported an even higher incidence of metastases in children younger than 5 years (57.9%) compared to those 5 years and older (8.5%) [14].

Treatment of skull base chordomas in the pediatric population does not differ much from the adult population. The value of a complete surgical excision in treatment is well established for all ages. However, Borba *et al.* [31] reported that there was no significant survival difference between radical or conservative surgery in atypical cases. They also reported a significantly better prognosis in pediatric patients with chordoma when they received adjuvant radiotherapy, regardless of the completeness of the surgical intervention [73].

## Conclusions

- Chordomas are rare, slow growing tumors of the axial skeleton, derive from the remnants of the fetal notochord and occur most commonly in the sacral area, skull base and less commonly in the spine.
- Patients commonly present with headaches and diplopia and can be readily diagnosed with current neuroradiological methods.
- Chordomas have a benign histopathology but exhibit malignant clinical behavior with invasive, destructive and metastatic potential. There are 3 pathological subtypes: classic, chondroid and dedifferentiated.
- Chondrosarcomas are distinct from chordomas, respond better to treatment and have a better prognosis. Preoperative differential diagnosis form chordoma is not reliable.
- There are at least two subsets of chordomas, one with a benign and another with an aggressive course.
- The eventual prognosis is determined by intrinsic tumor biology. To date we only have a limited understanding of this biology.
- Patients with chordomas benefit from surgical resection and postoperative high dose radiation treatment. Young patients likely benefit form the extent of surgery.
- Currently the most effective adjuvant therapy is charged particle radiation therapy. Radiosurgery may also be of value.
- Current chemotherapy has no role in the first line treatment of chordomas.

## References

1. (2000) Proton therapy for base of skull chordoma: a report for the Royal College of Radiologists. The Proton Therapy Working Party. Clin Oncol (R Coll Radiol) 12: 75–79
2. Abenoza P, Sibley RK (1986) Chordoma: an immunohistologic study. Hum Pathol 17: 744–747
3. Akimoto J, Takeda H, Hashimoto T, Haraoka J, Ito H (1996) A surgical case of ecchordosis physaliphora. No Shinkei Geka 24: 1021–1025
4. Al-Mefty O, Fox JL, Smith RR (1988) Petrosal approach for petroclival meningiomas. Neurosurgery 22: 510–517
5. Al-Mefty O, Borba LA (1997) Skull base chordomas: a management challenge. J Neurosurg 86: 182–189

6. Alezais MM, Peyron A (1914) Contrubution a letude des chordomes; chordomes de la region occipitale, Paris
7. Alezais MM, Peyron A (1914) Sur une tendence evolutive remarquable de certainc chordomes-passage de l'epitheliome au sarcome polymorphe, Paris
8. Alonso WA, Black P, Connor GH, Uematsu S (1971) Transoral transpalatal approach for resection of clival chordoma. Laryngoscope 81: 1626–1631
9. Arbit E, Patterson RH Jr (1981) Combined transoral and median labiomandibular glossotomy approach to the upper cervical spine. Neurosurgery 8: 672–674
10. Archer DJ, Young S, Uttley D (1987) Basilar aneurysms: a new transclival approach via maxillotomy. J Neurosurg 67: 54–58
11. Arnautovic KI, Al-Mefty O (2001) Surgical seeding of chordomas. Neurosurg Focus 10: E7
12. Arnold H, Herrmann HD (1986) Skull base chordoma with cavernous sinus involvement. Partial or radical tumour-removal? Acta Neurochir (Wien) 83: 31–37
13. Aszodi A, Chan D, Hunziker E, Bateman JF, Fassler R (1998) Collagen II is essential for the removal of the notochord and the formation of intervertebral discs. J Cell Biol 143: 1399–1412
14. Auger M, Raney B, Callender D, Eifel P, Ordonez NG (1994) Metastatic intracranial chordoma in a child with massive pulmonary tumor emboli. Pediatr Pathol 14: 763–770
15. Austin-Seymour M, Munzenrider J, Goitein M, Verhey L, Urie M, Gentry R, Birnbaum S, Ruotolo D, McManus P, Skates S, *et al* (1989) Fractionated proton radiation therapy of chordoma and low-grade chondrosarcoma of the base of the skull. J Neurosurg 70: 13–17
16. Aydin P, Ozek M, Kansu T (1994) Intermittent diplopia in chordoma. Ann Ophthalmol 26: 20–22
17. Azzarelli A, Quagliuolo V, Cerasoli S, Zucali R, Bignami P, Mazzaferro V, Dossena G, Gennari L (1988) Chordoma: natural history and treatment results in 33 cases. J Surg Oncol 37: 185–191
18. Babu RP, Sekhar LN, Wright DC (1994) Extreme lateral transcondylar approach: technical improvements and lessons learned. J Neurosurg 81: 49–59
19. Bailey SM, Murnane JP (2006) Telomeres, chromosome instability and cancer. Nucleic Acids Res 34: 2408–2417
20. Bayrakli F, Guney I, Kilic T, Ozek M, Pamir MN (2007) New candidate chromosomal regions for chordoma development. Surg Neurol 68(4): 425–430
21. Bayrakli FGI, Kilic T, Ozek MM, Pamir MN (accepted 1 November 2006) New candidate chromosomal regions for chordoma development. Surg Neurol (article in print)
22. Beck DW, Menezes AH (1987) Lesions in Meckel's cave: variable presentation and pathology. J Neurosurg 67: 684–689
23. Becker D, Ammirati M, Black K, Canalis R, Andrews J (1991) Transzygomatic approach to tumours of the parasellar region. Technical note. Acta Neurochir Suppl 53: 89–91
24. Bejjani GK, Sekhar LN, Riedel CJ (2000) Occipitocervical fusion following the extreme lateral transcondylar approach. Surg Neurol 54: 109–115; discussion 115–116
25. Benk V, Liebsch NJ, Munzenrider JE, Efird J, McManus P, Suit H (1995) Base of skull and cervical spine chordomas in children treated by high-dose irradiation. Int J Radiat Oncol Biol Phys 31: 577–581

26. Bergh P, Kindblom LG, Gunterberg B, Remotti F, Ryd W, Meis-Kindblom JM (2000) Prognostic factors in chordoma of the sacrum and mobile spine: a study of 39 patients. Cancer 88: 2122–2134
27. Bernstein M, Gutin PH (1985) Interstitial irradiation of skull base tumours. Can J Neurol Sci 12: 366–370
28. Berson AM, Castro JR, Petti P, Phillips TL, Gauger GE, Gutin P, Collier JM, Henderson SD, Baken K (1988) Charged particle irradiation of chordoma and chondrosarcoma of the base of skull and cervical spine: the Lawrence Berkeley Laboratory experience. Int J Radiat Oncol Biol Phys 15: 559–565
29. Bootz F, Keiner S, Schulz T, Scheffler B, Seifert V (2001) Magnetic resonance imaging – guided biopsies of the petrous apex and petroclival region. Otol Neurotol 22: 383–388
30. Borba L, Colli B, Al-Mefty O (2001) Skull base chordomas. Neurosurg Quart 11: 124–139
31. Borba LA, Al-Mefty O, Mrak RE, Suen J (1996) Cranial chordomas in children and adolescents. J Neurosurg 84: 584–591
32. Borgel J, Olschewski H, Reuter T, Miterski B, Epplen JT (2001) Does the tuberous sclerosis complex include clivus chordoma? A case report. Eur J Pediatr 160: 138
33. Bouropoulou V, Kontogeorgos G, Papamichales G, Bosse A, Roessner A, Vollmer E (1987) Differential diagnosis of chordoma immunohistochemical aspects. Arch Anat Cytol Pathol 35: 35–40
34. Bouvier D, Raghuveer CV (2001) Aspiration cytology of metastatic chordoma to the orbit. Am J Ophthalmol 131: 279–280
35. Bridge JA, Pickering D, Neff JR (1994) Cytogenetic and molecular cytogenetic analysis of sacral chordoma. Cancer Genet Cytogenet 75: 23–25
36. Brooks JJ, LiVolsi VA, Trojanowski JQ (1987) Does chondroid chordoma exist? Acta Neuropathol 72: 229–235
37. Brooks LJ, Afshani E, Hidalgo C, Fisher J (1981) Clivus chorodoma with pulmonary metastases appearing as failure to thrive. Am J Dis Child 135: 713–715
38. Brown RV, Sage MR, Brophy BP (1990) CT and MR findings in patients with chordomas of the petrous apex. Am J Neuroradiol 11: 121–124
39. Buchfelder M, Fahlbusch R, Ganslandt O, Stefan H, Nimsky C (2002) Use of intraoperative magnetic resonance imaging in tailored temporal lobe surgeries for epilepsy. Epilepsia 43: 864–873
40. Buonamici L, Roncaroli F, Fioravanti A, Losi L, Van den Berghe H, Calbucci F, Dal Cin P (1999) Cytogenetic investigation of chordomas of the skull. Cancer Genet Cytogenet 112: 49–52
41. Butler MG, Dahir GA, Hedges LK, Juliao HS, Sciadini M, Schwartz HS (1995) Cytogenetic, telomere, and telomerase studies in five surgically managed lumbosacral chordomas. Cancer Genet Cytogenet 85: 51–57
42. Butler MG, Sciadini M, Hedges LK, Schwartz HS (1996) Chromosome telomere integrity of human solid neoplasms. Cancer Genet Cytogenet 86: 50–53
43. Byrd SE, Harwood-Nash DC, Barry JF, Fitz CR, Boldt DW (1977) Coronal computed tomography of the skull and brain in infants and children. Part II. Clinical value. Radiology 124: 710–714
44. Cappabianca P, Cavallo LM, Colao A, Del Basso De Caro M, Esposito F, Cirillo S, Lombardi G, de Divitiis E (2002) Endoscopic endonasal transsphenoidal approach: outcome analysis of 100 consecutive procedures. Minim Invasive Neurosurg 45: 193–200

45. Casali PG, Messina A, Stacchiotti S, Tamborini E, Crippa F, Gronchi A, Orlandi R, Ripamonti C, Spreafico C, Bertieri R, Bertulli R, Colecchia M, Fumagalli E, Greco A, Grosso F, Olmi P, Pierotti MA, Pilotti S (2004) Imatinib mesylate in chordoma. Cancer 101: 2086–2097
46. Casson PR, Bananno PC, Converse JM (1974) The midface degloving procedure. Plast Reconst Surg 53: 102–103
47. Castro JR, Linstadt DE, Bahary JP, Petti PL, Daftari I, Collier JM, Gutin PH, Gauger G, Phillips TL (1994) Experience in charged particle irradiation of tumors of the skull base: 1977–1992. Int J Radiat Oncol Biol Phys 29: 647–655
48. Catton C, O'Sullivan B, Bell R, Laperriere N, Cummings B, Fornasier V, Wunder J (1996) Chordoma: long-term follow-up after radical photon irradiation. Radiother Oncol 41: 67–72
49. Cha ST, Jarrahy R, Yong WH, Eby T, Shahinian HK (2002) A rare symptomatic presentation of ecchordosis physaliphora and unique endoscope-assisted surgical management. Minim Invasive Neurosurg 45: 36–40
50. Chadduck WM (1973) Unusual lesions involving the sella turcica. South Med J 66: 948–955
51. Chadduck WM, Boop FA, Sawyer JR (1991) Cytogenetic studies of pediatric brain and spinal cord tumors. Pediatr Neurosurg 17: 57–65
52. Chambers PW, Schwinn CP (1979) Chordoma. A clinicopathologic study of metastasis. Am J Clin Pathol 72: 765–776
53. Chandler JP, Pelzer HJ, Bendok BB, Hunt Batjer H, Salehi SA (2005) Advances in surgical management of malignancies of the cranial base: the extended transbasal approach. J Neurooncol 73: 145–152
54. Chang S, Khoo C, DePinho RA (2001) Modeling chromosomal instability and epithelial carcinogenesis in the telomerase-deficient mouse. Semin Cancer Biol 11: 227–239
55. Chetty R, Levin CV, Kalan MR (1991) Chordoma: a 20-year clinicopathologic review of the experience at Groote Schuur Hospital, Cape Town. J Surg Oncol 46: 261–264
56. Chugh R, Dunn R, Zalupski MM, Biermann JS, Sondak VK, Mace JR, Leu KM, Chandler WF, Baker LH (2005) Phase II study of 9-nitro-camptothecin in patients with advanced chordoma or soft tissue sarcoma. J Clin Oncol 23: 3597–3604
57. Claus EB, Horlacher A, Hsu L, Schwartz RB, Dello-Iacono D, Talos F, Jolesz FA, Black PM (2005) Survival rates in patients with low-grade glioma after intraoperative magnetic resonance image guidance. Cancer 103: 1227–1233
58. Coffin CM, Swanson PE, Wick MR, Dehner LP (1993) Chordoma in childhood and adolescence. A clinicopathologic analysis of 12 cases. Arch Pathol Lab Med 117: 927–933
59. Colli B, Al-Mefty O (2001) Chordomas of the craniocervical junction: follow-up review and prognostic factors. J Neurosurg 95: 933–943
60. Colli BO, Al-Mefty O (2001) Chordomas of the skull base: follow-up review and prognostic factors. Neurosurg Focus 10: Article 1
61. Congdon CC (1952) Proliferative lesions resembling chordoma following puncture of nucleus pulposus in rabbits. J Nat Cancer Inst 12: 893–907
62. Couldwell WT, Sabit I, Weiss MH, Giannotta SL, Rice D (1997) Transmaxillary approach to the anterior cavernous sinus: a microanatomic study. Neurosurgery 40: 1307–1311
63. Couldwell WT, Weiss MH, Rabb C, Liu JK, Apfelbaum RI, Fukushima T (2004) Variations on the standard transsphenoidal approach to the sellar region, with emphasis on the extended approaches and parasellar approaches: surgical experience in 105 cases. Neurosurgery 55: 539–547; discussion 547–550

64. Crapanzano JP, Ali SZ, Ginsberg MS, Zakowski MF (2001) Chordoma: a cytologic study with histologic and radiologic correlation. Cancer 93: 40–51
65. Crockard A (1996) Chordomas and chondrosarcomas of the cranial base: results and follow-up of 60 patients. Neurosurgery 38: 420
66. Crockard A, Macaulay E, Plowman PN (1999) Stereotactic radiosurgery. VI. Posterior displacement of the brainstem facilitates safer high dose radiosurgery for clival chordoma. Br J Neurosurg 13: 65–70
67. Crockard HA, Calder I, Ransford AO (1990) One-stage transoral decompression and posterior fixation in rheumatoid atlanto-axial subluxation. J Bone Joint Surg Br 72: 682–685
68. Crockard HA, Cheeseman A, Steel T, Revesz T, Holton JL, Plowman N, Singh A, Crossman J (2001) A multidisciplinary team approach to skull base chondrosarcomas. J Neurosurg 95: 184–189
69. Crockard HA, Steel T, Plowman N, Singh A, Crossman J, Revesz T, Holton JL, Cheeseman A (2001) A multidisciplinary team approach to skull base chordomas. J Neurosurg 95: 175–183
70. Crumley RL, Gutin PH (1989) Surgical access for clivus chordoma. The University of California, San Francisco, experience. Arch Otolaryngol Head Neck Surg 115: 295–300
71. Cummings BJ, Hodson DI, Bush RS (1983) Chordoma: the results of megavoltage radiation therapy. Int J Radiat Oncol Biol Phys 9: 633–642
72. Cushing H (1912) The pituitary body and its disorders, clinical states produced by disorders of the hypophysis cerebri. J. B. Lippincott Company, Philadelphia, London
73. Dalpra L, Malgara R, Miozzo M, Riva P, Volonte M, Larizza L, Fuhrman Conti AM (1999) First cytogenetic study of a recurrent familial chordoma of the clivus. Int J Cancer 81: 24–30
74. de Divitiis E, Cappabianca P, Cavallo LM (2002) Endoscopic transsphenoidal approach: adaptability of the procedure to different sellar lesions. Neurosurgery 51: 699–705; discussion 705–707
75. DeBoer JM, Neff JR, Bridge JA (1992) Cytogenetics of sacral chordoma. Cancer Genet Cytogenet 64: 95–96
76. Debus J, Hug EB, Liebsch NJ, O'Farrel D, Finkelstein D, Efird J, Munzenrider JE (1997) Brainstem tolerance to conformal radiotherapy of skull base tumors. Int J Radiat Oncol Biol Phys 39: 967–975
77. Debus J, Schulz-Ertner D, Schad L, Essig M, Rhein B, Thillmann CO, Wannenmacher M (2000) Stereotactic fractionated radiotherapy for chordomas and chondrosarcomas of the skull base. Int J Radiat Oncol Biol Phys 47: 591–596
78. Delgado TE, Garrido E, Harwick RD (1981) Labiomandibular, transoral approach to chordomas in the clivus and upper cervical spine. Neurosurgery 8: 675–679
79. Deniz ML, Kilic T, Almaata I, Kurtkaya O, Sav A, Pamir MN (2002) Expression of growth factors and structural proteins in chordomas: basic fibroblast growth factor, transforming growth factor alpha, and fibronectin are correlated with recurrence. Neurosurgery 51: 753–760; discussion 760
80. Derome P (1972) Les tumeurs spheno-ethmoidales. Possibilites d'exerese et de reparation chirurgicale Neurochirurgie 18: 1–164
81. Derome PJ (1985) Surgical management of tumours invading the skull base. Can J Neurol Sci 12: 345–347
82. Dolenc VV, Skrap M, Sustersic J, Skrbec M, Morina A (1987) A transcavernous-transsellar approach to the basilar tip aneurysms. Br J Neurosurg 1: 251–259

83. Dolenc VV (1994) Frontotemporal epidural approach to trigeminal neurinomas. Acta Neurochir (Wien) 130: 55–65
84. Dolenc VV (1997) Transcranial epidural approach to pituitary tumors extending beyond the sella. Neurosurgery 41: 542–550; discussion 551–552
85. Dorfman HD, Czerniak B (1995) Bone cancers. Cancer 75: 203–210
86. Dort JC, Sutherland GR (2001) Intraoperative magnetic resonance imaging for skull base surgery. Laryngoscope 111: 1570–1575
87. Doucet V, Peretti-Viton P, Figarella-Branger D, Manera L, Salamon G (1997) MRI of intracranial chordomas. Extent of tumour and contrast enhancement: criteria for differential diagnosis. Neuroradiology 39: 571–576
88. Dow GR, Robson DK, Jaspan T, Punt JA (2003) Intradural cerebellar chordoma in a child: a case report and review of the literature. Childs Nerv Syst 19: 188–191
89. Dreghorn CR, Newman RJ, Hardy GJ, Dickson RA (1990) Primary tumors of the axial skeleton. Experience of the leeds regional bone tumor registry. Spine 15: 137–140
90. Eisenberg MB, Woloschak M, Sen C, Wolfe D (1997) Loss of heterozygosity in the retinoblastoma tumor suppressor gene in skull base chordomas and chondrosarcomas. Surg Neurol 47: 156–160; discussion 160–161
91. Ekinci G, Akpinar IN, Baltacioglu F, Erzen C, Kilic T, Elmaci I, Pamir MN (2003) Early-postoperative magnetic resonance imaging in glial tumors: prediction of tumor regrowth and recurrence. Eur J Radiol 45: 99–107
92. El-Kalliny M, van Loveren H, Keller JT, Tew JM Jr (1992) Tumors of the lateral wall of the cavernous sinus. J Neurosurg 77: 508–514
93. Enin IP (1964) Chordoma of the nasopharynx in 2 members of a family. Vestn Otorinolaringol 26: 88–90
94. Erbengi A, Tekkok IH, Acikgoz B (1991) Posterior fossa chordomas – with special reference to transoral surgery. Neurosurg Rev 14: 23–28
95. Erdem E, Angtuaco EC, Van Hemert R, Park JS, Al-Mefty O (2003) Comprehensive review of intracranial chordoma. Radiographics 23: 995–1009
96. Eriksson B, Gunterberg B, Kindblom LG (1981) Chordoma. A clinicopathologic and prognostic study of a Swedish national series. Acta Orthop Scand 52: 49–58
97. Fagundes MA, Hug EB, Liebsch NJ, Daly W, Efird J, Munzenrider JE (1995) Radiation therapy for chordomas of the base of skull and cervical spine: patterns of failure and outcome after relapse. Int J Radiat Oncol Biol Phys 33: 579–584
98. Fahlbusch R, Ganslandt O, Buchfelder M, Schott W, Nimsky C (2001) Intraoperative magnetic resonance imaging during transsphenoidal surgery. J Neurosurg 95: 381–390
99. Falconer MA, Bailey IC, Duchen LW (1968) Surgical treatment of chordoma and chondroma of the skull base. J Neurosurg 29: 261–275
100. Feigl GC, Bundschuh O, Gharabaghi A, Safavi-Abassi S, El Shawarby A, Samii M, Horstmann GA (2005) Evaluation of a new concept for the management of skull base chordomas and chondrosarcomas. J Neurosurg Suppl 102: 165–170
101. Ferry AP, Haddad HM, Goldman JL (1981) Orbital invasion by an intracranial chordoma. Am J Ophthalmol 92: 7–12
102. Fisch U (1978) Infratemporal fossa approach to tumours of the temporal bone and base of the skull. J Laryngol Otol 92: 949–967
103. Fischbein NJ, Kaplan MJ, Holliday RA, Dillon WP (2000) Recurrence of clival chordoma along the surgical pathway. Am J Neuroradiol 21: 578–583

104. Fleming GF, Heimann PS, Stephens JK, Simon MA, Ferguson MK, Benjamin RS, Samuels BL (1993) Dedifferentiated chordoma. Response to aggressive chemotherapy in two cases. Cancer 72: 714–718
105. Foote RF, Ablin G, Hall WW (1958) Chordoma in siblings. Calif Med 88: 383–386
106. Forsyth PA, Cascino TL, Shaw EG, Scheithauer BW, O'Fallon JR, Dozier JC, Piepgras DG (1993) Intracranial chordomas: a clinicopathological and prognostic study of 51 cases. J Neurosurg 78: 741–747
107. Fowler J (1989) The linear quadratic formula and progress in fractionated radiotherapy. Br J Radiol 62: 679–694
108. Fraioli B, Esposito V, Santoro A, Iannetti G, Giuffre R, Cantore G (1995) Transmaxillosphenoidal approach to tumors invading the medial compartment of the cavernous sinus. J Neurosurg 82: 63–69
109. Frank G, Sciarretta V, Calbucci F, Farneti G, Mazzatenta D, Pasquini E (2006) The endoscopic transnasal transsphenoidal approach for the treatment of cranial base chordomas and chondrosarcomas. Neurosurgery 59: ONS50–ONS57; discussion ONS50–ONS57
110. Franquemont DW, Katsetos CD, Ross GW (1989) Fatal acute pontocerebellar hemorrhage due to an unsuspected spheno-occipital chordoma. Arch Pathol Lab Med 113: 1075–1078
111. Fujita N, Miyamoto T, Imai J, Hosogane N, Suzuki T, Yagi M, Morita K, Ninomiya K, Miyamoto K, Takaishi H, Matsumoto M, Morioka H, Yabe H, Chiba K, Watanabe S, Toyama Y, Suda T (2005) CD24 is expressed specifically in the nucleus pulposus of intervertebral discs. Biochem Biophys Res Commun 338: 1890–1896
112. Fuller DB, Bloom JG (1988) Radiotherapy for chordoma. Int J Radiat Oncol Biol Phys 15: 331–339
113. Gadwal SR, Fanburg-Smith JC, Gannon FH, Thompson LD (2000) Primary chondrosarcoma of the head and neck in pediatric patients: a clinicopathologic study of 14 cases with a review of the literature. Cancer 88: 2181–2188
114. Gay E, Sekhar LN, Rubinstein E, Wright DC, Sen C, Janecka IP, Snyderman CH (1995) Chordomas and chondrosarcomas of the cranial base: results and follow-up of 60 patients. Neurosurgery 36: 887–896; discussion 896–897
115. Gehanne C, Delpierre I, Damry N, Devroede B, Brihaye P, Christophe C (2005) Skull base chordoma: CT and MRI features. Jbr-Btr 88: 325–327
116. George B, Dematons C, Cophignon J (1988) Lateral approach to the anterior portion of the foramen magnum. Application to surgical removal of 14 benign tumors: technical note. Surg Neurol 29: 484–490
117. George B, Ferrario CA, Blanquet A, Kolb F (2003) Cavernous sinus exenteration for invasive cranial base tumors. Neurosurgery 52: 772–780; discussion 780–782
118. Gibas Z, Miettinen M, Sandberg AA (1992) Chromosomal abnormalities in two chordomas. Cancer Genet Cytogenet 58: 169–173
119. Gil Z, Fliss DM, Voskoboinik N, Leider-Trejo L, Spektor S, Yaron Y, Orr-Urtreger A (2004) Cytogenetic analysis of three variants of clival chordoma. Cancer Genet Cytogen 154: 124–130
120. Glosser G, McManus P, Munzenrider J, Austin-Seymour M, Fullerton B, Adams J, Urie MM (1997) Neuropsychological function in adults after high dose fractionated radiation therapy of skull base tumors. Int J Radiat Oncol Biol Phys 38: 231–239

121. Goel A (1995) Extended middle fossa approach for petroclival lesions. Acta Neurochir (Wien) 135: 78–83
122. Goel A (1995) Chordoma and chondrosarcoma: relationship to the internal carotid artery. Acta Neurochir (Wien) 133: 30–35
123. Goel A, Muzumdar DP, Nitta J (2001) Surgery on lesions involving cavernous sinus. J Clin Neurosci 8 Suppl 1: 71–77
124. Gollin SM, Janecka IP (1994) Cytogenetics of cranial base tumors. J Neurooncol 20: 241–254
125. Gormley WB, Beckman ME, Ho KL, Boyd SB, Rock JP (1995) Primary craniofacial chordoma: case report. Neurosurgery 36: 1196–1199
126. Gottschalk D, Fehn M, Patt S, Saeger W, Kirchner T, Aigner T (2001) Matrix gene expression analysis and cellular phenotyping in chordoma reveals focal differentiation pattern of neoplastic cells mimicking nucleus pulposus development [see comment]. Am J Pathol 158: 1571–1578
127. Gutin PH, Leibel SA, Hosobuchi Y, Crumley RL, Edwards MS, Wilson CB, Lamb S, Weaver KA (1987) Brachytherapy of recurrent tumors of the skull base and spine with iodine-125 sources. Neurosurgery 20: 938–945
128. Gwak HS, Yoo HJ, Youn SM, Chang U, Lee DH, Yoo SY, Rhee CH (2005) Hypofractionated stereotactic radiation therapy for skull base and upper cervical chordoma and chondrosarcoma: preliminary results. Stereotact Funct Neurosurg 83: 233–243
129. Habrand JL, Mammar H, Ferrand R, Pontvert D, Bondiau PY, Kalifa C, Zucker JM (1999) Proton beam therapy (PT) in the management of CNS tumors in childhood. Strahlenther Onkol 175 (Suppl 2): 91–94
130. Haeckel C, Krueger S, Kuester D, Ostertag H, Samii M, Buehling F, Broemme D, Czerniak B, Roessner A (2000) Expression of cathepsin K in chordoma. Hum Pathol 31: 834–840
131. Hakuba A, Nishimura S, Inoue Y (1985) Transpetrosal-transtentorial approach and its application in the therapy of retrochiasmatic craniopharyngiomas. Surg Neurol 24: 405–415
132. Hakuba A, Tanaka K, Suzuki T, Nishimura S (1989) A comined orbitozygomatic infratemporal epidural and subdural approach for lesions involving the entire cavernous sinus'. J Neurosurg 71: 699–704
133. Halperin EC (1997) Why is female sex an independent predictor of shortened overall survival after proton/photon radiation therapy for skull base chordomas? Int J Radiat Oncol Biol Phys 38: 225–230
134. Handa J, Suzuki F, Nioka H, Koyama T (1987) Clivus chordoma in childhood. Surg Neurol 28: 58–62
135. Hara T, Kawahara N, Tsuboi K, Shibahara J, Ushiku T, Kirino T (2006) Sarcomatous transformation of clival chordoma after charged-particle radiotherapy. Report of two cases. J Neurosurg 105: 136–141
136. Hardy J, Vezina JL (1976) Transsphenoidal neurosurgery of intracranial neoplasm. Adv Neurol 15: 261–273
137. Harsh G, Ojemann R, Varvares M, Swearingen B, Cheney M, Joseph M (2001) Pedicled rhinotomy for clival chordomas invaginating the brainstem. Neurosurg Focus 10: E8
138. Harvey WF, Dawson EK (1941) Chordoma. Edinburgh Med J 48: 713–721
139. Hasse H (1857) Ein neuer Fall von Schleimgeschwulst am Clivus. Virch Arch 11

140. Hazarika D, Kumar RV, Muniyappa GD, Mukherjee G, Rao CR, Narasimhamurthy NK, Shenoy AM, Nanjundappa (1995) Diagnosis of clival chordoma by fine needle aspiration of an oropharyngeal mass. A case report. Acta Cytol 39: 507–510
141. Heffelfinger MJ, Dahlin DC, MacCarty CS, Beabout JW (1973) Chordomas and cartilaginous tumors at the skull base. Cancer 32: 410–420
142. Higinbotham NL, Phillips RF, Farr HW, Hustu HO (1967) Chordoma. Thirty-five-year study at Memorial Hospital. Cancer 20: 1841–1850
143. Ho KL (1985) Ecchordosis physaliphora and chordoma: a comparative ultrastructural study. Clin Neuropathol 4: 77–86
144. Hoch BL, Nielsen GP, Liebsch NJ, Rosenberg AE (2006) Base of skull chordomas in children and adolescents: a clinicopathologic study of 73 cases. Am J Surg Pathol 30: 811–818
145. Honeybul S, Neil-Dwyer D, Lang DA, Evans BT (2001) Extended transbasal approach with preservation of olfaction: ananatomical study. Br J Oral Maxillofac Surg 39: 149–157
146. Horiguchi H, Sano T, Qian ZR, Hirokawa M, Kagawa N, Yamaguchi T, Hirose T, Nagahiro S (2004) Expression of cell adhesion molecules in chordomas: an immunohistochemical study of 16 cases. Acta Neuropathol (Berl) 107: 91–96
147. Horten BC, Montague SR (1976) In vitro characteristics of a sacrococcygeal chordoma maintained in tissue and organ culture systems. Acta Neuropathologica 35: 13–25
148. Horten BC, Montague SR (1976) Human ecchordosis physaliphora and chick embryonic notochord. A comparative electron microscopic study. Virchows Arch A Pathol Anat Histol 371: 295–303
149. House WF, Shelton C (1992) Middle fossa approach for acoustic tumor removal. Otolaryngol Clin 25: 347–359
150. Hruban RH, Traganos F, Reuter VE, Huvos AG (1990) Chordomas with malignant spindle cell components. A DNA flow cytometric and immunohistochemical study with histogenetic implications. Am J Pathol 137: 435–447
151. Hug EB, Loredo LN, Slater JD, DeVries A, Grove RI, Schaefer RA, Rosenberg AE, Slater JM (1999) Proton radiation therapy for chordomas and chondrosarcomas of the skull base. J Neurosurg 91: 432–439
152. Hug EB (2001) Review of skull base chordomas: prognostic factors and long-term results of proton-beam radiotherapy. Neurosurg Focus 10: E11
153. Hug EB, Sweeney RA, Nurre PM, Holloway KC, Slater JD, Munzenrider JE (2002) Proton radiotherapy in management of pediatric base of skull tumors. Int J Radiat Oncol Biol Phys 52: 1017–1024
154. Igaki H, Tokuuye K, Okumura T, Sugahara S, Kagei K, Hata M, Ohara K, Hashimoto T, Tsuboi K, Takano S, Matsumura A, Akine Y (2004) Clinical results of proton beam therapy for skull base chordoma. Int J Radiat Oncol Biol Phys 60: 1120–1126
155. Jackson IT (1990) Craniofacial osteotomies to facilitate the resection of the tumors of the skull base. McGraw-Hill, Health Professions Division, New York
156. Jeffrey PB, Davis RL, Biava C, Rosenblum M (1993) Microtubule aggregates in a clival chordoma. Arch Pathol Lab Med 117: 1055–1057
157. Jeffrey PB, Biava CG, Davis RL (1995) Chondroid chordoma. A hyalinized chordoma without cartilaginous differentiation. Am J Clin Pathol 103: 271–279
158. Jho HD, Carrau RL, McLaughlin ML, Somaza SC (1996) Endoscopic transsphenoidal resection of a large chordoma in the posterior fossa. Case report. Neurosurg Focus 1: e3; discussion 1p following e3

159. Jho HD, Carrau RL (1997) Endoscopic endonasal transsphenoidal surgery: experience with 50 patients. J Neurosurg 87: 44–51
160. Jho HD, Carrau RL, McLaughlin MR, Somaza SC (1997) Endoscopic transsphenoidal resection of a large chordoma in the posterior fossa. Acta Neurochir (Wien) 139: 343–347; discussion 347–348
161. Kakuno Y, Yamada T, Hirano H, Mori H, Narabayashi I (2002) Chordoma in the sella turcica. Neurol Med Chir (Tokyo) 42: 305–308
162. Kamrin RP, Potanos JN, Pool JL (1964) An evaluation of the diagnosis and treatment of chordoma. J Neurol Neurosurg Psychiatry 27: 157–165
163. Kassam A, Snyderman CH, Mintz A, Gardner P, Carrau RL (2005) Expanded endonasal approach: the rostrocaudal axis. Part II. Posterior clinoids to the foramen magnum. Neurosurg Focus 19: E4
164. Kawase T (1990) Skull base approaches for clival tumors. No Shinkei Geka 18: 121–128
165. Kawase T (1997) Anatomical strategy of parasellar tumor surgery. No Shinkei Geka 25: 681–688
166. Kelley MJ, Korczak JF, Sheridan E, Yang X, Goldstein AM, Parry DM (2001) Familial chordoma, a tumor of notochordal remnants, is linked to chromosome 7q33. Am J Hum Genet 69: 454–460
167. Kerr WA, Allen KL, Haynes DR, Sellars SL (1975) Letter: familial nasopharyngeal chordoma. S Afr Med J 49: 1584
168. Kilgore S, Prayson RA (2002) Apoptotic and proliferative markers in chordomas: a study of 26 tumors. Ann Diagn Pathol 6: 222–228
169. Kilic T, Ekinci G, Seker A, Elmaci I, Erzen C, Pamir MN (2001) Determining optimal MRI follow-up after transsphenoidal surgery for pituitary adenoma: scan at 24 hours post-surgery provides reliable information. Acta Neurochir (Wien) 143: 1103–1126
170. Kimura F, Kim KS, Friedman H, Russell EJ, Breit R (1990) MR imaging of normal and abnormal clivus. Am J Neuroradiol 11: 1015–1021
171. Kitano M, Taneda M (2001) Extended transsphenoidal approach with submucosal posterior ethmoidectomy for parasellar tumors: technical note. J Neurosurg 94: 999–1004
172. Klebs E (1864) Ein Fall von Ecchondrosis spheno-occipitalise amylacea. Virchows Arch Path Anat 31: 396–399
173. Kleihues P, Louis DN, Scheithauer BW, Rorke LB, Reifenberger G, Burger PC, Cavenee WK (2002) The WHO classification of tumors of the nervous system. J Neuropathol Exp Neurol 61: 215–225; discussion 226–229
174. Klingler L, Shooks J, Fiedler PN, Marney A, Butler MG, Schwartz HS (2000) Microsatellite instability in sacral chordoma. J Surg Oncol 73: 100–103
175. Knisely JP, Linskey ME (2006) Less common indications for stereotactic radiosurgery or fractionated radiotherapy for patients with benign brain tumors. Neurosurg Clin N Am 17: 149–167, vii
176. Knutsen T, Gobu V, Knaus R, Padilla-Nash H, Augustus M, Strausberg RL, Kirsch IR, Sirotkin K, Ried T (2005) The interactive online SKY/M-FISH & CGH database and the Entrez cancer chromosomes search database: linkage of chromosomal aberrations with the genome sequence. Genes Chromosomes Cancer 44: 52–64
177. Kölliker A (1860) Über die Beziehungen der Chorda dorsalis zur Bildung der Wirbel der Selachier und einiger andern Fische. Verhandl. phys. med. Gesellsch. Würzburg 10: 193–242

178. Kombogiorgas D, St George EJ, Chapman S, English M, Solanki GA (2006) Infantile clivus chordoma without clivus involvement: case report and review of the literature. Childs Nerv Syst 22(10): 1369–1374
179. Kondziolka D, Lunsford LD, Flickinger JC (1991) The role of radiosurgery in the management of chordoma and chondrosarcoma of the cranial base. Neurosurgery 29: 38–45; discussion 45–46
180. Kouri JG, Chen MY, Watson JC, Oldfield EH (2000) Resection of suprasellar tumors by using a modified transsphenoidal approach. Report of four cases. J Neurosurg 92: 1028–1035
181. Koybasioglu F, Simsek GG, Onal BU, Han U, Adabag A (2005) Oropharyngeal chordoma diagnosed by fine needle aspiration: a case report. Acta Cytol 49: 173–176
182. Krayenbühl H, Yasargil MG (1975) Cranial chordomas. Progr Neurol Surg 6: 380–434
183. Krishnan S, Foote RL, Brown PD, Pollock BE, Link MJ, Garces YI (2005) Radiosurgery for cranial base chordomas and chondrosarcomas. Neurosurgery 56: 777–784; discussion 777–784
184. Kumar PP, Good RR, Leibrock LG, Mawk JR, Yonkers AJ, Ogren FP (1988) High activity iodine 125 endocurietherapy for recurrent skull base tumors. Cancer 61: 1518–1527
185. Kumar PP, Good RR, Skultety FM, Leibrock LG (1988) Local control of recurrent clival and sacral chordoma after interstitial irradiation with iodine-125: new techniques for treatment of recurrent or unresectable chordomas. Neurosurgery 22: 479–483
186. Kurokawa H, Miura S, Goto T (1988) Ecchordosis physaliphora arising from the cervical vertebra, the CT and MRI appearance. Neuroradiology 30: 81–83
187. Kurtsoy A, Menku A, Tucer B, Suat Oktem I, Akdemir H, Kemal Koc R (2004) Transbasal approaches: surgical details, pitfalls and avoidances. Neurosurg Rev 27: 267–273
188. Kuzniacka A, Mertens F, Strombeck B, Wiegant J, Mandahl N (2004) Combined binary ratio labeling fluorescence in situ hybridization analysis of chordoma. Cancer Genet Cytogenet 151: 178–181
189. Kyoshima K, Matsuo K, Kushima H, Oikawa S, Idomari K, Kobayashi S (2002) Degloving transfacial approach with Le Fort I and nasomaxillary osteotomies: alternative transfacial approach. Neurosurgery 50: 813–821
190. Lalwani AK, Kaplan MJ, Gutin PH (1992) The transsphenoethmoid approach to the sphenoid sinus and clivus. Neurosurgery 31: 1008–1014; discussion 1014
191. Lam R (1990) The nature of cytoplasmic vacuoles in chordoma cells. A correlative enzyme and electron microscopic histochemical study. Pathol Res Pract 186: 642–650
192. Lanzino G, Hirsch WL, Pomonis S, Sen CN, Sekhar LN (1992) Cavernous sinus tumors: neuroradiologic and neurosurgical considerations on 150 operated cases. J Neurosurg Sci 36: 183–196
193. Lanzino G, Sekhar LN, Hirsch WL, Sen CN, Pomonis S, Snyderman CH (1993) Chordomas and chondrosarcomas involving the cavernous sinus: review of surgical treatment and outcome in 31 patients. Surg Neurol 40: 359–371
194. Lanzino G, Dumont AS, Lopes MB, Laws ER Jr (2001) Skull base chordomas: overview of disease, management options, and outcome. Neurosurg Focus 10: E12
195. Larson TC 3rd, Houser OW, Laws ER Jr (1987) Imaging of cranial chordomas. Mayo Clin Proc 62: 886–893
196. Laws ER Jr, Trautmann JC, Hollenhorst RW Jr (1977) Transsphenoidal decompression of the optic nerve and chiasm. Visual results in 62 patients. J Neurosurg 46: 717–722

197. Laws ER Jr (1984) Transsphenoidal surgery for tumors of the clivus. Otolaryngol Head Neck Surg 92: 100–101
198. Laws ER Jr, Fode NC, Redmond MJ (1985) Transsphenoidal surgery following unsuccessful prior therapy. An assessment of benefits and risks in 158 patients. J Neurosurg 63: 823–829
199. Laws ER Jr (2001) Skull base chordomas: overview of disease, management options, and outcome. Neurosurg Focus 10(3): Article 12
200. Layfield LJ, Liu K, Dodd LG, Olatidoye BA (1998) "Dedifferentiated" chordoma: a case report of the cytomorphologic findings on fine-needle aspiration. Diagn Cytopathol 19: 378–381
201. Lee-Jones L, Aligianis I, Davies PA, Puga A, Farndon PA, Stemmer-Rachamimov A, Ramesh V, Sampson JR (2004) Sacrococcygeal chordomas in patients with tuberous sclerosis complex show somatic loss of TSC1 or TSC2. Genes Chromosomes Cancer 41: 80–85
202. Lee HJ, Kalnin AJ, Holodny AI, Schulder M, Grigorian A, Sharer LR (1998) Hemorrhagic chondroid chordoma mimicking pituitary apoplexy. Neuroradiology 40: 720–723
203. Leproux F, de Toffol B, Aesch B, Cotty P (1993) MRI of cranial chordomas: the value of gadolinium. Neuroradiology 35: 543–545
204. Lim GH (1975) Clivus chordoma with unusual bone sclerosis and brainstem invasion. A case report with review of the radiology of cranial chordomas. Australas Radiol 19: 242–250
205. Linck (1909) Chordoma malignum. Zieglers Beitr 46
206. Linsenmayer TF, Gibney E, Schmid TM (1986) Segmental appearance of type X collagen in the developing avian notochord. Dev Biol 113: 467–473
207. Losi L, Tomasich G (1996) Dedifferentiated (sarcomatoid) chordoma in the base of the skull. Report of a case. Pathologica 88: 514–518
208. Luschka H (1857) Über gallertartige Auswüchse am Clivus Blumenbachii. Virch Arch 11: 8–12
209. Mabrey R (1935) Chordoma: a study of 150 cases. Am J Cancer 25: 501–517
210. Macdonald RL, Deck JH (1990) Immunohistochemistry of ecchordosis physaliphora and chordoma. Can J Neurol Sci 17: 420–423
211. Magrini SM, Papi MG, Marletta F, Tomaselli S, Cellai E, Mungai V, Biti G (1992) Chordoma-natural history, treatment and prognosis. The Florence Radiotherapy Department experience (1956–1990) and a critical review of the literature. Acta Oncol 31: 847–851
212. Maira G, Pallini R, Anile C, Fernandez E, Salvinelli F, La Rocca LM, Rossi GF (1996) Surgical treatment of clival chordomas: the transsphenoidal approach revisited. J Neurosurg 85: 784–792
213. Makhmudov UB, Tcherekayev VA, Tanyashin SV (1992) Transoral approach to tumors of the clivus: report of two cases. J Craniofac Surg 3: 35–38
214. Mandahl N, Heim S, Arheden K, Rydholm A, Willen H, Mitelman F (1990) Chromosomal rearrangements in chondromatous tumors. Cancer 65: 242–248
215. Mapstone TB, Kaufman B, Ratcheson RA (1983) Intradural chordoma without bone involvement: nuclear magnetic resonance (NMR) appearance. Case report. J Neurosurg 59: 535–537
216. Marshman LA, Gunasekera L, Rose PE, Olney JS (2001) Primary intracerebral mesenchymal chondrosarcoma with rhabdomyosarcomatous differentiation: case report and literature review. Br J Neurosurg 15: 419–424

217. Matsumoto J, Towbin RB, Ball WS Jr (1989) Cranial chordomas in infancy and childhood. A report of two cases and review of the literature. Pediatr Radiol 20: 28–32
218. Matsumoto K, Tamesa N, Tomita S, Tamiya T, Furuta T, Ohmoto T (1997) Stereotactic brachytherapy for clival chordoma. No Shinkei Geka 25: 919–925
219. McDermott MW, Gutin PH (1996) Image-guided surgery for skull base neoplasms using the ISG viewing wand. Anatomic and technical considerations. Neurosurg Clin N Am 7: 285–295
220. McMaster ML, Goldstein AM, Bromley CM, Ishibe N, Parry DM (2001) Chordoma: incidence and survival patterns in the United States, 1973–1995. Cancer Causes Control 12: 1–11
221. Mehnert F, Beschorner R, Kuker W, Hahn U, Nagele T (2004) Retroclival ecchordosis physaliphora: MR imaging and review of the literature. Am J Neuroradiol 25: 1851–1855
222. Meis JM, Raymond AK, Evans HL, Charles RE, Giraldo AA (1987) "Dedifferentiated" chordoma. A clinicopathologic and immunohistochemical study of three cases. Am J Surg Pathol 11: 516–525
223. Meis JM, Giraldo AA (1988) Chordoma. An immunohistochemical study of 20 cases. Arch Pathol Lab Med 112: 553–556
224. Menezes AH, VanGilder JC (1988) Transoral-transpharyngeal approach to the anterior craniocervical junction. Ten-year experience with 72 patients. J Neurosurg 69: 895–903
225. Menezes AH, Gantz BJ, Traynelis VC, McCulloch TM (1997) Cranial base chordomas. Clin Neurosurg 44: 491–509
226. Mertens F, Kreicbergs A, Rydholm A, Willen H, Carlen B, Mitelman F, Mandahl N (1994) Clonal chromosome aberrations in three sacral chordomas. Cancer Genet Cytogenet 73: 147–151
227. Meyer JE, Oot RF, Lindfors KK (1986) CT appearance of clival chordomas. J Comput Assist Tomogr 10: 34–38
228. Meyers SP, Hirsch WL Jr, Curtin HD, Barnes L, Sekhar LN, Sen C (1992) Chondrosarcomas of the skull base: MR imaging features. Radiology 184: 103–108
229. Meyers SP, Hirsch WL Jr, Curtin HD, Barnes L, Sekhar LN, Sen C (1992) Chordomas of the skull base: MR features. Am J Neuroradiol 13: 1627–1636
230. Mills RP (1984) Chordomas of the skull base. J R Soc Med 77: 10–16
231. Miozzo M, Dalpra L, Riva P, Volonta M, Macciardi F, Pericotti S, Tibiletti MG, Cerati M, Rohde K, Larizza L, Fuhrman Conti AM (2000) A tumor suppressor locus in familial and sporadic chordoma maps to 1p36. Int J Cancer 87: 68–72
232. Mitchell A, Scheithauer BW, Unni KK, Forsyth PJ, Wold LE, McGivney DJ (1993) Chordoma and chondroid neoplasms of the spheno-occiput. An immunohistochemical study of 41 cases with prognostic and nosologic implications. Cancer 72: 2943–2949
233. Miyagi A, Maeda K, Sugawara T (1998) Usefulness of neuroendoscopy and a neuronavigator for removal of clival chordoma. No Shinkei Geka 26: 169–175
234. Mondal A, Mukherjee PK (1988) Cytological and cytochemical diagnosis of chordoma by fine needle aspiration biopsy – a case report. Indian J Pathol Microbiol 31: 64–66
235. Moreira-Gonzalez A, Pieper DR, Balaguer Cambra J, Simman R, Jackson IT (2005) Skull base tumors: a comprehensive review of transfacial swing osteotomy approaches. Plast Reconstr Surg 115: 711–720

236. Mortini P, Roberti F, Kalavakonda C, Nadel A, Sekhar LN (2003) Endoscopic and microscopic extended subfrontal approach to the clivus: a comparative anatomical study. Skull Base 13: 139–147
237. Müller H (1858) Über das Vorkommen von Resten des Chorda dorsalis bei Menschen nach der Geburt und über ihr Verhältniss zu den Gallertgeschwülesten am Clivus. Z Ration Med 2: 202–229
238. Munzenrider JE, Liebsch NJ (1999) Proton therapy for tumors of the skull base. Strahlenther Onkol 175 Suppl 2: 57–63
239. Muthukumar N, Kondziolka D, Lunsford LD, Flickinger JC (1998) Stereotactic radiosurgery for chordoma and chondrosarcoma: further experiences. Int J Radiat Oncol Biol Phys 41: 387–392
240. Nagib MG, Wisiol ES, Simonton SC, Levinson RM (1990) Transoral labiomandibular approach to basiocciput chordomas in childhood. Childs Nerv Syst 6: 126–130
241. Naka T, Boltze C, Samii A, Herold C, Ostertag H, Iwamoto Y, Oda Y, Tsuneyoshi M, Kuester D, Roessner A (2003) Skull base and nonskull base chordomas: clinicopathologic and immunohistochemical study with special reference to nuclear pleomorphism and proliferative ability. Cancer 98: 1934–1941
242. Naka T, Boltze C, Kuester D, Schulz TO, Samii A, Herold C, Ostertag H, Roessner A (2004) Expression of matrix metalloproteinase (MMP)-1, MMP-2, MMP-9, cathepsin B, and urokinase plasminogen activator in non-skull base chordoma. Am J Clin Pathol 122: 926–930
243. Naka T, Boltze C, Kuester D, Samii A, Herold C, Ostertag H, Iwamoto Y, Oda Y, Tsuneyoshi M, Roessner A (2005) Intralesional fibrous septum in chordoma: a clinicopathologic and immunohistochemical study of 122 lesions. Am J Clin Pathol 124: 288–294
244. Naka T, Boltze C, kuester D, Schulz T, Schneider-Stock R, Kellner A, Samii A, Herold C, Ostertag H, Roessner A (2005) Alterations of G1-S checkpoint in chordoma: the prognostic impact of p53 overexpression. Cancer 104: 1255–1263
245. Ng SH, Ko SF, Wan YL, Tang LM, Ho YS (1998) Cervical ecchordosis physaliphora: CT and MR features. Br J Radiol 71: 329–331
246. Nijhawan VS, Rajwanshi A, Das A, Jayaram N, Gupta SK (1989) Fine-needle aspiration cytology of sacrococcygeal chordoma. Diagn Cytopathol 5: 404–407
247. Nimsky C, Ganslandt O, Von Keller B, Romstock J, Fahlbusch R (2004) Intraoperative high-field-strength MR imaging: implementation and experience in 200 patients. Radiology 233: 67–78
248. Nimsky C, Ganslandt O, Buchfelder M, Fahlbusch R (2006) Intraoperative visualization for resection of gliomas: the role of functional neuronavigation and intraoperative 1.5 T MRI. Neurol Res 28: 482–487
249. Noel G, Habrand JL, Jauffret E, de Crevoisier R, Dederke S, Mammar H, Haie-Meder C, Pontvert D, Hasboun D, Ferrand R, Boisserie G, Beaudre A, Gaboriaud G, Guedea F, Petriz L, Mazeron JJ (2003) Radiation therapy for chordoma and chondrosarcoma of the skull base and the cervical spine. Prognostic factors and patterns of failure. Strahlenther Onkol 179: 241–248
250. Noel G, Feuvret L, Calugaru V, Dhermain F, Mammar H, Haie-Meder C, Ponvert D, Hasboun D, Ferrand R, Nauraye C, Boisserie G, Beaudre A, Gaboriaud G, Mazal A, Habrand JL, Mazeron JJ (2005) Chordomas of the base of the skull and upper cervical spine. One hundred patients irradiated by a 3D conformal technique combining photon and proton beams. Acta Oncol 44: 700–708

251. O'Neill P, Bell BA, Miller JD, Jacobson I, Guthrie W (1985) Fifty years of experience with chordomas in southeast Scotland. Neurosurgery 16: 166–170
252. Ogi H, Kiryu H, Hori Y, Fukui M (1995) Cutaneous metastasis of CNS chordoma. Am J Dermatopathol 17: 599–602
253. Oikawa S, Kyoshima K, Goto T, Iwashita T, Takizawa T, Kobayashi S, Ito M (2001) Histological study on local invasiveness of clival chordoma. Case report of autopsy. Acta Neurochir (Wien) 143: 1065–1069
254. Okada Y, Aoki S, Barkovich AJ, *et al* (1989) Cranial bone marrow in children: assessment of normal development with mr imaging. Radiology 171: 161–164
255. Oot RF, Melville GE, New PF, Austin-Seymour M, Munzenrider J, Pile-Spellman J, Spagnoli M, Shoukimas GM, Momose KJ, Carroll R, *et al* (1988) The role of MR and CT in evaluating clival chordomas and chondrosarcomas. AJR Am J Roentgenol 151: 567–575
256. Paavolainen P, Teppo L (1976) Chordoma in Finland. Acta Orthop Scand 47: 46–51
257. Pai HH, Thornton A, Katznelson L, Finkelstein DM, Adams JA, Fullerton BC, Loeffler JS, Leibsch NJ, Klibanski A, Munzenrider JE (2001) Hypothalamic/pituitary function following high-dose conformal radiotherapy to the base of skull: demonstration of a dose-effect relationship using dose-volume histogram analysis. Int J Radiat Oncol Biol Phys 49: 1079–1092
258. Pallini R, Maira G, Pierconti F, Falchetti ML, Alvino E, Cimino-Reale G, Fernandez E, D'Ambrosio E, Larocca LM (2003) Chordoma of the skull base: predictors of tumor recurrence. J Neurosurg 98: 812–822
259. Pamir MN, Kilic T, Ture U, Ozek MM (2004) Multimodality management of 26 skull-base chordomas with 4-year mean follow-up: experience at a single institution. Acta Neurochir (Wien) 146: 343–354; discusion 354
260. Pamir MN, Kilic T, Ozek MM, Ozduman K, Ture U (2006) Non-meningeal tumours of the cavernous sinus: a surgical analysis. J Clin Neurosci 13: 626–635
261. Pamir MN, Ozduman K (2006) Analysis of radiological features relative to histopathology in 42 skull-base chordomas and chondrosarcomas. Eur J Radiol 58: 461–470
262. Pamir MN, Peker S, Ozek MM, Dincer A (2006) Intraoperative MR imaging: preliminary results with 3 tesla MR system. Acta Neurochir Suppl 98: 97–100
263. Parkinson D (2000) Extradural neural axis compartment. J Neurosurg 92: 585–588
264. Patten BM (1968) Human ebryology. McGraw Hill, New York, pp 430–431
265. Pearlman AW, Friedman M (1970) Radical radiation therapy of chordoma. Am J Roentgenol Radium Ther Nucl Med 108: 332–341
266. Peker S, Kurtkaya-Yapicier O, Kilic T, Pamir MN (2005) Microsurgical anatomy of the lateral walls of the pituitary fossa. Acta Neurochir (Wien) 147: 641–648; discussion 649
267. Persons DL, Bridge JA, Neff JR (1991) Cytogenetic analysis of two sacral chordomas. Cancer Genet Cytogenet 56: 197–201
268. Petti PL (1996) Evaluation of a pencil-beam dose calculation technique for charged particle radiotherapy. Int J Radiat Oncol Biol Phys 35: 1049–1057
269. Placzek M (1995) The role of the notochord and floor plate in inductive interactions. Curr Opin Genet Dev 5: 499–506
270. Price CH, Jeffree GM (1977) Incidence of bone sarcoma in SW England, 1946–74, in relation to age, sex, tumour site and histology. Br J Cancer 36: 511–522
271. Probst EN, Zanella FE, Vortmeyer AO (1993) Congenital clivus chordoma. Am J Neuroradiol 14: 537–539

272. Rabadan A, Conesa H (1992) Transmaxillary-transnasal approach to the anterior clivus: a microsurgical anatomical model. Neurosurgery 30: 473–481; discussion 482
273. Radner H, Katenkamp D, Reifenberger G, Deckert M, Pietsch T, Wiestler OD (2001) New developments in the pathology of skull base tumors. Virchows Arch 438: 321–335
274. Raffel C, Wright DC, Gutin PH, Wilson CB (1985) Cranial chordomas: clinical presentation and results of operative and radiation therapy in twenty-six patients. Neurosurgery 17: 703–710
275. Raso JL, Gusmao S (2006) Transbasal approach to skull base tumors: evaluation and proposal of classification. Surg Neurol 65 (Suppl 1) S1: 33-1:37; discussion 1: 37-1:38
276. Reifenberger G, Weber T, Weber RG, Wolter M, Brandis A, Kuchelmeister K, Pilz P, Reusche E, Lichter P, Wiestler OD (1999) Chordoid glioma of the third ventricle: immunohistochemical and molecular genetic characterization of a novel tumor entity. Brain Pathol 9: 617–626
277. Rengachary SS, Grotte DA, Swanson PE (1997) Extradural ecchordosis physaliphora of the thoracic spine: case report. Neurosurgery 41: 1198–1201; discussion 1201–1202
278. Rhomberg W, Eiter H, Bohler F, Dertinger S (2006) Combined radiotherapy and razoxane in the treatment of chondrosarcomas and chordomas. Anticancer Res 26: 2407–2411
279. Ribbert H (1895) Über die experimentelle Erzeugung einer Ecchondrosis physalifora. Verhandl. d. XIII. Kongr f inn Med 13: 455–464
280. Ribbert H (1904) Geschwülstlehre für Arzte und studierende, Bonn
281. Ribbert H, Virchow R (1959) Chordoma
282. Rich TA, Schiller A, Suit HD, Mankin HJ (1985) Clinical and pathologic review of 48 cases of chordoma. Cancer 56: 182–187
283. Richardson MS (2001) Pathology of skull base tumors. Otolaryngol Clin North Am 34: 1025–1042
284. Riva P, Crosti F, Orzan F, Dalpra L, Mortini P, Parafioriti A, Pollo B, Fuhrman Conti AM, Miozzo M, Larizza L (2003) Mapping of candidate region for chordoma development to 1p36.13 by LOH analysis. Int J Cancer 107: 493–497
285. Roche PH, Malca SA, Payan MJ, Pellet W (1995) Chondrosarcoma of the skull base. Apropos of sphenotemporal localization and review of the literature. Neurochirurgie 41: 353–358
286. Rodriguez L, Colina J, Lopez J, Molina O, Cardozo J (1999) Intradural prepontine growth: giant ecchordosis physaliphora or extraosseous chordoma? Neuropathology 19: 336–340
287. Romero J, Cardenes H, la Torre A, Valcarcel F, Magallon R, Regueiro C, Aragon G (1993) Chordoma: results of radiation therapy in eighteen patients. Radiother Oncol 29: 27–32
288. Rone R, Ramzy I, Duncan D (1986) Anaplastic sacrococcygeal chordoma. Fine needle aspiration cytologic findings and embryologic considerations. Acta Cytol 30: 183–188
289. Rosenberg AE, Brown GA, Bhan AK, Lee JM (1994) Chondroid chordoma – a variant of chordoma. A morphologic and immunohistochemical study. Am J Clin Pathol 101: 36–41
290. Rosenberg AE, Nielsen GP, Keel SB, Renard LG, Fitzek MM, Munzenrider JE, Liebsch NJ (1999) Chondrosarcoma of the base of the skull: a clinicopathologic study of 200 cases with emphasis on its distinction from chordoma. Am J Surg Pathol 23: 1370–1378
291. Rosenberg AE, Nielsen GP, Keel SB (2000) Lipoid chordoma. Mod Pathol 13: 15a
292. Saad AG, Collins MH (2005) Prognostic value of MIB-1, E-cadherin, and CD44 in pediatric chordomas. Pediatr Dev Pathol 8: 362–368

293. Sabit I, Schaefer SD, Couldwell WT (2000) Extradural extranasal combined transmaxillary transsphenoidal approach to the cavernous sinus: a minimally invasive microsurgical model. Laryngoscope 110: 286–291
294. Saito A, Hasegawa T, Shimoda T, Toda G, Hirohashi S, Tajima G, Moriya Y (1998) Dedifferentiated chordoma: a case report. Jpn J Clin Oncol 28: 766–771
295. Salisbury JR, Isaacson PG (1985) Demonstration of cytokeratins and an epithelial membrane antigen in chordomas and human fetal notochord. Am J Surg Pathol 9: 791–797
296. Salisbury JR (1993) The pathology of the human notochord. J Pathol 171: 253–255
297. Salisbury JR, Deverell MH, Cookson MJ, Whimster WF (1993) Three-dimensional reconstruction of human embryonic notochords: clue to the pathogenesis of chordoma. J Pathol 171: 59–62
298. Samii M, Ammirati M (1988) The combined supra-infratentorial pre-sigmoid sinus avenue to the petro-clival region. Surgical technique and clinical applications. Acta Neurochir (Wien) 95: 6–12
299. Sandberg AA, Bridge JA (2003) Updates on the cytogenetics and molecular genetics of bone and soft tissue tumors: chondrosarcoma and other cartilaginous neoplasms. Cancer Genet Cytogenet 143: 1–31
300. Santoni R, Liebsch N, Finkelstein DM, Hug E, Hanssens P, Goitein M, Smith AR, O'Farrell D, Efird JT, Fullerton B, Munzenrider JE (1998) Temporal lobe (TL) damage following surgery and high-dose photon and proton irradiation in 96 patients affected by chordomas and chondrosarcomas of the base of the skull. Int J Radiat Oncol Biol Phys 41: 59–68
301. Sautner D, Saeger W, Ludecke DK (1993) Tumors of the sellar region mimicking pituitary adenomas. Exp Clin Endocrinol 101: 283–289
302. Sawamura Y, Terasaka S, Fukushima T (1999) Extended transsphenoidal approach with sigma-shape osteotomy of the maxilla: technical note. Skull Base Surg 9: 119–125
303. Sawyer JR, Husain M, Al-Mefty O (2001) Identification of isochromosome 1q as a recurring chromosome aberration in skull base chordomas: a new marker for aggressive tumors? Neurosurg Focus 10: E6
304. Scheil S, Bruderlein S, Liehr T, Starke H, Herms J, Schulte M, Moller P (2001) Genome-wide analysis of sixteen chordomas by comparative genomic hybridization and cytogenetics of the first human chordoma cell line, U-CH1. Genes Chromosomes Cancer 32: 203–211
305. Schisano G, Tovi D (1962) Clivus chordomas. Neurochirurgia (Stuttg) 5: 99–120
306. Schonegger K, Gelpi E, Prayer D, Dieckmann K, Matula C, Hassler M, Hainfellner JA, Marosi C (2005) Recurrent and metastatic clivus chordoma: systemic palliative therapy retards disease progression. Anticancer Drugs 16: 1139–1143
307. Schulz-Ertner D, Haberer T, Jakel O, Thilmann C, Kramer M, Enghardt W, Kraft G, Wannenmacher M, Debus J (2002) Radiotherapy for chordomas and low-grade chondrosarcomas of the skull base with carbon ions. Int J Radiat Oncol Biol Phys 53: 36–42
308. Schulz-Ertner D, Nikoghosyan A, Thilmann C, Haberer T, Jakel O, Karger C, Scholz M, Kraft G, Wannenmacher M, Debus J (2003) Carbon ion radiotherapy for chordomas and low-grade chondrosarcomas of the skull base. Results in 67 patients. Strahlenther Onkol 179: 598–605
309. Sefiani S, Amarti A, Maher M, Benkiran L, Saidi A (2002) Dedifferentiated chordoma of the skull base. A case report. Neurochirurgie 48: 436–439

310. Seifert G, Donath K (1998) [Cranial and cervical chordomas. A differential diagnostic problem]. Mund Kiefer Gesichtschir 2: 153–159
311. Seifert V, Laszig R (1991) Transoral transpalatal removal of a giant premesencephalic clivus chordoma. Acta Neurochir (Wien) 112: 141–146
312. Sekhar LN, Moller AR (1986) Operative management of tumors involving the cavernous sinus. J Neurosurg 64: 879–889
313. Sekhar LN, Nanda A, Sen CN, Snyderman CN, Janecka IP (1992) The extended frontal approach to tumors of the anterior, middle, and posterior skull base. J Neurosurg 76: 198–206
314. Sekhar LN, Janecka IP (1993) Surgery of cranial base tumors. Raven Press, New York
315. Sekhar LN, Pranatartiharan R, Chanda A, Wright DC (2001) Chordomas and chondrosarcomas of the skull base: results and complications of surgical management. Neurosurg Focus 10: E2
316. Sen C, Triana A (2001) Cranial chordomas: results of radical excision. Neurosurg Focus 10: E3
317. Sen CN, Sekhar LN, Schramm VL, Janecka IP (1989) Chordoma and chondrosarcoma of the cranial base: an 8-year experience. Neurosurgery 25: 931–940; discussion 940–941
318. Sepehrnia A, Samii M, Tatagiba M (1991) Management of intracavernous tumours: an 11-year experience. Acta Neurochir Suppl 53: 122–126
319. Shugar JM, Som PM, Krespi YP, Arnold LM, Som ML (1980) Primary chordoma of the maxillary sinus. Laryngoscope 90: 1825–1830
320. Sibley RK, Day DL, Dehner LP, Trueworthy RC (1987) Metastasizing chordoma in early childhood: a pathological and immunohistochemical study with review of the literature. Pediatr Pathol 7: 287–301
321. Slater JM, Slater JD, Archambeau JO (1995) Proton therapy for cranial base tumors. J Craniofac Surg 6: 24–26
322. Spallone A, Tcherekarjev VA, Korshunov AG (1996) Chondrosarcoma of the anterior cranial fossa. Report of two cases. J Neurosurg Sci 40: 115–120
323. Spetzler RF, Herman JM, Beals S, Joganic E, Milligan J (1993) Preservation of olfaction in anterior craniofacial approaches. J Neurosurg 79: 48–52
324. Spiro RH, Gerold FP, Strong EW (1981) Mandibular "swing" approach for oral and oropharyngeal tumors. Head Neck Surg 3: 371
325. Steiner and Fischer (1907) Über ein malignes chordom der Schaedel-Rückgradshöhle. Beitr Path Anat 40: 109–119
326. Stemple DL (2005) Structure and function of the notochord: an essential organ for chordate development. Development 132: 2503–2512
327. Stepanek J, Cataldo SA, Ebersold MJ, Lindor NM, Jenkins RB, Unni K, Weinshenker BG, Rubenstein RL (1998) Familial chordoma with probable autosomal dominant inheritance. Am J Med Genet 75: 335–336
328. Stewart M, Morin J (1926) Chordoma: a review, with report of a new sacrococcygeal case. J Pathol Bacterial 29: 41–60
329. Stough DR, Hartzog JT, Fisher RG (1971) Unusual intradural spinal metastasis of a cranial chordoma. Case report. J Neurosurg 34: 560–562
330. Sundaresan N (1986) Chordomas. Clin Orthop Relat Res: 135–142
331. Sweet MB, Thonar EJ, Berson SD, Skikne MI, Immelman AR, Kerr WA (1979) Biochemical studies of the matrix of craniovertebral chordoma and a metastasis. Cancer 44: 652–660

332. Sze G, Uichanco LS 3rd, Brant-Zawadzki MN, Davis RL, Gutin PH, Wilson CB, Norman D, Newton TH (1988) Chordomas: MR imaging. Radiology 166: 187–191
333. Tai PT, Craighead P, Bagdon F (1995) Optimization of radiotherapy for patients with cranial chordoma. A review of dose-response ratios for photon techniques. Cancer 75: 749–756
334. Tallini G, Dorfman H, Brys P, Dal Cin P, De Wever I, Fletcher CD, Jonson K, Mandahl N, Mertens F, Mitelman F, Rosai J, Rydholm A, Samson I, Sciot R, Van den Berghe H, Vanni R, Willen H (2002) Correlation between clinicopathological features and karyotype in 100 cartilaginous and chordoid tumours. A report from the Chromosomes and Morphology (CHAMP) Collaborative Study Group. J Pathol 196: 194–203
335. Tamaki N, Nagashima T, Ehara K, Motooka Y, Barua KK (2001) Surgical approaches and strategies for skull base chordomas. Neurosurg Focus 10: E9
336. Taniguchi K, Tateishi A, Higaki S, Igarashi M, Hayashi V, Inoue S, Shoji H (1984) Type of collagen in chordoma. Nippon Seikeigeka Gakkai Zasshi 58: 829–834
337. Terahara A, Niemierko A, Goitein M, Finkelstein D, Hug E, Liebsch N, O'Farrell D, Lyons S, Munzenrider J (1999) Analysis of the relationship between tumor dose inhomogeneity and local control in patients with skull base chordoma. Int J Radiat Oncol Biol Phys 45: 351–358
338. Tewfik HH, McGinnis WL, Nordstrom DG, Latourette HB (1977) Chordoma: evaluation of clinical behavior and treatment modalities. Int J Radiat Oncol Biol Phys 2: 959–962
339. Thodou E, Kontogeorgos G, Scheithauer BW, Lekka I, Tzanis S, Mariatos P, Laws ER Jr (2000) Intrasellar chordomas mimicking pituitary adenoma. J Neurosurg 92: 976–982
340. Toda H, Kondo A, Iwasaki K (1998) Neuroradiological characteristics of ecchordosis physaliphora. Case report and review of the literature. J Neurosurg 89: 830–834
341. Tomlinson FH, Scheithauer BW, Forsythe PA, Unni KK, Meyer FB (1992) Sarcomatous transformation in cranial chordoma. Neurosurgery 31: 13–18
342. Tsai EC, Santoreneos S, Rutka JT (2002) Tumors of the skull base in children: review of tumor types and management strategies. Neurosurg Focus 12: e1
343. Tuite GF, Veres R, Crockard HA (1996) Pediatric transoral surgery: indications, complications, and long-term outcome. J Neurosurg 84: 573–583
344. Ture U, Pamir MN (2002) Extreme lateral-transatlas approach for resection of the dens of the axis. J Neurosurg 96: 73–82
344a. Ture U, Pamir MN (2004) Small petrosal approach to the middle portion of the mediobasal temporal region: technical case report. Surg Neurol 61(1): 60–67
345. Tzortzidis F, Elahi F, Wright D, Natarajan SK, Sekhar LN (2006) Patient outcome at long-term follow-up after aggressive microsurgical resection of cranial base chordomas. Neurosurgery 59: 230–237; discussion 230–237
346. Tzortzidis F, Elahi F, Wright DC, Temkin N, Natarajan SK, Sekhar LN (2006) Patient outcome at long-term follow-up after aggressive microsurgical resection of cranial base chondrosarcomas. Neurosurgery 58: 1090–1098; discussion 1090–1098
347. Uggowitzer MM, Kugler C, Groell R, Lindbichler F, Radner H, Sutter B, Ranner G (1999) Drop metastases in a patient with a chondroid chordoma of the clivus. Neuroradiology 41: 504–507
348. Ulich TR, Mirra JM (1982) Ecchordosis physaliphora vertebralis. Clin Orthop Relat Res 163: 282–289

349. Unni KK (1996) Dahlin's bone tumors: general aspects and data on 11087 cases, 5 edn. Lippincot-Raven, Phhiladelphia, PA
350. Urie MM, Fullerton B, Tatsuzaki H, Birnbaum S, Suit HD, Convery K, Skates S, Goitein M (1992) A dose response analysis of injury to cranial nerves and/or nuclei following proton beam radiation therapy. Int J Radiat Oncol Biol Phys 23: 27–39
351. Utne JR, Pugh DG (1955) The roentgenologic aspects of chordoma. Am J Roentgenol Radium Ther Nucl Med 74: 593–608
352. Uttley D, Moore A, Archer DJ (1989) Surgical management of midline skull-base tumors: a new approach. J Neurosurg 71: 705–710
353. Valderrama E, Kahn LB, Lipper S, Marc J (1983) Chondroid chordoma. Electron-microscopic study of two cases. Am J Surg Pathol 7: 625–632
354. Van Loveren HR, Fernandez PM, Keller JT, Tew JM Jr, Shumrick K (1994) Neurosurgical applications of Le Fort I-type osteotomy. Clin Neurosurg 41: 425–443
355. Verma K, Murthy L, Kapila K (1986) Cytologic diagnosis of chordoma by fine needle aspiration. Indian J Pathol Microbiol 29: 189–191
356. Virchow RLK (1857) Untersuchungen über die Entwickelung des Schädelgrundes im gesunden und krankhaften Zustande, und über den Einfluss derselben auf Schädelform, Gesichtsbildung und Gehirnbau. G. Reimer, Berlin
357. Volpe NJ, Liebsch NJ, Munzenrider JE, Lessell S (1993) Neuro-ophthalmologic findings in chordoma and chondrosarcoma of the skull base. Am J Ophthalmol 115: 97–104
358. Volpe R, Mazabraud A (1983) A clinicopathologic review of 25 cases of chordoma (a pleomorphic and metastasizing neoplasm). Am J Surg Pathol 7: 161–170
359. Vougioukas VI, Hubbe U, Schipper J, Spetzger U (2003) Navigated transoral approach to the cranial base and the craniocervical junction: technical note. Neurosurgery 52: 247–250; discussion 251
360. Walaas L, Kindblom LG (1991) Fine-needle aspiration biopsy in the preoperative diagnosis of chordoma: a study of 17 cases with application of electron microscopic, histochemical, and immunocytochemical examination. Hum Pathol 22: 22–28
361. Watanabe A, Yanagita M, Ishii R, Shirabe T (1994) Magnetic resonance imaging of ecchordosis physaliphora – case report. Neurol Med Chir (Tokyo) 34: 448–450
361a. Watkins L, Khudados ES, Kaleoglu M, et al. (1993) Skull base chordomas: a review of 38 patients, 1958–1988. Br J Neurosurg 7: 241–248
362. Weber AL, Liebsch NJ, Sanchez R, Sweriduk ST Jr (1994) Chordomas of the skull base. Radiologic and clinical evaluation. Neuroimaging Clin N Am 4: 515–527
363. Weber DC, Rutz HP, Pedroni ES, Bolsi A, Timmermann B, Verwey J, Lomax AJ, Goitein G (2005) Results of spot-scanning proton radiation therapy for chordoma and chondrosarcoma of the skull base: the Paul Scherrer Institut experience. Int J Radiat Oncol Biol Phys 63: 401–409
364. Weinberger P, Yu Z, Kowalski D, Joe J, Manger P, Psyrri A, Sasaki C (2005) Differential expression of epidermal growth factor receptor, c-Met, and HER2/neu in chordoma compared with 17 other malignancies. Arch Otolaryngol Head Neck Surg 131: 707–711
365. Wojno KJ, Hruban RH, Garin-Chesa P, Huvos AG (1992) Chondroid chordomas and low-grade chondrosarcomas of the craniospinal axis. An immunohistochemical analysis of 17 cases. Am J Surg Pathol 16: 1144–1152

366. Wold LE, Laws ER Jr (1983) Cranial chordomas in children and young adults. J Neurosurg 59: 1043–1047
367. Wolfe JT 3rd, Scheithauer BW (1987) "Intradural chordoma" or "giant ecchordosis physaliphora"? Report of two cases. Clin Neuropathol 6: 98–103
368. Wyatt RB, Schochet SS Jr, McCormick WF (1971) Ecchordosis physaliphora. An electron microscopic study. J Neurosurg 34: 672–677
369. Yamada T, Placzek M, Tanaka H, Dodd J, Jessell TM (1991) Control of cell pattern in the developing nervous system: polarizing activity of the floor plate and notochord. Cell 64: 635–647
370. Yamaguchi T, Yamato M, Saotome K (2002) First histologically confirmed case of a classic chordoma arising in a precursor benign notochordal lesion: differential diagnosis of benign and malignant notochordal lesions. Skeletal Radiol 31: 413–418
371. Yamaguchi T, Suzuki S, Ishiiwa H, Shimizu K, Ueda Y (2004) Benign notochordal cell tumors: a comparative histological study of benign notochordal cell tumors, classic chordomas, and notochordal vestiges of fetal intervertebral discs. Am J Surg Pathol 28: 756–761
372. Yamaguchi T, Suzuki S, Ishiiwa H, Ueda Y (2004) Intraosseous benign notochordal cell tumours: overlooked precursors of classic chordomas? Histopathology 44: 597–602
373. Yamaguchi T, Watanabe-Ishiiwa H, Suzuki S, Igarashi Y, Ueda Y (2005) Incipient chordoma: a report of two cases of early-stage chordoma arising from benign notochordal cell tumors. Mod Pathol 18: 1005–1010
374. Yang XR, Beerman M, Bergen AW, Parry DM, Sheridan E, Liebsch NJ, Kelley MJ, Chanock S, Goldstein AM (2005) Corroboration of a familial chordoma locus on chromosome 7q and evidence of genetic heterogeneity using single nucleotide polymorphisms (SNPs). Int J Cancer 116: 487–491
375. Yasargil MG (1996) Microneurosurgery. Thieme Verlag, Stuttgart, NewYork
376. Zenker FA (1857) Ueber die gallertgeschwülste des Clivus Blumenbachii (Ecchondrosis prolifera, Virchow). Virch Arch 12: 108–110
377. Zhou L, Guo H, Li S, Ji Y, Huang F (1995) An extensive subfrontal approach to the lesions involving the skull base. Chin Med J (Engl) 108: 407–412
378. Zorlu F, Gurkaynak M, Yildiz F, Oge K, Atahan IL (2000) Conventional external radiotherapy in the management of clivus chordomas with overt residual disease. Neurol Sci 21: 203–207
379. Zülch KJ, Christensen E (1956) Pathologische Anatomie der raumbeengenden intrakraniellen Prozesse. Springer, Berlin, Heidelberg New York

# The influence of genetics on intracranial aneurysm formation and rupture: current knowledge and its possible impact on future treatment

B. KRISCHEK and M. TATAGIBA

Department of Neurosurgery, University of Tuebingen, Tuebingen, Germany

## Contents



## Abstract

The etiology of intracranial aneurysm formation and rupture remains mostly unknown, but lately several studies have increasingly supported the role of genetic factors. In reports so far, genome-wide linkage studies suggest several susceptibility loci that may contain one or more predisposing genes. Depending on the examined ethnic population, several different non-matching chromosomal regions have been found. Studies of several candidate genes report association with intracranial aneurysms. To date, no single gene has been identified as responsible for intracranial aneurysm formation or rupture.

In addition to the well-published environmental factors, such as alcohol intake, hypertension and smoking, only the recent progress in molecular genetics enables us to investigate the possible genetic determinants of this disease. Although a familial predisposition is the strongest risk factor for the development of intracranial aneurysms, the mode of Mendelian inheritance is uncertain in most families. Therefore, multiple genetic susceptibilities in conjunction with the environmental factors are considered to act together in the disease's etiology. Accordingly, researchers performed linkage studies and case-control association studies for the genetic analysis and have identified several genes to be susceptible to intracranial aneurysms. The identification of susceptible genes may lead to the understanding of the mechanism of formation and rupture and possibly lead to the development of a pharmacological therapy. Furthermore, should it be possible to identify a genetic marker associated with an increased risk of formation and rupture of an intracranial aneurysm, the necessity for screening and urgency of treatment could be determined more easily.

In this review we summarize the current knowledge of intracranial aneurysm genetics and also discuss the method to detect the causalities. In view of the recent advances made in this field, we also give an outlook on possible future genetically engineered therapies, whose development are well underway.

*Keywords:* Cerebral aneurysms; subarachnoid hemorrhage; genetic; intracerebral hemorrhage.

## Introduction

Although the incidence of other kinds of stroke has declined in the last three decades the frequency of subarachnoid hemorrhage due to a ruptured intracranial aneurysm has remained the same. The peak incidence of suffering from a subarachnoid hemorrhage is in persons 55–60 years of age [26], whereas there is a preponderance of the female ratio of around 2:1 [76, 83]. Recent technical advances have changed intracranial aneurysm (IA) treatment dramatically. According to availability, coiling has taken over a large part of IA treatment in industrialized countries [75]. Nevertheless, mortality of individuals remains around 50% of patients who had suffered an intracranial aneurysm [44], while the survivors have a 30% danger of developing a persisting neurological deficit. Environmental factors associated with intracranial aneurysms such as hypertension, alcohol intake and smoking have all been well documented [20] but they alone can not be held responsible for IA formation and rupture. It has been shown that the risk of ruptured IA in first-degree relatives of patients with aneurysmal SAH is four times higher, and the relative risk in siblings is six times higher, than that in the general population [77, 81]. According to the period of follow-up the risk of rupture is between 0.6 and 1.3% per year [63, 95]. As the relative risk (RR) for rupture is 2.0 in patients above the age of 60, it is also increased in the female gender (RR1.6) and in patients of Japanese and Finnish descent (RR3.4) [95].

## Different epidemiology in different countries

Rupture rates in highly industrialized countries have been determined to be between 11/100,000 in the USA and 96/100,000 in distinct regions in Japan, which may again reflect the genetic component that plays a role in formation and/or rupture [39, 50, 63]. Even within Japan the incidence varies from 20 to 96/100,000 [36, 50, 90]. As of now, still little is known about the rates in highly populated countries such as India and China [38]. The increasingly wide-spread use of digital communication between IA treating departments that are in different locations allows easy access to each others documentation within different countries and will hopefully lead to further insight into the globally differing epidemiological data of IA.

A widely cited figure for the prevalence for asymptomatic unruptured intracranial aneurysms is 5% although the prevalence in the general population is unclear. The prevalence for all cerebral aneurysms according to autopsy procedures ranges from 0.2 to 9%, with a prevalence of 0.6 to 4.2% for unruptured aneurysms alone [96]. As an example, one of the largest autopsy studies of 1230 Japanese cases over a period of 30 years revealed a prevalance of incidental intracranial aneurysms to be 4.6% [41].

The increasingly sophisticated and susceptible means of non-invasive diagnostic imaging will further change early treatment modalities. Nowadays 3 Tesla MRIs can detect IAs with diameters as small as 2–3 mm. With health care systems providing extensive check-ups, e.g. – prophylactic brain MR scan in Japan [63, 101], the very early detection and treatment of IAs is bound to change.

## Etiology of intracranial aneurysm formation and rupture

The detailed causes for intracranial aneurysm formation and rupture have not been elucidated, but there have been several studies on possible etiological causes. Inflammatory mechanisms [12], hypertension [37] and hormonal influence in the female gender [31, 42, 43] have all been connected to IA formation and rupture.

The typical intracranial artery is made up of three histological layers: 1) the inner layer (tunica intima) consisting of an endothelial layer and smooth muscle cells, 2) the muscular layer (tunica media) made up of the internal elastic lamina and SMCs and 3) the outer loose connective tissue layer (tunica adventitia) [78]. At bifurcation sites they have a gap in the continuity of the muscular media layer which are called medial gaps or raphés. This particular gap has often been cited as a predisposing weakness to the formation of intracranial aneurysms due to a possible decrease in tensile strength. But ultrastructural examination at these sites has revealed a tendon-like organization of collagen fibers increasing the resistency to mechanical stretching [22, 85, 86]. In intracranial aneurysms the layers are often not clearly defined [24]. A lack of elastic lamina, disorganized smooth muscle cells, neointimal and myointimal hyperplasia as well as early atherosclerotic changes are common features [45, 51]. Structural abnormalities in structural proteins of the extracellular matrix have been identified in the arterial wall at a distance from the aneurysm itself. Reticular fibers were significantly decreased in the Tunica media of intracranial aneurysms as compared to those of control arteries [13].

Continuous pressure exerted at points of bifurcation around the circle of Willis are subject to aneurysm formation [18]. This leads to the conclusion that a vessel wall weakness predisposes an outpouching. Furthermore, structural weaknesses seen in connective tissue disorders are associated with the presence of IA and their rupture. Among them are diseases such as the autosomal dominant polycystic kidney disease, Ehlers-Danlos Syndrome, pseudoxanthoma elasticum and fibromuscular dysplasia [80]. Hereditary hemorrhagic telangiectasia (HHT) or Osler-Weber-Rendu syndrome is an autosomal dominant vascular disorder characterized by telangiectases, internal arteriovenous malformations and intracranial aneurysms. Endoglin gene mutations are responsible for HHT type 1 and ACVRL1 (activin receptor like kinase 1) mutations cause HHT type 2 [21]. A polymorphism of the endoglin gene has been correlated with intracranial aneurysm formation in a Japanese population but could not be replicated by others [54, 69, 89]. Several genes of the extracellular matrix have been examined regarding their immediate role in the vessel wall formation. Most recent reports have shown that irregularities in the elastin gene [2], the collagen gene [100] and the lysl oxidase like family gene 2 (LOXL 2), which cross links collagen and elastin [1], play a role in IA formation although replication studies in patients of different ethnic origin did not always reach the same conclusions [56].

Whether or not genetic susceptibilities play a role in the rupture of IA in combination with the well-known environmental factors, remains to be seen. In an article comparing a group of ruptured and unruptured intracranial aneurysm patients of Caucasian ethnicity it was found that three polymorphisms in the endothelial nitric oxide synthase gene (eNOS) could possibly indicate an enheightened risk of rupture [47]. In a larger study of Japanese patients none of the aforementioned polymorphisms of the eNOS gene could be verified [57].

Aside from the strucutral differences several findings of infiltrating inflammatory cells have been reported [12, 45, 92]. Macrophages and T-cells infiltrate all layers of the aneurysm vessel wall. Comparison between ruptured and unruptured aneurysm tissue has demonstrated similar histological findings indicating a restrucuring process to have begun before the aneurysm's rupture [12, 15, 25, 51].

## Vascular and cerebrovascular diseases associated with a genetic component

Family history studies and the results from studies of twins have shown a tendency for different types of stroke to cluster within families. Several mendelian and mitochondrial disorders cause cerebrovascular malformations, ischemic stroke as well as hemorrhagic stroke [62]. As an example, among the most intensively genetically researched cerebral vascular malformations are the cerebral cavernous malformations (CCM). Three linkage regions have been described: CCM1 on chromosome locus 7q21–q22, CCM2 on 7p13–15 and CCM3 on 3q25.2–q27. The genetic defects for CCM 1 are due to various mutations in the gene Krit1, which encodes for the Krev interaction Trapped 1 (Krit1) protein. CCM2 encodes the MGC4607 protein, also called malcavernin, and CCM3 the programmed cell death 10 (PDCD10) protein [60]. Other cerebrovascular malformations in which multiple genetic components are likely to play a role include brain arteriovenous malformations and Moyamoya disease [66]. Recently there have been reports on the association of polymorphisms of Interleukin-6 [8] and ACVRL1 [82] with arteriovenous malformations of the central nervous system.

Abdominal aortic aneurysms have been examined extensively, revealing similar results of a multigenic origin [67]. Comparative studies between aortic and intracranial aneurysms have yet to yield identical findings [49], but similar mechanisms of formation seem fathomable.

## Approaches to genetic research of intracranial aneurysms

There are two major approaches for the identification of possible intracranial aneurysm genes. They are not mutually exclusive, but more complementary. One is to perform a **linkage** analysis which locates the locus of disease using DNA and clinical information of families (including more than one member). The other is the **association** approach that may comprise the whole genome or single candidate genes. It identifies potential disease alleles in a case-control design.

While linkage analysis is arguably the most powerful method for identifying a locus involving rare, high-risk alleles in Mendelian diseases, as was the case for the Krit1 gene in cerebral cavernous malformation [30] and Notch3 for CADASIL (cerebral autosomal dominant arteriopathy with subcortical infarcts and leukoencephalopathy) [91], many consider genetic association analyses to be the best method for identifying genetic variants related to common and complex diseases, such as for IA. The HapMap project, in particular, has made genomewide association studies the most powerful tool for identification of common alleles to common diseases. The recently emerged hypothesis, the so called "rare variant-common disease hypothesis", implies that several rare variants in a gene may be involved in the causality of a common disease [14]. If this is the case, an association study (even one that is genome-wide with high-density genotyping of single nucleotide polymorphisms) may not be able to detect the disease gene because most of the SNPs in the database are common SNPs designed to map common alleles. Therefore, both family-based genetic linkage studies as well as association studies are required for the full understanding of the genetics of IA.

## Linkage analyses reveal chromosomal loci

Although the molecular basis of the disorder is not known, family studies strongly support genetic factors in the formation of IA [77]. Several studies of familial aneurysms have identified chromosomal loci showing suggestive evidence of linkage [56]. The mode of transmission for harboring an IA is not clear, and the genetics of the disorder appear to be complex, involving multiple loci and interaction of multiple genes [70]. In accordance with this, several genomewide scans and linkage studies have identified multiple chromosomal regions that may contain one or more susceptible genes. However, in some cases, results could not be replicated, even when examining patients of the same ethnic background [58, 70, 98, 99]. Onda *et al.* observed positive evidence of linkage on chromosome 5q22–31 (MLS 2.24), 7q11 (MLS 3.22) and 14q22 (MLS 2.31) with 104 affected sib-pairs. Yamada *et al.* observed positive evidence of linkage on chromosome 17cen (MLS 3.00), 19q13 (MLS 2.15) and Xp22 (MLS 2.16) with 29 extended families [98]. The inconsistency must be interpreted with caution. Discrepancies are possibly due to genetic heterogeneity and differences of patient cohorts (affected sib-pairs vs. extensive nuclear families). Further studies comprising larger sample sizes are undoubtedly needed, as multiple interacting genes and environmental factors contribute to the phenotype. Three regions that were confirmed in samples of patients of different ethnic origin are on chromosome 7q [19, 68, 70], 19q [19, 68, 98] and 14q [70, 72]. All regions were verified once using affected sib-pairs and once using extended pedigrees.

Alternatively, the rare Mendelian forms of disease might lead to the identification of genes or pathways that play a key role in the pathogenesis of the common form of the disease. Nahed *et al.* identified a large family of IA (six living patients and four deceased) showing autosomal dominant inheritance and detected a single locus with a LOD score of 4.2 at chromosome 1p34.3–36.13 [65]. Positional (candidate) cloning might be underway in the locus.

## Candidate gene association analyses: positional and functional

Association studies and the selection of target genes and sequence variants have often been limited to the investigation of candidate genes selected because of a priori hypotheses about their etiological role in a disease. These studies depended on the ability to predict functional candidate genes and polymorphisms [88]. Positional candidate genes can be selected from regions that have been identified by linkage analyses or genome wide scans [27, 28, 33].

More than 25 different candidate genes have been examined in case-control studies by different groups using the DNA of patients with different ethnic backgrounds. Selection of these genes were usually either of functional or positional nature. After identifying several susceptibility loci on different chromosomes, many **positional candidate genes** have been looked at that are located in the found regions. On the other hand, many of the examined **functional candidate genes** play a role in connective tissue formation, such as the collagen gene [100], the elastin gene [2], the matrix metalloproteinases and their tissue inhibitor genes [52, 53] and the endoglin gene [89]. Only a few have shown moderate positive association. Considering the genetic role in the formation of IAs, some of the examined candidate genes potentially possess both attributes of function and position (e.g., the elastin gene [2] which makes up part of the extracellular matrix of the vessel wall and is located in the linkage region of chromosome 7q11 found in a Japanese sibpair linkage study and replicated in a group of white patients in Utah). Detailed contemporary descriptions and tables of all examined candidate genes and chromosomal loci have been published in recent articles [56, 64, 79]. Conflicting results have been obtained, and no single gene has been consistently identified as a candidate gene. Possible reasons for these inconsistencies are false-positive studies, false-negative studies and differences between populations. Inadequate sample size is a major cause for false-positive and false-negative results [40]. Other causes include population stratification, misclassification (genotyping or phenotyping errors), and inappropriate statistical methods.

Variability in the association between different populations may be due to the frequency of disease-causing alleles, the pattern of association between disease causing alleles or interacting genetic or environmental factors. Therefore, failure to replicate does not necessarily mean lack of causality but possibly point to the need for additional studies [17]. As mentioned most of the association studies to date have focussed on single polymorphisms, but recently joint effects of single markers on a haplotype level have been examined [2]. Haplotypes are a set of markers that are physically close to each other on the DNA strand and are therefore inherited as a unit (a set of alleles in strong linkage disequilibrium (LD)). Association between a polymorphism and a trait, such as intracranial aneurysm, does not necessarily imply causality. Instead, the polymorphism/haplotype under investigation may be in LD with the causative sequence variant, requiring more detailed studies to identify the causative sequence alteration. Thus far, numerous association studies have been performed, some showing positive associations, some negative. But the majority of studies only examined small sample sizes and thus are mostly preliminary.

Many tested variants are single-nucleotide polymorphisms (SNPs) that change an amino acid and are therefore more likely to have a functional consequence. However, based on the successful positional cloning of disease genes for several common diseases, including schizophrenia [84], osteoporosis [87], myocardial infarction [33], ischemic stroke [28] and asthma [3], the most important variants are noncoding variants that affect the expression and/or efficiency of splicing. A large percentage of many organisms' total genome sizes is comprised of noncoding DNA. Some noncoding DNA is involved in regulating the activity of coding regions. However, much of this DNA has no known function and is sometimes referred to as "junk DNA". Recent evidence suggests that "junk DNA" may in fact be employed by proteins created from coding DNA [6].

## Gene expression microarray analyses

One of the newer genetic research techniques is the microarray which allows examination of several thousand genes at once. Although its deployment is related to substantial costs, its efficiency can hardly be beaten. No other methodological approach has transformed molecular biology more in recent years than the use of microarrays. Microarray technology has led the way from studies of the individual biological functions of a few related genes, proteins or, at best, pathways towards more global investigations of cellular activity. The development of this technology immediately yielded new and interesting information, and has produced more data than can be currently dealt with. To many, the term microarray analysis is equivalent to transcript analysis. Although transcriptional profiling is unquestionably the most widely used application at present, it might become less important in future because it focuses on a biological intermediate. Currently a whole battery of sophisticated applications for this technology are being developed, e.g. for epigenetic studies, expanding RNA studies and probing with genomic sequences [35].

Concerning intracranial aneurysms there are several studies with this technique that are being completed worldwide. Analysis of the results of those genes differentially expressed within IA tissue will again shift focus towards hitherto unexamined targets.

## Application of genetic findings to novel diagnostic tests and future therapies

Nowadays, there is a wide array of over-the-counter commercially available tests which, for example, lets users find out whether they are prone to develop cardiovascular disease or are the carriers of Factor V Leiden, a single mutation that raises the risk for thrombophilia, or abnormal blood clotting. The results of these kinds of tests have to be interpreted with caution, as in some cases they could lead to false behaviour after negative results [16, 97]. Nevertheless, with increasing availability of such non-invasive diagnostic procedures, a wider spectrum of people can be screened at a relative cost-efficient basis, which in turn, in the case of intracranial aneurysms, could lead to timely prophylactic measures.

An early diagnosis through a genetic test, such as available for BRCA [4], could potentially spare patients from needless dangerous invasive diagnostic procedures or treatment. Furthermore, a precise diagnosis of an underlying genetic component could permit rational family counseling. Genetic markers showing an increased risk of rupture in patients harboring intracranial aneurysms that are of a smaller size (<7 mm) could facilitate the decision for immediate treatment. Genes, such as the above mentioned eNOS, could be possible candidates. Such kinds of genetic tests could easily be performed during a visit to the outpatient clinic during which a simple blood withdrawal for the extraction of DNA could take place.

Although a few publications have reported on ultrastructural findings of skin biopsies possibly being able to indicate the risk of developing an intracranial aneurysm this hypothesis has not been further substantiated. Mostly these findings were linked to connective tissue disease such as Ehlers Danlos Syndrome Type IV [29, 46, 55, 59, 93].

The goal of gene therapy is either to introduce a gene that is deficient in patients, to overexpress a therapeutic gene, or to silence a gene that is detrimental. Several studies have reported the feasibility of transferring genes to blood vessels to alter vascular function [10]. An alternative is to transfer the genes to the liver or the skeletal muscle so that the released protein from the transgene binds to blood vessels to alter vascular function [32]. The gene transfer, either direct or indirect by vector, is achieved with DNA or RNA. The transgene then expresses RNA or a protein.

Naked DNA, for direct transfection, is the safest approach but inefficient for transduction of cells and tissues [11]. Several recombinant viruses are used as vectors: Adenoviruses are efficient but the transfection period is short, as the viruses also induce an inflammatory response. Retroviruses provide long-term expression but may lead to insertional mutagenesis. Leukemia has been induced in children during retroviral transfer. Adeno-associated viruses provide long-term expression without inflammation, however it is difficult to produce large amounts of recombinant viruses [23]. So widespread use of gene therapy is being held back by the fact that a safe and efficient vector for delivery of genes has not been developed yet [32]. Cerebrovascular diseases have been the target of experimental gene therapy in animal models. Such as cerebral vasospasm, chronic cerebral ischaemia with poor collateral circulation and restenosis of the extracranial artery.

Although lately drug eluting stents have been strongly criticized for a possible increase of restenosis after deployment [5], they or coils may be an effective method of administering genetically engineered treatment to the site of an intracranial aneurysm. For this kind of topically administered gene therapy, newer developments such as endovascular devices carrying vectors [74] and techniques of delivering genetically modified autologous fibroblasts are being pursued [61, 74].

A further approach and challenge is the direct administration of vectors into the carotid artery which unfortunately still requires an interruption of the blood flow for 10–30 min so that the virus can infect the endothelium [94]. Further techniques being studied are perivascular approaches, e.g., by administering adenoviral vectors into the CSF [7, 71] and by paintbrush technique [48]. An intravenous application could lead to the entrapment of the virus in the liver [34] where a secretable protein could then be released into the circulation. Similarly subcutaneous/intramuscular injections could deploy the same mechanism [9, 73].

Even though intracranial aneurysms may be considered as an irreversible process possibly genetic therapy can lead to a regression. A recent publication of an abdominal aortic aneurysm (AAA) mouse model has shown that an intraperitoneal application of a JNK inhibitor led to the regression of the aneurysm's diameter. In the case of AAA the diseased aorta seems to have the potential to regress if exacerbating factors are eliminated and/or the tissue repair is reinforced [102].

## Conclusion and proposals for the future

Several reports have substantiated the fact that intracranial aneurysms and their rupture are associated with a strong genetic component. Overall, the results point to a multigenic disease in which environmental factors interact in the etiology.

It will be necessary to perform multicenter studies to 1) substantially increase the number of affected patients, 2) substratisfy the different regions and ethnicities of the patients and 3) to approach the genetic research from several angles. Positive results in candidate gene association studies as well as positive linkage regions need to be compared among cohorts of different ethnicity. The publications so far have shown the different influence in different countries. With the advent of ever increasing sophistication of computational analyses programs gene-gene interaction and gene-environment action will be scrutinized, leading to possible novel therapeutic approaches.

## References

1. Akagawa H, Narita A, Yamada H, Tajima A, Krischek B, Kasuya H, Hori T, Kubota M, Saeki N, Hata A, Mizutani T, Inoue I (2007) Systematic screening of lysyl oxidase-like (LOXL) family genes demonstrates that LOXL2 is a susceptibility gene to intracranial aneurysms. Hum Genet 121(3–4): 377–387
2. Akagawa H, Tajima A, Sakamoto Y, Krischek B, Yoneyama T, Kasuya H, Onda H, Hori T, Kubota M, Machida T, Saeki N, Hata A, Hashiguchi K, Kimura E, Kim CJ, Yang TK, Lee JY, Kimm K, Inoue I (2006) A haplotype spanning two genes, ELN and LIMK1, decreases their transcripts and confers susceptibility to intracranial aneurysms. Hum Mol Genet 15: 1722–1734
3. Allen M, Heinzmann A, Noguchi E, Abecasis G, Broxholme J, Ponting CP, Bhattacharyya S, Tinsley J, Zhang Y, Holt R, Jones EY, Lench N, Carey A, Jones H, Dickens NJ, Dimon C, Nicholls R, Baker C, Xue L, Townsend E, Kabesch M, Weiland SK, Carr D, von Mutius E, Adcock IM, Barnes PJ, Lathrop GM, Edwards M, Moffatt MF, Cookson WO (2003) Positional cloning of a novel gene influencing asthma from chromosome 2q14. Nat Genet 35: 258–263
4. Armstrong K, Eisen A, Weber B (2000) Assessing the risk of breast cancer. N Engl J Med 342: 564–571
5. Camenzind E, Steg PG, Wijns W (2007) Stent thrombosis late after implantation of first-generation drug-eluting stents: a cause for concern. Circulation 115: 1440–1455
6. Castillo-Davis CI (2005) The evolution of noncoding DNA: how much junk, how much func? Trends Genet 21: 533–536
7. Chen AF, Jiang SW, Crotty TB, Tsutsui M, Smith LA, O'Brien T, Katusic ZS (1997) Effects of in vivo adventitial expression of recombinant endothelial nitric oxide synthase gene in cerebral arteries. Proc Natl Acad Sci USA 94: 12568–12573
8. Chen Y, Pawlikowska L, Yao JS, Shen F, Zhai W, Achrol AS, Lawton MT, Kwok PY, Yang GY, Young WL (2006) Interleukin-6 involvement in brain arteriovenous malformations. Ann Neurol 59: 72–80
9. Chu Y, Iida S, Lund DD, Weiss RM, DiBona GF, Watanabe Y, Faraci FM, Heistad DD (2003) Gene transfer of extracellular superoxide dismutase reduces arterial pressure in spontaneously hypertensive rats: role of heparin-binding domain. Circ Res 92: 461–468
10. Chu Y, Miller JD, Heistad DD (2007) Gene therapy for stroke: 2006 overview. Curr Hypertens Rep 9: 19–24
11. Chu Y, Weintraub N, Heistad DD (2005) Gene therapy and cardiovascular diseases. In: Runge M, Patterson C (eds) Principles of molecular cardiology. Humana Press, Totowa, New Jersey
12. Chyatte D, Bruno G, Desai S, Todor DR (1999) Inflammation and intracranial aneurysms. Neurosurgery 45: 1137–1146
13. Chyatte D, Reilly J, Tilson MD (1990) Morphometric analysis of reticular and elastin fibers in the cerebral arteries of patients with intracranial aneurysms. Neurosurgery 26: 939–943
14. Cohen JC, Kiss RS, Pertsemlidis A, Marcel YL, McPherson R, Hobbs HH (2004) Multiple rare alleles contribute to low plasma levels of HDL cholesterol. Science 305: 869–872
15. Crompton MR (1966) The comparative pathology of cerebral aneurysms. Brain 89: 789–796
16. De Francesco L (2006) Genetic profiteering. Nat Biotechnol 24: 888–890

17. Dichgans M, Markus HS (2005) Genetic association studies in stroke: methodological issues and proposed standard criteria. Stroke 36: 2027–2031
18. Ellegala DB, Day AL (2005) Ruptured cerebral aneurysms. N Engl J Med 352: 121–124
19. Farnham JM, Camp NJ, Neuhausen SL, Tsuruda J, Parker D, MacDonald J, Cannon-Albright LA (2004) Confirmation of chromosome 7q11 locus for predisposition to intracranial aneurysm. Hum Genet 114: 250–255
20. Feigin VL, Rinkel GJ, Lawes CM, Algra A, Bennett DA, van Gijn J, Anderson CS (2005) Risk factors for subarachnoid hemorrhage: an updated systematic review of epidemiological studies. Stroke 36: 2773–2780
21. Fernandez-Lopez A, Garrido-Martin EM, Sanz-Rodriguez F, Pericacho M, Rodriguez-Barbero A, Eleno N, Lopez-Novoa JM, Duwell A, Vega MA, Bernabeu C, Botella LM (2007) Gene expression fingerprinting for human hereditary hemorrhagic telangiectasia. Hum Mol Gen 16: 1515–1533
22. Finlay HM, Whittaker P, Canham PB (1998) Collagen organization in the branching region of human brain arteries. Stroke 29: 1595–1601
23. Flotte TR, Carter BJ (1995) Adeno-associated virus vectors for gene therapy. Gene Ther 2: 357–362
24. Frosch M, Anthony D, De Girolami U (2004) The central nervous system. In: Kumar V, Fausto N, Abbas A (eds) Robbins & Cotran pathologic basis of disease. Elsevier Saunders, Philadelphia
25. Frosen J, Piippo A, Paetau A, Kangasniemi M, Niemela M, Hernesniemi J, Jaaskelainen J (2004) Remodeling of saccular cerebral artery aneurysm wall is associated with rupture: histological analysis of 24 unruptured and 42 ruptured cases. Stroke 35: 2287–2293
26. Greenberg M (2000) SAH and aneurysms. In: Greenberg M (ed) Handbook of neurosurgery. Thieme Medical, New York
27. Gretarsdottir S, Sveinbjornsdottir S, Jonsson HH, Jakobsson F, Einarsdottir E, Agnarsson U, Shkolny D, Einarsson G, Gudjonsdottir HM, Valdimarsson EM, Einarsson OB, Thorgeirsson G, Hadzic R, Jonsdottir S, Reynisdottir ST, Bjarnadottir SM, Gudmundsdottir T, Gudlaugsdottir GJ, Gill R, Lindpaintner K, Sainz J, Hannesson HH, Sigurdsson GT, Frigge ML, Kong A, Gudnason V, Stefansson K, Gulcher JR (2002) Localization of a susceptibility gene for common forms of stroke to 5q12. Am J Hum Genet 70: 593–603
28. Gretarsdottir S, Thorleifsson G, Reynisdottir ST, Manolescu A, Jonsdottir S, Jonsdottir T, Gudmundsdottir T, Bjarnadottir SM, Einarsson OB, Gudjonsdottir HM, Hawkins M, Gudmundsson G, Gudmundsdottir H, Andrason H, Gudmundsdottir AS, Sigurdardottir M, Chou TT, Nahmias J, Goss S, Sveinbjornsdottir S, Valdimarsson EM, Jakobsson F, Agnarsson U, Gudnason V, Thorgeirsson G, Fingerle J, Gurney M, Gudbjartsson D, Frigge ML, Kong A, Stefansson K, Gulcher JR (2003) The gene encoding phosphodiesterase 4D confers risk of ischemic stroke. Nat Genet 35: 131–138
29. Grond-Ginsbach C, Schnippering H, Hausser I, Weber R, Werner I, Steiner HH, Luttgen N, Busse O, Grau A, Brandt T (2002) Ultrastructural connective tissue aberrations in patients with intracranial aneurysms. Stroke 33: 2192–2196
30. Gunel M, Awad IA, Anson J, Lifton RP (1995) Mapping a gene causing cerebral cavernous malformation to 7q11.2-q21. Proc Natl Acad Sci USA 92: 6620–6624
31. Harrod CG, Batjer HH, Bendok BR (2005) Deficiencies in estrogen-mediated regulation of cerebrovascular homeostasis may contribute to an increased risk of cerebral aneurysm

pathogenesis and rupture in menopausal and postmenopausal women. Med Hypotheses 66: 736–756
32. Heistad DD (2006) Gene therapy for vascular disease. Vascul Pharmacol 45: 331–333
33. Helgadottir A, Manolescu A, Thorleifsson G, Gretarsdottir S, Jonsdottir H, Thorsteinsdottir U, Samani NJ, Gudmundsson G, Grant SF, Thorgeirsson G, Sveinbjornsdottir S, Valdimarsson EM, Matthiasson SE, Johannsson H, Gudmundsdottir O, Gurney ME, Sainz J, Thorhallsdottir M, Andresdottir M, Frigge ML, Topol EJ, Kong A, Gudnason V, Hakonarson H, Gulcher JR, Stefansson K (2004) The gene encoding 5-lipoxygenase activating protein confers risk of myocardial infarction and stroke. Nat Genet 36: 233–239
34. Herz J, Gerard RD (1993) Adenovirus-mediated transfer of low density lipoprotein receptor gene acutely accelerates cholesterol clearance in normal mice. Proc Natl Acad Sci USA 90: 2812–2816
35. Hoheisel JD (2006) Microarray technology: beyond transcript profiling and genotype analysis. Nat Rev 7: 200–210
36. Inagawa T, Ishikawa S, Aoki H, Takahashi M, Yoshimoto H (1988) Aneurysmal subarachnoid hemorrhage in Izumo City and Shimane Prefecture of Japan. Incidence. Stroke 19: 170–175
37. Inci S, Spetzler RF (2000) Intracranial aneurysms and arterial hypertension: a review and hypothesis. Surg Neurol 53: 530–540
38. Ingall T, Asplund K, Mahonen M, Bonita R (2000) A multinational comparison of subarachnoid hemorrhage epidemiology in the WHO MONICA stroke study. Stroke 31: 1054–1061
39. Ingall TJ, Whisnant JP, Wiebers DO, O'Fallon WM (1989) Has there been a decline in subarachnoid hemorrhage mortality? Stroke 20: 718–724
40. Ioannidis JP, Ntzani EE, Trikalinos TA, Contopoulos-Ioannidis DG (2001) Replication validity of genetic association studies. Nat Genet 29: 306–309
41. Iwamoto H, Kiyohara Y, Fujishima M, Kato I, Nakayama K, Sueishi K, Tsuneyoshi M (1999) Prevalence of intracranial saccular aneurysms in a Japanese community based on a consecutive autopsy series during a 30-year observation period. The Hisayama study. Stroke 30: 1390–1395
42. Jamous MA, Nagahiro S, Kitazato KT, Satomi J, Satoh K (2005a) Role of estrogen deficiency in the formation and progression of cerebral aneurysms. Part I: experimental study of the effect of oophorectomy in rats. J Neurosurg 103: 1046–1051
43. Jamous MA, Nagahiro S, Kitazato KT, Tamura T, Kuwayama K, Satoh K (2005b) Role of estrogen deficiency in the formation and progression of cerebral aneurysms. Part II: experimental study of the effects of hormone replacement therapy in rats. J Neurosurg 103: 1052–1057
44. Juvela S (2002) Natural history of unruptured intracranial aneurysms: risks for aneurysm formation, growth, and rupture. Acta Neurochir Suppl 82: 27–30
45. Kataoka K, Taneda M, Asai T, Kinoshita A, Ito M, Kuroda R (1999) Structural fragility and inflammatory response of ruptured cerebral aneurysms. A comparative study between ruptured and unruptured cerebral aneurysms. Stroke 30: 1396–1401
46. Kato T, Hattori H, Yorifuji T, Tashiro Y, Nakahata T (2001) Intracranial aneurysms in Ehlers-Danlos syndrome type IV in early childhood. Pediatr Neurol 25: 336–339
47. Khurana VG, Meissner I, Sohni YR, Bamlet WR, McClelland RL, Cunningham JM, Meyer FB (2005) The presence of tandem endothelial nitric oxide synthase gene polymorphisms identifying brain aneurysms more prone to rupture. J Neurosurg 102: 526–531

48. Khurana VG, Weiler DA, Witt TA, Smith LA, Kleppe LS, Parisi JE, Simari RD, O'Brien T, Russell SJ, Katusic ZS (2003) A direct mechanical method for accurate and efficient adenoviral vector delivery to tissues. Gene Ther 10: 443–452
49. Kim DH, Van Ginhoven G, Milewicz DM (2005) Familial aggregation of both aortic and cerebral aneurysms: evidence for a common genetic basis in a subset of families. Neurosurgery 56: 655–661
50. Kiyohara Y, Ueda K, Hasuo Y, Wada J, Kawano H, Kato I, Sinkawa A, Ohmura T, Iwamoto H, Omae T, *et al.* (1989) Incidence and prognosis of subarachnoid hemorrhage in a Japanese rural community. Stroke 20: 1150–1155
51. Kosierkiewicz TA, Factor SM, Dickson DW (1994) Immunocytochemical studies of atherosclerotic lesions of cerebral berry aneurysms. J Neuropathol Exp Neurol 53: 399–406
52. Krex D, Kotteck K, Konig IR, Ziegler A, Schackert HK, Schackert G (2004) Matrix metalloproteinase-9 coding sequence single-nucleotide polymorphisms in caucasians with intracranial aneurysms. Neurosurgery 55: 207–212
53. Krex D, Rohl H, Konig IR, Ziegler A, Schackert HK, Schackert G (2003) Tissue inhibitor of metalloproteinases-1, -2, and -3 polymorphisms in a white population with intracranial aneurysms. Stroke 34: 2817–2821
54. Krex D, Ziegler A, Schackert HK, Schackert G (2001) Lack of association between endoglin intron 7 insertion polymorphism and intracranial aneurysms in a white population: evidence of racial/ethnic differences. Stroke 32: 2689–2694
55. Krischek B, Inoue I, Kasuya H (2005) Response to letter: collagen morphology is not associated with the Ala549Pro polymorphism of the COL1A2 gene. Stroke 36: 2068–2955
56. Krischek B, Inoue I (2006a) The genetics of intracranial aneurysms. J Hum Genet 51: 587–594
57. Krischek B, Kasuya H, Akagawa H, Tajima A, Narita A, Onda H, Hori T, Inoue I (2006b) Using endothelial nitric oxide synthase gene polymorphisms to identify intracranial aneurysms more prone to rupture in Japanese patients. J Neurosurg 105: 717–722
58. Krischek B, Narita A, Akagawa H, Kasuya H, Tajima A, Onda H, Yoneyama T, Hori T, Inoue I (2006c) Is there any evidence for linkage on chromosome 17cen in affected Japanese sib-pairs with an intracranial aneurysm? J Hum Genet 51: 491–494
59. Kuivaniemi H, Prockop DJ, Wu Y, Madhatheri SL, Kleinert C, Earley JJ, Jokinen A, Stolle C, Majamaa K, Myllyla VV, Norrgard O, Schievink WI, Mokri B, Fukawa O, ter Berg JWM, De Paepe A, Lozano AM, Leblanc R, Ryynanen M, Baxter BT, Shikata H, Ferrell RE, Tromp G (1993) Exclusion of mutations in the gene for type III collagen (COL3A1) as a common cause of intracranial aneurysms or cervical artery dissections: results from sequence analysis of the coding sequences of type III collagen from 55 unrelated patients. Neurology 43: 2652–2658
60. Labauge P, Denier C, Bergametti F, Tournier-Lasserve E (2007) Genetics of cavernous angiomas. Lancet Neurol 6: 237–244
61. Mazighi M, Tchetche D, Goueffic Y, San Juan A, Louedec L, Henin D, Michel JB, Jacob MP, Feldman LJ (2006) Percutaneous transplantation of genetically-modified autologous fibroblasts in the rabbit femoral artery: a novel approach for cardiovascular gene therapy. J Vasc Surg 44: 1067–1075
62. Meschia JF, Brott TG, Brown RD Jr (2005) Genetics of cerebrovascular disorders. Mayo Clin Proc 80: 122–132

63. Morita A, Fujiwara S, Hashi K, Ohtsu H, Kirino T (2005) Risk of rupture associated with intact cerebral aneurysms in the Japanese population: a systematic review of the literature from Japan. J Neurosurg 102: 601–606
64. Nahed BV, Bydon M, Ozturk AK, Bilguvar K, Bayrakli F, Gunel M (2007) Genetics of intracranial aneurysms. Neurosurgery 60: 213–225
65. Nahed BV, Seker A, Guclu B, Ozturk AK, Finberg K, Hawkins AA, DiLuna ML, State M, Lifton RP, Gunel M (2005) Mapping a Mendelian form of intracranial aneurysm to 1p34.3-p36.13. Am J Hum Genet 76: 172–179
66. Nanba R, Kuroda S, Tada M, Ishikawa T, Houkin K, Iwasaki Y (2006) Clinical features of familial moyamoya disease. Childs Nerv Syst 22: 258–262
67. NY Cp (2006) The abdominal aortic aneurysm. Genetics, pathophysiology, and molecular biology. Proceedings of a conference. April 3–5, 2006. New York, USA. Ann NY Acad Sci 1085: 1–408
68. Olson JM, Vongpunsawad S, Kuivaniemi H, Ronkainen A, Hernesniemi J, Ryynanen M, Kim LL, Tromp G (2002) Search for intracranial aneurysm susceptibility gene(s) using Finnish families. BMC Med Genet 3: 7
69. Onda H, Kasuya H, Yoneyama T, Hori T, Nakajima T, Inoue I (2003) Endoglin is not a major susceptibility gene for intracranial aneurysm among Japanese. Stroke 34: 1640–1644
70. Onda H, Kasuya H, Yoneyama T, Takakura K, Hori T, Takeda J, Nakajima T, Inoue I (2001) Genomewide-linkage and haplotype-association studies map intracranial aneurysm to chromosome 7q11. Am J Hum Genet 69: 804–819
71. Ooboshi H, Welsh MJ, Rios CD, Davidson BL, Heistad DD (1995) Adenovirus-mediated gene transfer in vivo to cerebral blood vessels and perivascular tissue. Circ Res 77: 7–13
72. Ozturk AK, Nahed BV, Bydon M, Bilguvar K, Goksu E, Bademci G, Guclu B, Johnson MH, Amar A, Lifton RP, Gunel M (2006) Molecular genetic analysis of two large kindreds with intracranial aneurysms demonstrates linkage to 11q24-25 and 14q23-31. Stroke 37: 1021–1027
73. Pradat PF, Kennel P, Naimi-Sadaoui S, Finiels F, Orsini C, Revah F, Delaere P, Mallet J (2001) Continuous delivery of neurotrophin 3 by gene therapy has a neuroprotective effect in experimental models of diabetic and acrylamide neuropathies. Hum Gene Ther 12: 2237–2249
74. Ribourtout E, Raymond J (2004) Gene therapy and endovascular treatment of intracranial aneurysms. Stroke 35: 786–793
75. Richling B (2006) History of endovascular surgery: personal accounts of the evolution. Neurosurgery 59: S30–S38
76. Rinkel GJ, Djibuti M, Algra A, van Gijn J (1998) Prevalence and risk of rupture of intracranial aneurysms: a systematic review. Stroke 29: 251–256
77. Ronkainen A, Hernesniemi J, Puranen M, Niemitukia L, Vanninen R, Ryynanen M, Kuivaniemi H, Tromp G (1997) Familial intracranial aneurysms. Lancet 349: 380–384
78. Ross M, Pawlina W (2006) Histology: text & atlas. Lippincott Williams & Wilkins, Baltimore
79. Ruigrok YM, Rinkel GJ, Wijmenga C (2005) Genetics of intracranial aneurysms. Lancet Neurol 4: 179–189
80. Schievink WI, Michels VV, Piepgras DG (1994) Neurovascular manifestations of heritable connective tissue disorders. A review. Stroke 25: 889–903

81. Schievink WI, Schaid DJ, Michels VV, Piepgras DG (1995) Familial aneurysmal subarachnoid hemorrhage: a community-based study. J Neurosurg 83: 426–429
82. Simon M, Franke D, Ludwig M, Aliashkevich AF, Koster G, Oldenburg J, Bostrom A, Ziegler A, Schramm J (2006) Association of a polymorphism of the ACVRL1 gene with sporadic arteriovenous malformations of the central nervous system. J Neurosurg 104: 945–949
83. Stapf C, Mohr J (2004) Aneurysms and subarachnoid hemorrhage – epidemiology. In: Le Roux P, Winn H, Newell D (eds) Management of cerebral aneurysms. Saunders, Philadelphia
84. Stefansson H, Sigurdsson E, Steinthorsdottir V, Bjornsdottir S, Sigmundsson T, Ghosh S, Brynjolfsson J, Gunnarsdottir S, Ivarsson O, Chou TT, Hjaltason O, Birgisdottir B, Jonsson H, Gudnadottir VG, Gudmundsdottir E, Bjornsson A, Ingvarsson B, Ingason A, Sigfusson S, Hardardottir H, Harvey RP, Lai D, Zhou M, Brunner D, Mutel V, Gonzalo A, Lemke G, Sainz J, Johannesson G, Andresson T, Gudbjartsson D, Manolescu A, Frigge ML, Gurney ME, Kong A, Gulcher JR, Petursson H, Stefansson K (2002) Neuregulin 1 and susceptibility to schizophrenia. Am J Hum Genet 71: 877–892
85. Stehbens WE (1989) Etiology of intracranial berry aneurysms. J Neurosurg 70: 823–831
86. Stehbens WE (1999) Relationship of cerebral aneurysms and medial raphes. Surg Neurol 52: 536–538
87. Styrkarsdottir U, Cazier JB, Kong A, Rolfsson O, Larsen H, Bjarnadottir E, Johannsdottir VD, Sigurdardottir MS, Bagger Y, Christiansen C, Reynisdottir I, Grant SF, Jonasson K, Frigge ML, Gulcher JR, Sigurdsson G, Stefansson K (2003) Linkage of osteoporosis to chromosome 20p12 and association to BMP2. PLoS Biol 1: E69
88. Tabor HK, Risch NJ, Myers RM (2002) Candidate-gene approaches for studying complex genetic traits: practical considerations. Nat Rev 3: 391–397
89. Takenaka K, Sakai H, Yamakawa H, Yoshimura S, Kumagai M, Nakashima S, Nozawa Y, Sakai N (1999) Polymorphism of the endoglin gene in patients with intracranial saccular aneurysms. J Neurosurg 90: 935–938
90. Tanaka H, Ueda Y, Date C, Baba T, Yamashita H, Hayashi M, Shoji H, Owada K, Baba KI, Shibuya M, Kon T, Detels R (1981) Incidence of stroke in Shibata, Japan: 1976–1978. Stroke 12: 460–466
91. Tournier-Lasserve E, Joutel A, Melki J, Weissenbach J, Lathrop GM, Chabriat H, Mas JL, Cabanis EA, Baudrimont M, Maciazek J, Bach MA, Bousser MG (1993) Cerebral autosomal dominant arteriopathy with subcortical infarcts and leukoencephalopathy maps to chromosome 19q12. Nat Genet 3: 256–259
92. Tulamo R, Frosen J, Junnikkala S, Paetau A, Pitkaniemi J, Kangasniemi M, Niemela M, Jaaskelainen J, Jokitalo E, Karatas A, Hernesniemi J, Meri S (2006) Complement activation associates with saccular cerebral artery aneurysm wall degeneration and rupture. Neurosurgery 59: 1069–1076
93. van den Berg JS, Pals G, Arwert F, Hennekam RC, Albrecht KW, Westerveld A, Limburg M (1999) Type III collagen deficiency in saccular intracranial aneurysms. Defect in gene regulation? Stroke 30: 1628–1631
94. von der Leyen HE, Gibbons GH, Morishita R, Lewis NP, Zhang L, Nakajima M, Kaneda Y, Cooke JP, Dzau VJ (1995) Gene therapy inhibiting neointimal vascular lesion: in vivo transfer of endothelial cell nitric oxide synthase gene. Proc Natl Acad Sci USA 92: 1137–1141

95. Wermer MJ, van der Schaaf IC, Algra A, Rinkel GJ (2007) Risk of rupture of unruptured intracranial aneurysms in relation to patient and aneurysm characteristics. An updated meta-analysis. Stroke 38: 1404–1410
96. Winn HR, Jane JA Sr, Taylor J, Kaiser D, Britz GW (2002) Prevalence of asymptomatic incidental aneurysms: review of 4568 arteriograms. J Neurosurg 96: 43–49
97. Wolfberg AJ (2006) Genes on the Web – direct-to-consumer marketing of genetic testing. N Engl J Med 355: 543–545
98. Yamada S, Utsunomiya M, Inoue K, Nozaki K, Inoue S, Takenaka K, Hashimoto N, Koizumi A (2004) Genome-wide scan for Japanese familial intracranial aneurysms: linkage to several chromosomal regions. Circulation 110: 3727–3733
99. Yamada S, Utsunomiya M, Inoue K, Nozaki K, Miyamoto S, Hashimoto N, Takenaka K, Yoshinaga T, Koizumi A (2003) Absence of linkage of familial intracranial aneurysms to 7q11 in highly aggregated Japanese families. Stroke 34: 892–900
100. Yoneyama T, Kasuya H, Onda H, Akagawa H, Hashiguchi K, Nakajima T, Hori T, Inoue I (2004) Collagen type I alpha2 (COL1A2) is the susceptible gene for intracranial aneurysms. Stroke 35: 443–448
101. Yoshimoto T, Mizoi K (1997) Importance of management of unruptured cerebral aneurysms. Surg Neurol 47: 522–525
102. Yoshimura K, Aoki H, Ikeda Y, Fujii K, Akiyama N, Furutani A, Hoshii Y, Tanaka N, Ricci R, Ishihara T, Esato K, Hamano K, Matsuzaki M (2005) Regression of abdominal aortic aneurysm by inhibition of c-Jun N-terminal kinase. Nat Med 11: 1330–1338

# Technical standards

# Extended endoscopic endonasal approach to the midline skull base: the evolving role of transsphenoidal surgery

P. Cappabianca, L. M. Cavallo, F. Esposito, O. de Divitiis, A. Messina, and E. de Divitiis

Division of Neurosurgery, Department of Neurological Sciences,
Università degli Studi di Napoli Federico II, Naples, Italy

With 30 Figures

## Contents

## Abstract

The evolution of the endoscopic endonasal transsphenoidal technique, which was initially reserved only for sellar lesions through the sphenoid sinus cavity, has lead in the last decades to a progressive possibility to access the skull base from the nose. This route allows midline access and visibility to the suprasellar, retrosellar and parasellar space while obviating brain retraction, and makes possible to treat transsphenoidally a variety of relatively small midline skull base and parasellar lesions traditionally approached transcranially.

We report our current knowledge of the endoscopic anatomy of the midline skull base as seen from the endonasal perspective, in order to describe the surgical path and structures whose knowledge is useful during the operation. Besides, we describe the step-by-step surgical technique to access the different compartments, the "dangerous landmarks" to avoid in order to minimize the risks of complications and how to manage them, and our paradigm and techniques for dural and bony reconstruction. Furthermore, we report a brief description of the useful instruments and tools for the extended endoscopic approaches.

Between January 2004 and April 2006 we performed 33 extended endonasal approaches for lesions arising from or involving the sellar region and the surrounding areas. The most representative pathologies of this series were the ten craniopharyngiomas, the six giant adenomas and the five meningiomas; we also used this procedure in three cases of chordomas, three of Rathke's cleft cysts and three of meningo-encephaloceles, one case of optic nerve glioma, one olfactory groove neuroendocrine tumor and one case of fibro-osseous dysplasia.

Tumor removal, as assessed by post-operative MRI, revealed complete removal of the lesion in 2/6 pituitary adenomas, 7/10 craniopharyngiomas, 4/5 meningiomas, 3/3 Rathke's cleft cyst, 3/3 meningo-encephalocele.

Surgical complications have been observed in 3 patients, two with a craniopharyngioma, one with a clival meningioma and one with a recurrent giant pituitary macroadenoma involving the entire left cavernous sinus, who developed a CSF leak and a second operation was necessary in order to review the cranial base reconstruction and seal the leak. One of them developed a bacterial meningitis, which resolved after a cycle of intravenous antibiotic therapy with no permanent neurological deficits. One patient with an intra-suprasellar non-functioning adenoma presented with a generalized epileptic seizure a few hours after the surgical procedure, due to the intraoperative massive CSF loss and consequent presence of intracranial air. We registered one surgical mortality.

In three cases of craniopharyngioma and in one case of meningioma a new permanent diabetes insipidus was observed. One patient developed a sphenoid sinus mycosis, cured with antimycotic therapy. Epistaxis and airway difficulties were never observed.

It is difficult today to define the boundaries and the future limits of the extended approaches because the work is still in progress. Such extended endoscopic approaches, although at a first glance might be considered something that everyone can do, require an advanced and specialized training.

*Keywords:* Endoscope; transsphenoidal surgery; extended approach; anatomy; surgical technique; skull base.

## Introduction

The base of the skull is amongst the most fascinating and complex anatomical areas, either from the anatomical and surgical perspectives. It can be involved in a variety of lesions, either neoplastic or not and the successful treatment of such pathologies may be extremely difficult to achieve, without paying an high cost in terms of invasiveness, morbidity and mortality, specially for those lesions located in the midline. For most of the lesions of the skull base area, a variety of innovative skull base cranio-facial approaches including anterior, antero-lateral and and postero-lateral routes, have been developed [1, 27, 28, 53, 62–64, 68, 69, 76, 77, 79, 92, 98, 100, 109, 113, 115, 124, 127, 130, 134, 136, 146]. Most large tumors often require combinations of multiple approaches or staged operations, with extensive bone and tissue disruption, which can be aesthetically disfiguring, and a certain degree of neurovascular manipulation, with obvious repercussions on the perioperative morbidity and/or mortality rates, is a prerequisite step of the surgical action.

The evolution of surgical techniques has lead in the last decades to a progressive reduction of the invasiveness of these approaches, namely through the transcranial routes, but the possibility to access the skull base from the nose was initially reserved only for sellar lesions through the sphenoid sinus cavity. It was Weiss in 1987 [149] that termed and originally described the **extended transsphenoidal approach**, intending a transsphenoidal approach with removal of additional bone along the tuberculum sellae and the posterior planum sphenoidale between the optic canals, with subsequent opening of the dura mater above the diaphragma sellae. This route allows midline access and visibility to the suprasellar space while obviating brain retraction, and makes possible to treat transsphenoidally small midline suprasellar lesions traditionally approached transcranially, namely tuberculum sellae meningiomas and craniopharyngiomas. Initially, such operations were done with microsurgical technique [91, 97, 110, 149].

Perhaps, it has been the fundamental contribute brought by the endoscope in transsphenoidal surgery, together with the progress in diagnostic imaging techniques and the intraoperative neuronavigation systems, that have boosted the development of the extension of the transsphenoidal approach to the entire midline skull base. Furthermore, because of the increased visualization offered by the endoscope, a variety of modifications of the standard transsphenoidal approach have been described, which have created new surgical routes targeted for the extrasellar compartment from the anterior cranial base to the craniocervical junction [2, 3, 16, 17, 25, 31, 33, 38, 40, 41, 43, 45, 48, 54, 56, 58, 85, 86, 88, 91, 97, 106] As a matter of facts, endoscopy has caused a renewal of the interest for anatomic studies, which are essential to the comprehension of the approach itself, and has contributed to the more contemporary knowledge of the possibilities of the transsphenoidal approach also on clinical settings [3, 14, 25, 33, 40, 41, 78, 80, 82–84, 102, 107, 121, 122, 133, 140].

Such considerations give an idea of the extended endoscopic endonasal route as a versatile approach [40] that offers the possibility to expose the entire midline skull base from below, with the possibility to pass through a less noble structure (nasal cavity) in order to reach a more noble one (the brain with its neurovascular structures). Indeed, cases of suprasellar, retroclival, and intracavernous lesions treated by means of the transsphenoidal technique, either fully endoscopic or endo-microscopically assisted procedures are now routinely done in Centers dedicated to such type of surgery.

## Endoscopic anatomy of the midline skull base: the endonasal perspective

According to the surgical view, the anatomy of the midline skull base can be divided in three areas:

1) the midline anterior skull base: from the frontal sinus to the posterior ethmoidal artery;
2) the middle skull base: the sphenoid sinus cavity;
3) the posterior skull base: from the dorsum sellae to the cranio-vertebral junction.

### *The anterior skull base: from the frontal sinus to the posterior ethmoidal artery*

From the endonasal point of view the midline anterior skull base corresponds to the roof of the nasal cavities. After the removal of the anterior and posterior ethmoid cells and of the superior part of the septum (lamina perpendicularis), the anterior skull base appears as a rectangular area limited laterally by the medial surfaces of the orbital walls (lamina papyracea), posteriorly by the planum sphenoidale and anteriorly by the two frontal recesses (see Fig. 1a, b). This area is divided into two simmetrical parts by the lamina perpendicularis of the ethmoid bone. Each part is formed by the lamina cribrosa medially and ethmoid labyrinth laterally. The lamina cribrosa is a very thin osseous membrane crossed by olfactory nerves fibres, while the ethmoid labyrinth is formed by the anterior and posterior ethmoidal complexes. The anterior ethmoidal complex is constituted by the bullar and the suprabullar recesses and is separated from the posterior ethmoidal complex by the basal lamella of the middle turbinate [143]. The arterial supply of the dura mater of the ethmoidal planum

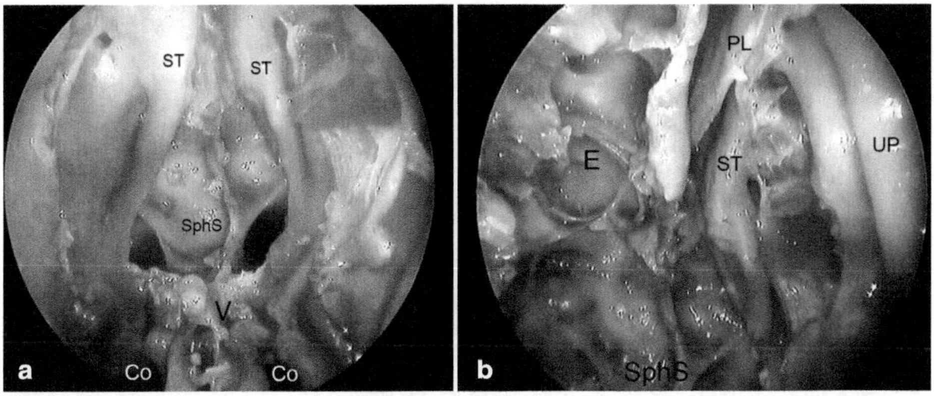


**Fig. 1.** Endoscopic endonasal anatomy of the anterior midline skull base. a) The superior portion of the nasal septum, the middle turbinate on both sides and the anterior wall of the sphenoid sinus have been removed. The superior turbinate and the ethmoid complex of both sides are visible. b) On the right side the anterior and posterior ethmoid cells have been opened. *SphS* Sphenoid sinus; *V* vomer; *Co* choana; *ST* superior turbinate; *E* ethmoid cells; *PL* perpendicularis lamina; *UP* uncinate process

is ensured by the anterior ethmoidal artery (AEA) and the posterior ethmoidal artery (PEA), that are branches of the oftalmic artery. These vessels send many small branches to the cribriform plate where they anastomize with the nasal branches of the sphenopalatine artery.

The AEA, after branching off, passes in the medial part of the optic nerve and in the lateral part of the superior oblique and medial rectus muscles to reach the anterior ethmoidal foramen at the lamina papyracea; it initially curves posteriorly and then anteriorly, in an anteromedial direction, running into the anterior ethmoidal canal (AEC) to reach the cribriform plate [47, 114, 150]. For the identification of the anterior ethmoidal artery (AEA) it is essential to expose the frontal recess. The frontal recess is constituted by the anterior part of the middle turbinate medially, by the lamina papyracea laterally and by the agger nasi cell anteriorly. The posterior ethmoidal artery, after its origin from the ophthalmic artery, runs between the rectus superior and the superior oblique muscle, then emerges from the orbit to enter the posterior ethmoidal canal (PEC) which courses horizontally the ethmoidal roof. It is useful to identify the carotid and optic protuberances and the opto-carotid recess located on the posterior wall of the sphenoid sinus in order to expose the PEA (see Fig. 2a, b). The posterior ethmoidal artery runs only few millimeters anteriorly to the roof of the sphenoid sinus cavity. Therefore its course has to be kept in mind during the transplanum approach, in order to avoid its accidental injury. Opening the dura of the anterior cranial fossa the olfactory nerves and the basal surface of the frontal lobes are visualized.

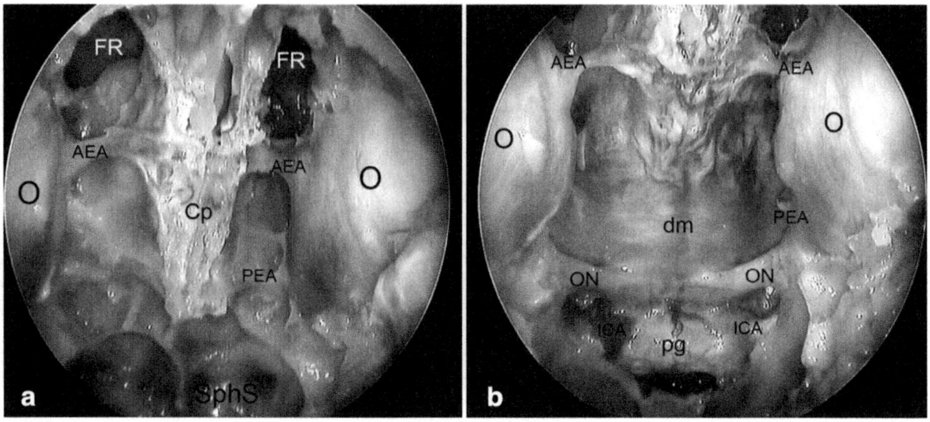


**Fig. 2.** Endoscopic endonasal anatomy of the anterior midline skull base. a) The anterior and posterior ethmoidal labyrinth on both side has been removed in order to visualize the anterior and posterior ethmoidal arteries in their bone canals. b) Panoramic view after the bilateral ethmoidectomy showing the dura mater of the anterior midline skull base from the frontal sinus till the sellar region. *FR* Frontal recess; *AEA* anterior ethmoidal artery; *PEA* posterior ethmoidal artery; *O* orbit; *Cp* cribiform plate; *ICA* internal carotid artery; *ON* optic nerve; *dm* dura mater; *pg* pituitary gland

## ***The middle skull base: the sphenoid sinus cavity*** [24]

Seen from the nasal cavity, the middle skull base corresponds to the posterior and lateral walls of the sphenoid sinus, where a series of protuberances and depressions are recognizable. The sellar floor is at the center, the spheno-ethmoid planum above it and the clival indentation below; lateral to the sellar floor the bony prominences of the intracavernous carotid artery (ICA) and the optic nerve can be seen and, between them, the lateral opto-carotid recess, moulded by the pneumatization of the optic strut of the anterior clinoid process (see Fig. 3a, b) [148]. The superior border of the lateral opto-carotid recess is covered by a thickening of the dura and periosteum which forms the distal dural ring, separating the optic nerve from the clinoidal segment of the internal carotid artery. The inferior border of the lateral opto-carotid recess is covered by a tickening of the dura and periosteum, which forms the proximal dural ring, which covers the third cranial nerve, the upper one inside the superior orbital fissure. Although rarely visible in the cavity of the sphenoid sinus, it is important to define the position of the medial opto-carotid recess since its removal on both sides significantly increases the surgical exposure over the suprasellar area. It corresponds intracranially to the medial clinoid process, which is present in about 50% of cases. The medial opto-carotid recess can be identified using as landmarks the lateral opto-carotid recess (see Fig. 4a–c).

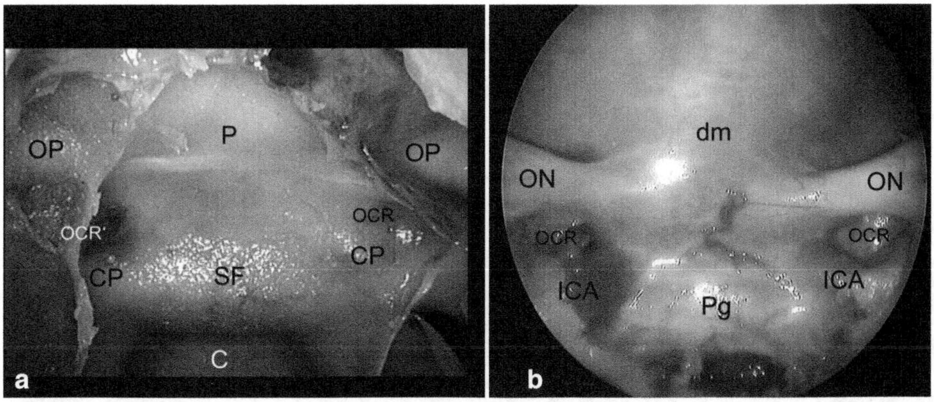


**Fig. 3.** Endoscopic endonasal anatomy of the middle skull base. a) The sphenoid septa have been removed allowing the identification of all the bone landmarks on the posterior wall of the sphenoid sinus. b) The posterior wall of the sphenoid sinus has been completely drilled out in order to expose the underlying anatomical structures. *P* Planum sphenoidale; *OP* optic protuberance; *OCR* opto-carotid recess; *CP* carotid protuberance; *SF* sellar floor; *C* clivus; *ON* optic nerve; *ICA* internal carotid artery; *dm* dura mater of the planum sphenoidale; *Pg* pituitary gland

Proceeding laterally other bony anatomical landmarks can be recognized, such as the cavernous sinus apex, the trigeminal maxillary and the trigeminal mandibulary protuberances, which is seen only in a well pneumatized sphenoid sinus. These bony bulges limit two main depressions, the first between the cavernous sinus apex and V2 protuberances and the other between V2 and V3 protuberances [3]. On the fllor of the sphenoid sinus cavity, specially when it is well pneumatized, it is possible to recognize the protuberance of the vidian nerve passing through the middle cranial fossa and foramen lacerum and entering the pterygopalatine fossa through the pterygoid canal, to reach the pterygopalatine ganglion.

Removing the bone and the dura over the sella, the tuberculum sellae and the posterior part of the planum sphenoidale it is possible to explore the suprasellar region. It has been divided in four areas using two ideal planes, one passing trough the inferior surface of the chiasm and the mammilary bodies, and one passing trough the posterior edge of chiasm and the dorsum sellae: supra-chiasmatic, sub-chiasmatic, retrosellar and ventricular (see Fig. 5).

In the **supra-chiasmatic area** the anterior margin of the chiasm and the medial portion of the optic nerves in the chiasmatic cistern, as well as the $A_1$ and $A_2$ segments and the anterior communicating artery in the lamina terminalis cistern are visualized (see Fig. 6a).

In the **sub-chiasmatic area** the first structure encountered is the pituitary stalk. The superior hypophyseal arteries and the branches for the inferior surface of the optic chiasm and nerves are visible (see Fig. 6a).

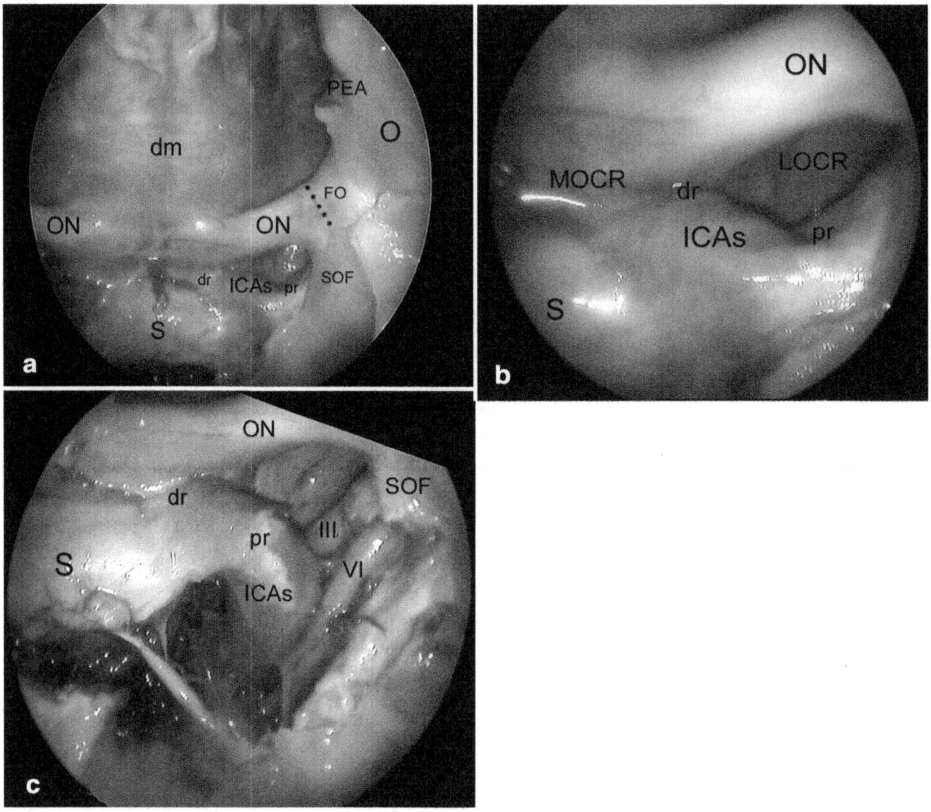


**Fig. 4.** Endoscopic endonasal anatomy of the middle skull base. a) After removal of the optic and carotid bone protuberances, it is possible to recognize the periostal dural layer covering the neurovascular structures. b) A close-up view of the lateral and medial opto-carotid recess. c) After opening of the cavernous sinus, the third and sixth cranial nerves converging towards the superior orbital fissure are visible. dm Dura mater; *PEA* posterior ethmoidal artery; *ON* optic nerve; *O* orbit; *S* sella; *ICAs* parasellar segment of the internal carotid artery; *dr* distal ring; *pr* proximal ring; *MOCR* medial opto-carotid recess; *LOCR* lateral opto-carotid recess; *III* oculomotor nerve; *VI* abducent nerve; *SOF* superior orbital fissure

The **retrosellar area** is reached passing between the pituitary stalk and the internal carotid artery, above the dorsum sellae. The upper third of the basilar artery, the pons, the superior cerebellar arteries, the oculomotor nerve and the posterior cerebral arteries are recognized. The mammillary bodies with the floor of the third ventricle are also visible (see Fig. 6b).

The opening of the floor of the third ventricle at the level of the tuber cinereum allows to explore the **ventricular area**. The lateral walls of the ventricle, formed by the medial portion of the talami, the interthalamic commissure, as well as the foramens of Monro are visible. On the posterior wall of

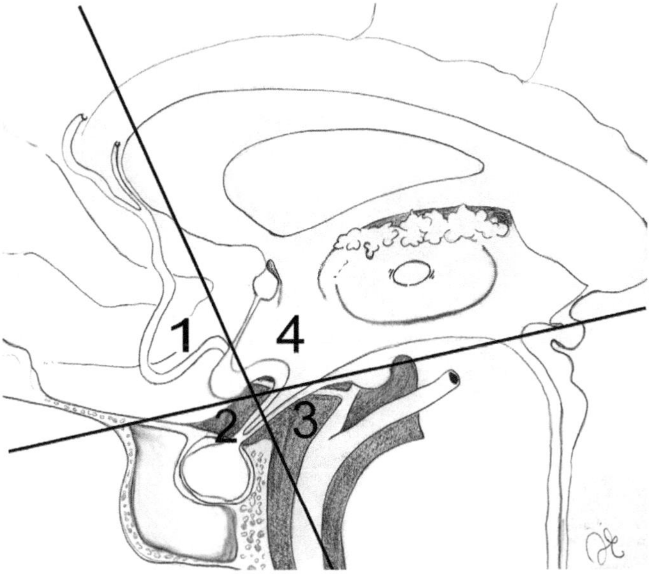


**Fig. 5.** Endoscopic endonasal anatomy of the middle skull base. Schematic drawing showing the areas explorable with the endoscope through the transtuberculum-transplanum sphenoidale approach. They have been divided in: *1* suprachiasmatic; *2* infrachiasmatic; *3* retrosellar; *4* intraventricular

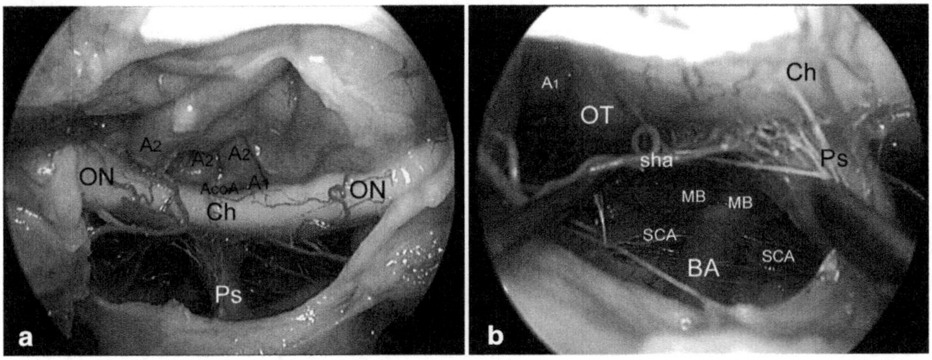


**Fig. 6.** Endoscopic endonasal anatomy of the middle skull base (intradural exploration). a) Endoscopic endonasal view of the suprachiasmatic and subchiasmatic areas. b) Endoscopic endonasal view of the retrosellar area. *ON* Optic nerve; *Ch* chiasm; *ps* pituitary stalk; *A1* anterior cerebral artery; *AcoA* anterior communicating artery; *A2* anterior cerebral artery; *MB* mammilary body; *sha* superior hypophyseal artery; *OT* optic tract; *SCA* superior cerebellar artery; *BA* basilar artery

the ventricle, it is possible to recognize the pineal and suprapineal recesses, the posterior commissure, the habenular commissure, the habenular trigona and the beginning of the aqueduct (see Fig. 7a–c).

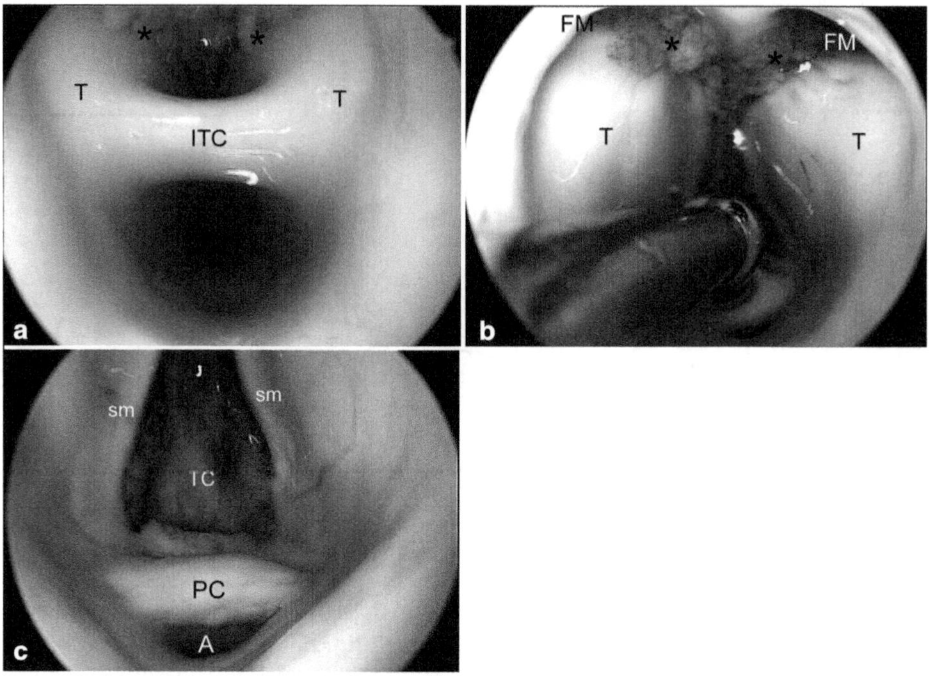


**Fig. 7.** Endoscopic endonasal view of the cavity of the III ventricle. a) Identification of the interthalamic commissure. b) Passing with the endoscope above the interthalamic adhesion, both the foramens of Monro and the choroids plexuses are visible. c) Passing below the interthalamic adhesion, the posterior portion of the third ventricle becomes visible. *T* Thalamus; *ICT* interthalamic commisure; * choroid plexus; *FM* foramen of Monro; *TC* tela choroidea; *PC* posterior commisure; *A* mesencephalic acqueduct; ** striae medullaris

The removal of the bone covering the lateral wall of the sphenoid sinus and the carotid protuberance permits the exposure of the neurovascular structures that form the anterior part of the cavernous sinus. After removing the fibrous trabecular structure of the medial wall of the cavernous sinus, the C-shaped parasellar segment of the internal carotid artery is immediately seen.

Displacing laterally the ICA, the meningohypophyseal artery and its branches, as well as the proximal portion of the oculomotor and trochlear nerves, can be visualized inside the C-shaped tract of the ICA.

Pushing medially the ICA it is possible to observe the lateral wall of the cavernous sinus from its interior surface. The origin of the infero-lateral trunk and its branches are detected. The oculomotor, the abducent nerves and the maxillary branch of the trigeminal nerve (V2) lie on an inner plane, compared with the trochlear nerve and the ophthalmic nerve (V1), thus the oculomotor nerve covers the trochelar nerve while the six nerve partially covers the first branch of the trigeminal nerve (see Fig. 8a, b). The oculomotor nerve passes at the level of the parasellar carotid artery, where it is usually joined by sympathetic

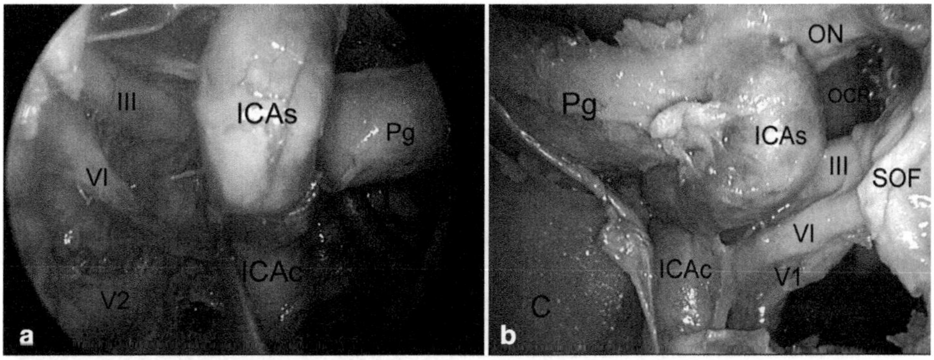


**Fig. 8.** Endoscopic endonasal anatomy of the cavernous sinus. a) Displacing medially the internal carotid artery, the third, the sixth and the maxillary branch of the trigeminal nerve are recognizable. b) After removal of the lateral wall of the cavernous sinus, the ophthalmic branch of the trigeminal nerve is also visible. *Pg* Pituitary gland; *OCR* opto-carotid recess; *III* oculomotor nerve; *VI* abducent nerve; *V1* ophthalmic branch of the trigeminal nerve; *ICAs* parasellar segment of the internal carotid artery; *ICAc* paraclival segment of the internal carotid artery; *ON* optic nerve; *C* clivus

fibers from the adventitia of ICA. The trochlear nerve lies parallel and just inferior to the oculomotor nerve. The abducens nerve crosses the ICA at the level of the rostral portion of the paraclival segment. The III, the IV and the ophthalmic nerve run upward to reach the superior orbital fissure, while the maxillary nerve runs caudally to reach the foramen rotundum. The oculomotor nerve superiorly, and the abducens nerve inferiorly limit a triangular area with the base represented by the lateral loop of the ICA. The surface of this area contains the throclear nerve and a part of V1. The abducens nerve superiorly and V2 inferiorly define a quadrangular area laterally delimited by the bone of the lateral wall of sphenoid sinus, from the superior orbital fissure to the foramen rotundum, and medially by the ICA. The ophthalmic branch of the trigeminal nerve and the artery of the inferior cavernous sinus run in this area. In case of a well pneumatized sphenoid sinus an inferior quadrangular area is identificable. Superiorly is delimited by V2 and inferiorly by the vidian nerve. The lesser base is formed by the intrapetrous segment and the caudal portion of the vertical tract of the ICA; the anterior edge is formed by the bone of the lateral wall of the sphenoid sinus from the foramen rotundum to the pterygoid canal [23].

## *The posterior skull base: from the dorsum sellae to the cranio-vertebral junction*

From an inferior route, the midline posterior cranial fossa is represented by the anterior surface of the clivus, from the dorsum sellae to the cranio-vertebral junction. The clivus is divided by the inferior wall of the sphenoid sinus in an

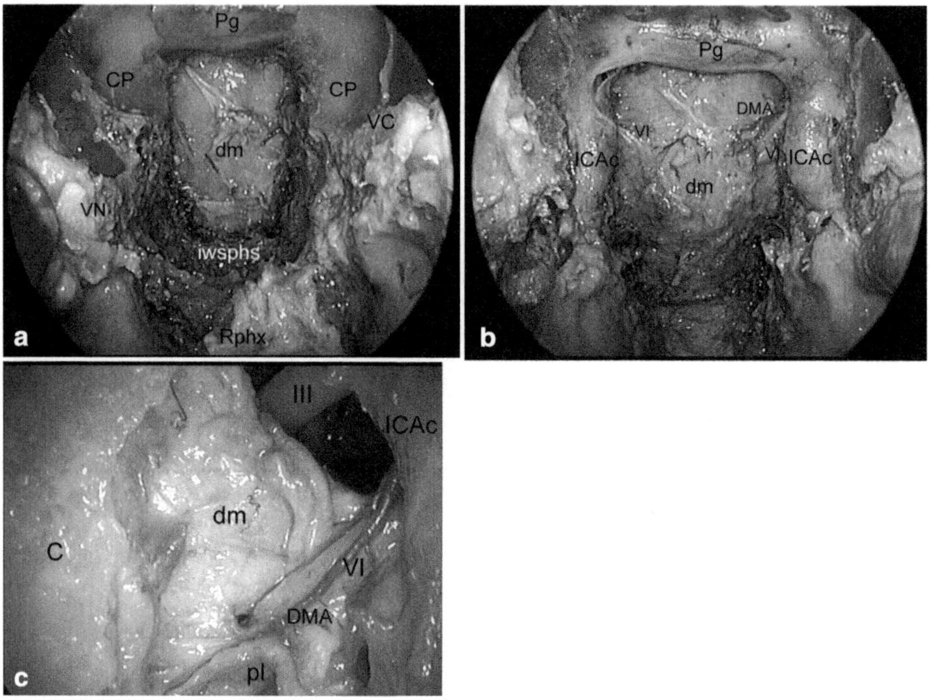


**Fig. 9.** Endoscopic endonasal anatomy of the clival area. a) The bone of the clivus and of the inferior wall of the sphenoid sinus have been removed up to identify the Vidian nerves. b) After complete removal of the bony protuberance of the intracavernous carotid arteries, the abducent nerve and its relationships with the dorsal meningeal artery are visible. c) Note the abducent nerve passing behind the the paraclival segment of the intracavernous carotid artery. *Pg* Pituitary gland; *CP* carotid protuberance; *ICAc* paraclival tract of the intracavernous carotid artery; *VN* Vidian nerve; *VC* vidian canal; *Rphx* rhinopharynx; *dm* dura mater; *DMA* dorsal meningeal artery; *III* oculomotor nerve; *VI* abducent nerve; *pl* periostial layer

upper part (sphenoid portion) and in a lower part (rhino-pharyngeal portion). Laterally on the sphenoid portion of the clivus the carotid protuberances are visible. After removal of the bone of the upper part of the clivus the periostium-dural layer is exposed; the opening of the carotid protuberance permits to identify the sixth cranial nerve, which passes together with the dorsal meningeal artery just medially to the paraclival carotid artery, thus representing the real lateral limit of the approach at this level (see Fig. 9a–c). After the opening of the dura, the basilar artery and its branches, as well as the upper cranial nerves, are well seen along their courses in the posterior cranial fossa (see Fig. 10a, b).

Extending the bone removal to the inferior wall of the sphenoid sinus the rhinopharynx is exposed. The lower third of the clivus is removed and both the *foramina lacera* are identified, representing them the lateral limit of the approach at this level. It is possible to further enlarge this opening by removing the

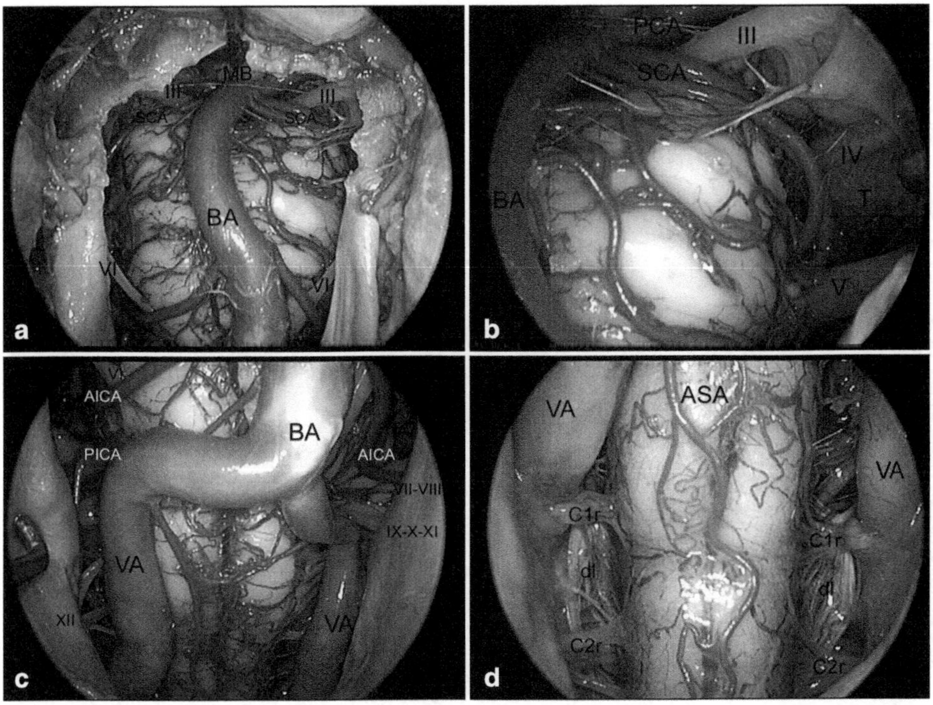


**Fig. 10.** Endoscopic endonasal anatomy of the clivus and cranio-vertebral junction (intradural exploration). a) After the opening of the dura, the basilar artery and the ventral surface of the brain stem become visible. b) With the endoscope in close-up view it is possible to see the entry zones of the oculomotor and the trigeminal nerves. c) The vertebral arteries, the spino-medullary junction and the lower cranial nerves are exposed. d) The entrance of the vertebral arteries in the vertebral canal as well as the ventral rootlets of the first two cervical nerves and the dentate ligaments, are visible. *SCA* Superior cerebellar artery; *BA* basilar artery; *III* oculomotor nerve; *IV* trochlear nerve; *T* tentorium; *V* trigeminal nerve; *VI* abducent nerve; *XII* hypoglossal nerve; *IX–XI* glossopharyngeal, vagus and accessory nerves; *VII, VIII*: acoustic-facial boundle; *PICA* posterior inferior cerebellar artery; *AICA* anterior inferior cerebellar artery; *VA* vertebral artery; *ASA* anterior spinal artery; *dm* dura mater; *C1r* ventral rootlets of the first cervical nerve; *C2r* ventral rootlets of the second cervical nerve; *dl* dentate ligament

anterior third of the occipital condyles, without entering in the hypoglossal canal, which is located at the junction of the anterior and middle third of each occipital condyle. Moreover the articular surface of the condyle is located on its lateral portion, so that the removal of its inner third, through an anterior route, does not involve the articular junction. The mucosa of the rhinopharynx is removed and the atlanto-occipital membrane, the longus capitis and colli muscles, the atlas and axis are exposed (see Fig. 11a, b). The anterior arch of the atlas is removed and the dens is exposed (see Fig. 11c). Using the microdrill the dens is thinned; it is then separated from the apical and alar ligamens and

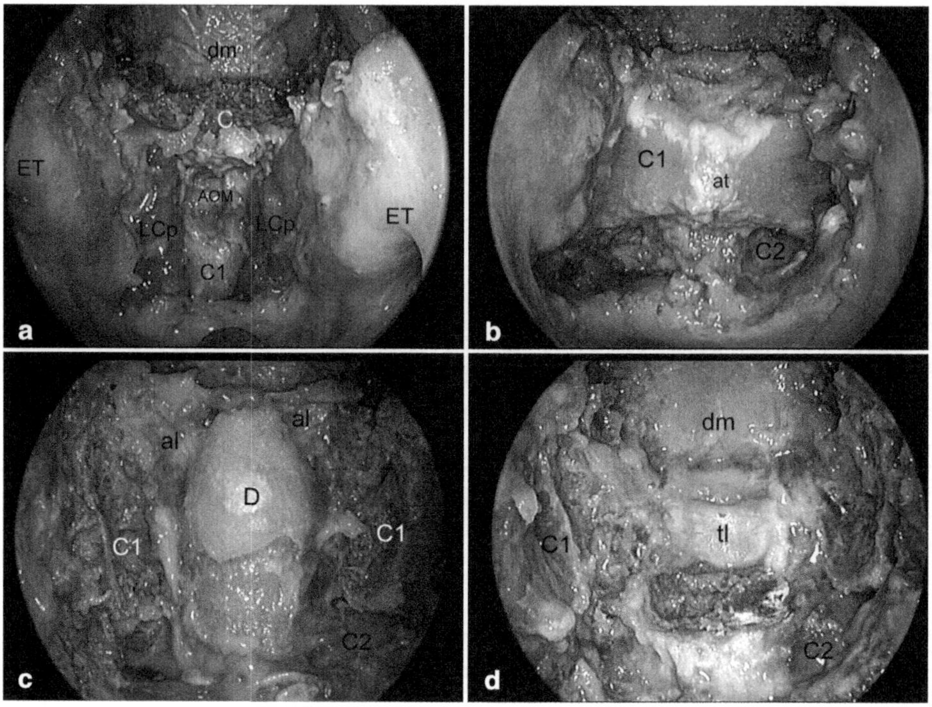


**Fig. 11.** Endoscopic endonasal anatomy of the cranio-vertebral junction. a, b) The mucosa of the rhinopharynx has been removed and the longus capitis and longus colli muscles have been elevated in order to expose the cranio-vertebral junction. c) The anterior arch of the atlas has been drilled out and the dens has been exposed. d) After removal of the dens, the transverse ligament is visible. *dm* Dura mater; *C* clivus; *LCp* longus capitis muscle; *AOM* anterior atlanto-occipital membrane; *C1* atlas; *at* anterior tubercle; *ET* Eustachian tube; *C2* axis; *tl* transverse ligament; *al* alar ligaments

finally dissected from the transverse ligament and removed (see Fig. 11d). The vertebral arteries can be explored from their dural entrance up to their confluence in the basilar artery. The posterior inferior cerebellar artery (PICA) and the anterior ventral spinal artery are also visible. Above and behind the vertebral artery the lower cranial nerves and the acoustic-facial boundle (VII–VIII), with the antero inferior cerebellar artery (AICA), are visible. The rootlets of the hypoglossal nerve as well as the ventral rootlets of C1 and C2, and the dentate ligament between them can be identified (see Fig. 10c, d).

## Instruments and tools for extended approaches

Extended endoscopic endonasal approaches to the skull base have been accompanied and facilitated by the design and development of dedicated endonasal instruments and tools, some of them following prior studies on the endoscopic transsphenoidal approach for sellar lesions [9, 12, 29].

As already noted, the extended endoscopic operations basically use the endonasal route to access the entire midline skull base. Such a corridor is more restricted when compared with the "open" approaches and, therefore, the handling of the instruments is not always easy, specially when trying to control bleeding. As a matter of fact, the control of bleeding, specially when arterial, may constitute one of the most cumbersome problems of endoscopic surgery. Even though monopolar coagulation can be easily employed inside the nose, its extensive use is not recommended because of the potential injury of neural fibers of the olfactory nerve in the posterior part of the nasal cavities.

Furthermore, monopolar coagulation must be avoided close to major neurovascular structures, such as on the posterior wall of the sphenoid sinus, in the intradural space or in proximity to nerve or vascular bony protuberances within the sphenoid sinus. Some endoscopic monopolars are combined with a suction cannula to aspirate the smoke during coagulation, which maintains a clear surgical field. For such reasons, bipolar coagulation should be preferred. Although the use through the nose of the classic microsurgical bipolar forceps is possible, their maneuverability is not always easy or secure due to their shape. Consequently, different endonasal bipolar forceps have been designed, with various diameters and lengths, which have proven to be quite effective in bipolar control of bleeding. The bipolar forceps for endoscopic surgery need to have some special features: i) they should have a shape to be easily introduced and manoeuvred in the nasal cavity; ii) the tips of the forceps have to be adequately isolated. For the purposes of the extended endonasal endoscopic surgery, the bipolar has the shape of forceps with ring handle like scissors. The movements of the handle causes the tips to open and close and, eventually, to coagulate. Furthermore, new coagulating instruments, either monopolar and bipolar, based on radiofrequency waves have been proposed in such types of operations (Ellman Innovations, Oceanside, NY, USA): they have the advantages that the spatial heat dispersion is minimal, with consequent minimal risk of heating injury to the neurovascular structures. Besides, the radiofrequency bipolar forceps do not need to be used with irrigation or to be cleaned every time.

Endoscopic endonasal skull base surgery demands the use of special instruments and devices that have proven to be quite helpful for the effectiveness and safety of the procedure, even though they are not absolutely needed.

Image guided neuronavigation systems are very useful for intraoperative identification of the limits of the lesion and of the bony, vascular and nervous structures, especially if they are encased by the tumor [46, 101, 117, 129]. In some select cases, the classic landmarks for endoscopic transsphenoidal surgery (sellar floor, clival indentation, carotid and optic nerve protuberances, optico-carotid recess) are not easily identifiable and neuronavigation can help to maintain the surgeon's orientation even in the presence of distorted anatomy. However, the use of such devices requires the head of the patient to be fixed in the three-pin skeletal fixation headrest in order to render the head of the patient fixed with the reference system. Some authors use the three-pin headrest not fixed to the surgical table but the head is actually put in the horseshoe headrest [45, 48]. The neuronavigation systems and the panoramic view provided by the endoscope also make it possible to do without the use of fluoroscopy, thus avoiding unnecessary radiation exposure to the patient and the surgical team.

High-speed low-profile drills may be very helpful for the opening the bony structures to gain access to the dural space [45, 48]. They are specifically designed for endonasal use and have some special characteristics: they are low-profile and also long enough but not too bulky, so they can be easily used together with the endoscope (The Anspach Efforts, Inc., Palm Beach Gardens, Florida, USA). The combined use of such drills and endonasal bony rongeurs have proven to be effective and time-saving during the extended approaches to the skull base, especially for access to the suprasellar or retroclival regions. It is important to find a good balance between the length of the tip and stability during fine drilling, as a too long tip may dangerously vibrate.

Prior to opening the dura mater and whenever the surgeon thinks it is appropriate (especially while working very close to vascular structures), it is of utmost importance to use the microDoppler probe to insonate the major arteries [4, 45, 48, 151]. The use of such a device is particularly useful while operating inside the cavernous sinus, in the retroclival prepontine area or in the suprasellar space.

## Endoscopic endonasal techniques

### *Basic steps for extended endonasal transsphenoidal approaches*

The procedure goes through the same basic steps of a standard transsphenoidal operation – i.e., vision of the surgical target areas by means of a rigid diagnostic endoscope (Karl Storz Endoscopy, Tuttlingen, Germany) and their exposure, followed by management and removal of the lesion and, finally, reconstruction of the approach route. All the extended endoscopic endonasal procedures have been performed in a fully integrated operating room (Karl Storz OR1$^{TM}$), centrally monitored and controlled, in which surgical processes and routine work are simultaneously streamlined and simplified. Such operating room is dedicated for minimally invasive procedures.

According with the concepts outlined by Perneczky [120], the approach could be considered a "key-hole" procedure, with a "door" – the sphenoid sinus – a "window" to be open on the skull base and different "corridors" to the different "rooms" – the various perisellar compartments.

In contrast to traditional transsphenoidal approach to the sellar region, where a horse-shoe headrest is used, in extended approaches a rigid three-pin head fixation is preferred because an image-guided system is required.

The head is turned 10–15° on the horizontal plane, towards the surgeon, who is on the patient's right side and in front of him and extended for about 10–15° for lesions located in the suprasellar area or on the cribiform plate and slightly flexed for those lesions located in the clival area. These changes of the head position are necessary to allow an optimal position of the endoscope during the surgical procedure: not too close to the thorax, nor perpendicular to the patient's head. The surgical corridor required for the extended approaches is wider in respect to that of the standard approach [11, 15, 39]. To increase the working space and the manoeuvrability of the instruments it is necessary: i) to remove the middle turbinate on one side; ii) tolateralize the middle turbinate in the other nostril; and iii) to remove the posterior portion of the nasal septum (see Fig. 12a, b). These surgical maneuvers allow the use of both nostrils, so that two or three instruments plus the endoscope can be inserted.

The procedure starts with the removal of the middle turbinate, which represents an important step of the procedure, since it allows the creation of a larger corridor through one nostril, thus permitting the easy introduction of the endoscope and of one instrument. Usually the right middle turbinate is removed. The areas just above the head of the middle turbinate and its tail are coagulated. The head of the middle turbinate is cut with nasal scissors and pushed downward in order to expose its tail. After completing hemostasis around the tail of the turbinate, the tail is cut and the turbinate is removed.

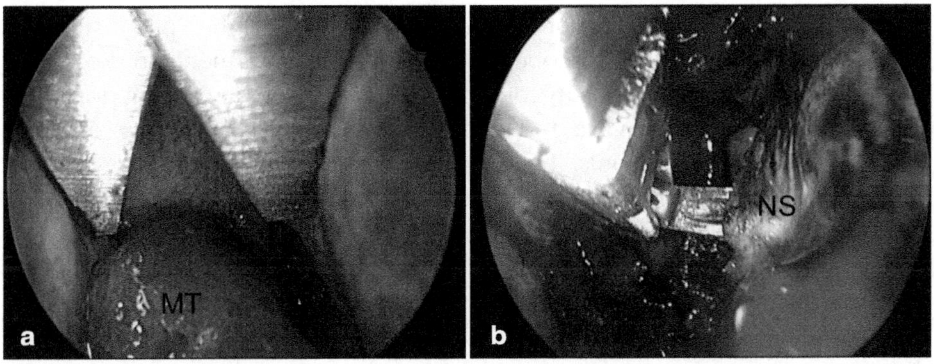


**Fig. 12.** Basic concepts for extended approaches. a) Right middle turbinectomy; b) removal of the posterior portion of the nasal septum with a retrograde bone punch. *NS* Nasal septum; *MT* middle turbinate

Such technique has been performed according with the guidelines of the Pittsburgh's group [86].

With a retrograde bone punch, the posterior nasal septum is then removed to a variable extent and the mucosal edges are accurately coagulated with the bipolar forceps. In this way, the nasal septum does not blur the endoscopic view when other instruments are inserted through the other nostril, this being a binostril technique. In those cases in which a wide osteo-dural opening is necessary over the planum or the clivus a mucopericondrial flap harvested from the nasal septum can be realized to render more effective the reconstruction at the end of the procedure. The flap is created cutting the septal mucosa along the inferior edge of the septum from the roof of the choana to the cartilaginous portion and superiorly at the level of the rostral portion of the middle turbinate. Then the mucoperichondrium flap is dissected from the septal bone and pedicted around the sphenopalatine foramen. During the operation, the flap is located in the choana and at the end of the procedure is used to cover the posterior wall of the sphenoid sinus, to support the reconstruction materials [66].

The middle turbinate of the contralateral nostril is pushed laterally with an elevator allowing a binasal route for the instruments. Up to this point, the surgical procedure is usually performed by one surgeon who holds the endoscope with one hand and one instrument with the other. From now on, the endoscope is held by the assistant and the surgeon can use both his hands [22]. The two nostril approach requires good collaboration between of two surgeons as if they were running a rally car race: one holds the endoscope and can be considered a sort of "navigator"; the second, the "pilot", handles two surgical instruments inside the surgical field, as in the traditional microsurgical technique. The "navigator" "dynamically" uses the endoscope during the surgical procedure. He is responsible of the visual control of the instruments, which constantly remain under direct endoscopic view. The endoscope follows the in-and-out movements of the instruments, so minimizing the risks of injury to the neurovascular structures, The other member of the team, the "pilot" surgeon, is free from holding the endoscope and can use two instruments in the operative field. Otherwise the first surgeon holds the endoscope in the non dominant hand and an instrument in the dominant hand, while the second surgeon helps with suction and other tools. In distinction to the microsurgical technique, where the microscope remains outside and the increased magnification narrows the visual field, in this endoscopic technique the "pilot" and the "navigator" continuously pass between the close-up view, as during the dissecting manoeuvres, and a panoramic view of the neurovascular structures.

The anterior sphenoidotomy is performed starting with the coagulation of the spheno-ethmoid recess 5 mm above the choana up to the sphenoid ostium. Using the microdrill with diamond burr the entire anterior wall of the sphenoid sinus is removed. The sphenoidotomy is enlarged more than in the standard approach, especially in lateral and superior direction where bony spurs are flattened in order to create an adequate space for the endoscope during the deeper steps of the procedure. All the septa inside the sphenoid sinus are removed including those attached on the bony protuberances and depressions on the posterior wall of the sphenoid sinus cavity.

## *The transtuberculum transplanum approach to the suprasellar area*

Traditionally surgical approaches for tumors located in the suprasellar region are transcranial and the most favoured are the pterional and the subfrontal routes. Although these procedures are well standardized and widely utilized, several authors have proposed different minicraniotomical approaches to reach the suprasellar area [5, 18, 42, 52, 63, 76, 125], and, even with these, there is the need for a certain degree of brain retraction. The transsphenoidal approach has been widely adopted for the surgical treatment of intrasellar and intra-suprasellar infradiaphragmatic lesions. However some Authors [52, 73, 103] have described successful transsphenoidal removal of suprasellar/supradiaphragmatic lesions. In these cases the access to the suprasellar area is obtained, after the resection of the intrasellar component of the tumor, through a wide opening of the diaphagma sellae (trans-sellar transdiaphragmatic approach). More recently some Authors [17, 31, 33, 40, 41, 45, 57, 82, 85, 91, 95, 97, 102, 105, 110, 149] have reported the successful removal of suprasellar/supradiaphragmatic lesions through a modified transsphenoidal microsurgical approach, the so-called *transsphenoidal transtuberculum approach*. This technique provides a direct access to the supradiaphragmatic space, allowing sufficient exposure for the removal of supradiaphragmatic tumors, regardless of the sellar size (even a not enlarged sella), and preserving normal pituitary tissue and function. This approach permits a direct view of the neurovascular structures of the suprasellar region lesion without any brain retraction.

### Surgical procedure

After the preliminary steps for extended transsphenoidal approaches have been performed, the bone removal over the sella starts with the drilling of the tuberculum sellae (see Fig. 13a) which, inside the sphenoid sinus cavity, corresponds to the angle formed by the planum sphenoidale with the sellar floor. The drilling is then extended bilaterally, towards both the medial opto-carotid recesses. The upper half of the sella is removed up to reach the superior intercavernous sinus. A Kerrison's rongeur is used to complete the bone removal from the planum (see Fig. 13b). The extension of the bone removal depends on the size of the lesion and is performed under the control of neuronavigator. Above the opto-carotid recess, the extension of the bone opening

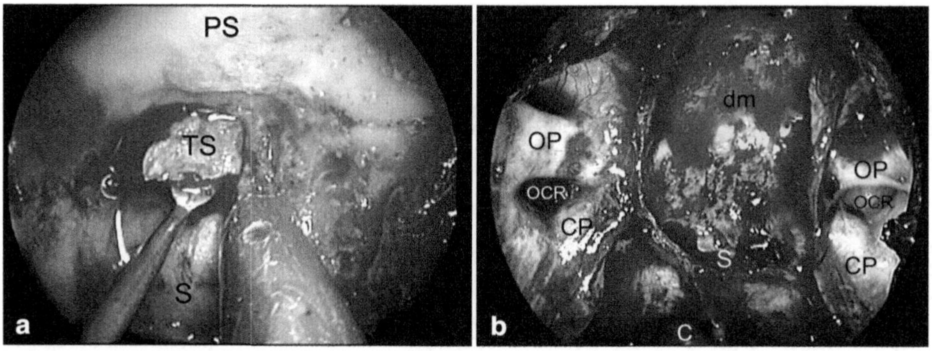


**Fig. 13.** Extended approach to the planum sphenoidale. a) Isolation and removal of the tuberculum sellae. b) Panoramic view after the bone removal. *PS* Planum sphenoidale; *TS* tuberculum sellae; *S* sella turcica; *OP* optic protuberance; *OCR* opto-carotid recess; *CP* carotid protuberance; *dm* dura mater; *C* clivus

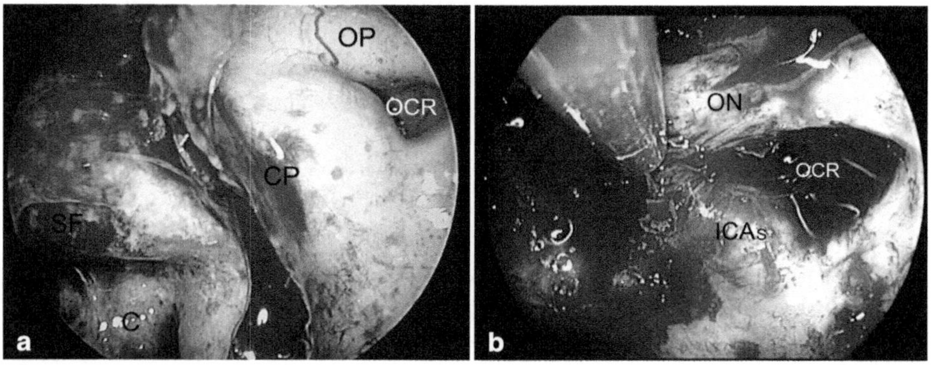


**Fig. 14.** Extended approach to the planum sphenoidale. a, b) The medial opto-carotid recess, pointed by the suction cannula in figure; b represents the lateral limit of the bone drilling. *SF* Sella turcica; *OP* optic protuberance; *OCR* opto-carotid recess; *CP* carotid protuberance; *C* clivus; *ICAs* parasellar segment of the internal carotid artery; *ON* optic nerve

is limited laterally by the protuberances of the optic nerves, which diverge towards the optic canal (see Fig. 14a, b). Thus, the opening over the planum has a trapezoidal shape, with the short bases at the level of the tuberculum sellae. During the bone opening, it is not so rare to cause bleeding of the superior intercavernous sinus. In such cases its management can be problematic and cause the operation to be longer, increase the blood loss and make more difficult the access to the intradural compartment. Apart the use of hemostatic agents, like Floseal® (Baxter, BioSciences, Vienna, Austria), it is preferable to close the sinus with the bipolar forceps instead of using the hemoclips, which narrows the dural opening. Two horizontal incisions are made just few millimetres above and below the superior intercavernous sinus. The sinus is then closed between the two tips of the bipolar forceps and coagulated in its median portion. It is incised with microscissors, and the two resulting dural flaps are coagulated to achieve their retraction and enlargement of the dural opening.

The dissection and the removal of the lesion in the suprasellar area follows the same principles of microsurgery and uses low-profile instruments and dedicated bipolar forceps. Also the strategy for tumor removal is tailored to each lesion, so that it will be different for giant pituitary adenomas, craniopharyngiomas or meningiomas.

- *Pituitary adenomas*

The transtuberculum transplanum approach for the removal of pituitary adenomas is required only for highly selected cases. In fact usually even for

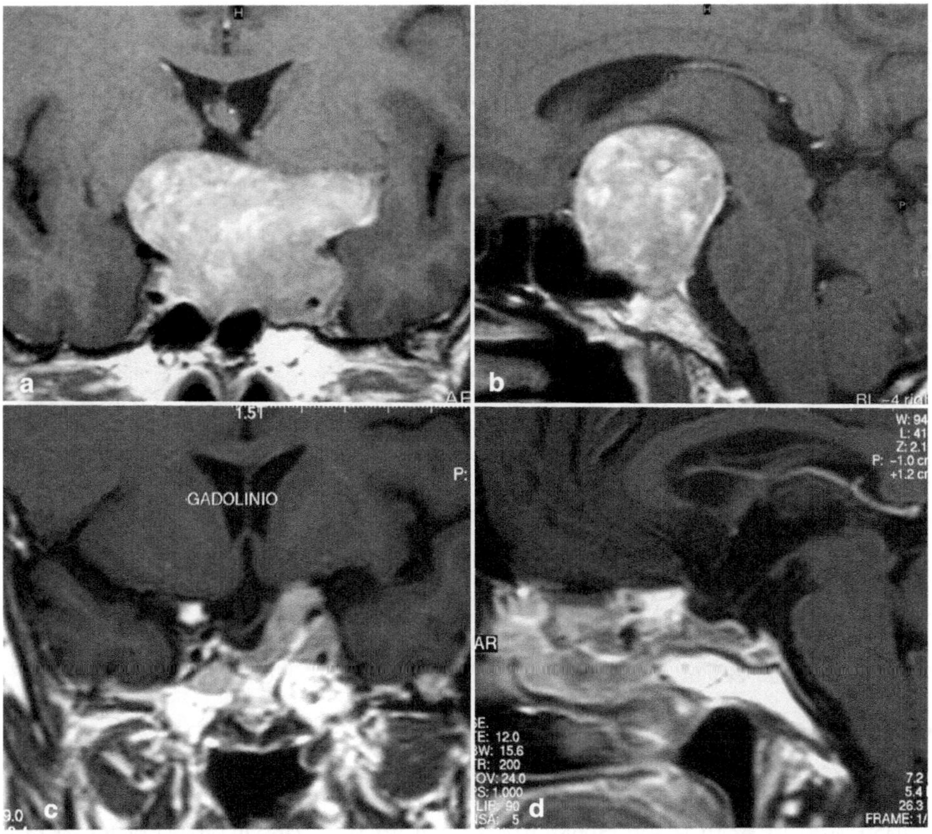


**Fig. 15.** a, b) Coronal and sagittal pre-operative MRI images showing a case of a giant adenoma. c, d) Coronal and sagittal post-operative MRI images of the same patient showing the subtotal removal of the lesion

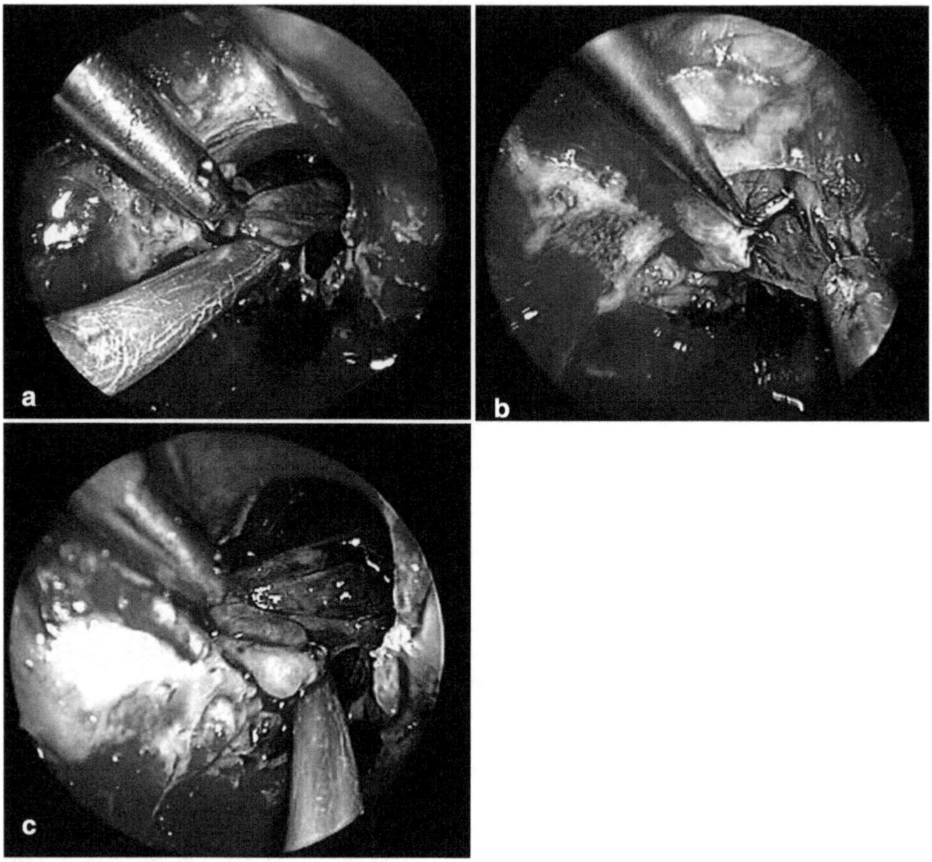

**Fig. 16.** Intraoperative pictures of the giant macroadenoma showed in Fig. 15. After the internal debulking (a), the tumor capsule (b, c) is dissected from the surrounding neurovascular structures and removed

very large intra-suprasellar pituitary adenomas, the trans-sellar approach allows the progressive descent of the suprasellar portion of the tumor and thence visualization of the suprasellar cistern.

In contrast, there are some conditions in which the extended approach can be used instead of the transcranial one, namely some purely suprasellar, or dumb-bell-shaped, and the giant pituitary adenomas (see Figs. 15 and 16).

- *Craniopharyngiomas*

Using the extended transplanar route in the cases of suprasellar craniopharyngiomas, the tumor is seen immediately after the dural opening, anterior to the chiasm and in front of the stalk. In contrast, in the case of intraventricular craniopharyngiomas, the tumor is not readily visible, because it is located behind the stalk and the chiasm and has to be approached passing laterally to the stalk. Working alternatively from both sides of the stalk, the dome of the tumor is

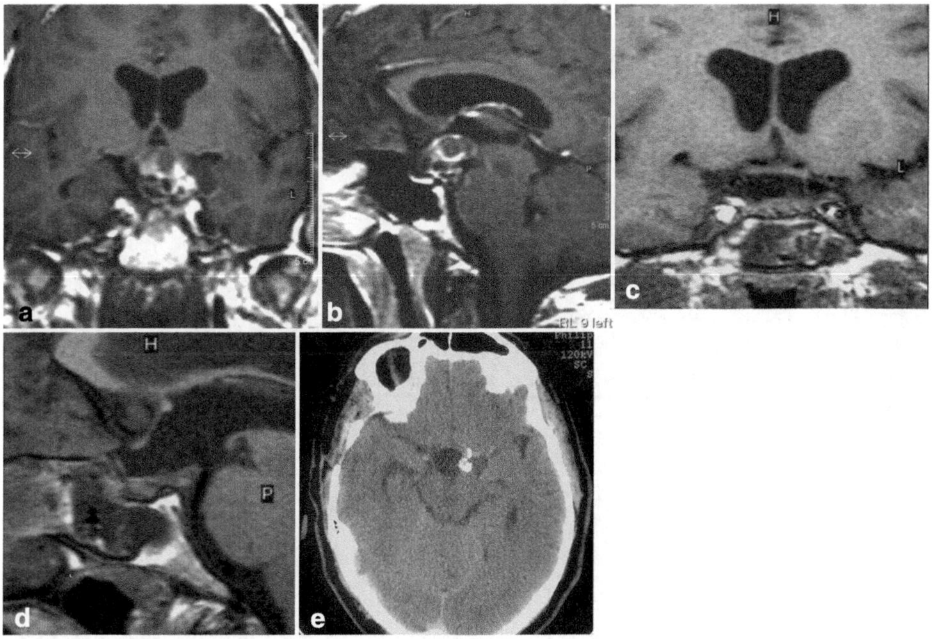


**Fig. 17.** a, b) Coronal and sagittal pre-operative MRI images showing a case of suprasellar craniopharyngioma already operated through a right pterional approach. c, d) Coronal and sagittal post-operative MRI images of the same patient showing the subtotal removal of the lesion. e) Early post-operative CT scan. Note the calcified remnant of the tumor

reached and manipulated. In this case the floor of the third ventricle is not early recognizable, because the lesion pushes it downward and behind, making it visible only after tumor removal and therefore care should be taken in preserving its integrity, specially at the level of the mammillary bodies. In cases of infundibular craniopharyngioma that had produced the swelling of the stalk, this was split allowing the removal of the craniopharyngioma. Tumor removal is performed according to the same paradigms of microsurgery: internal debulking of the solid part and/or cystic evacuation, avoiding the seeding of the craniopharyngioma tissue, followed by fine and meticulous dissection from the chiasm, the stalk and the superior hypophyseal arteries, while the AComA complex, located above the chiasm, andprotected by an arachnoidal sheath, is usually not involved in the procedure. The dissection is carried out under close-up view, with continuous and direct visual control of the neighbouring neurovascular structures.

At the end of the tumor resection, an inspection of the surgical cavity is made with 0 and 30 degrees endoscopes, in order to check the completeness of removal and to establish haemostasis (see Figs. 17 and 18).

Obviously this kind of approach presents some limits and contraindications for craniopharyngioma surgery. In cases of pre-sellar or conchal type of sinus,

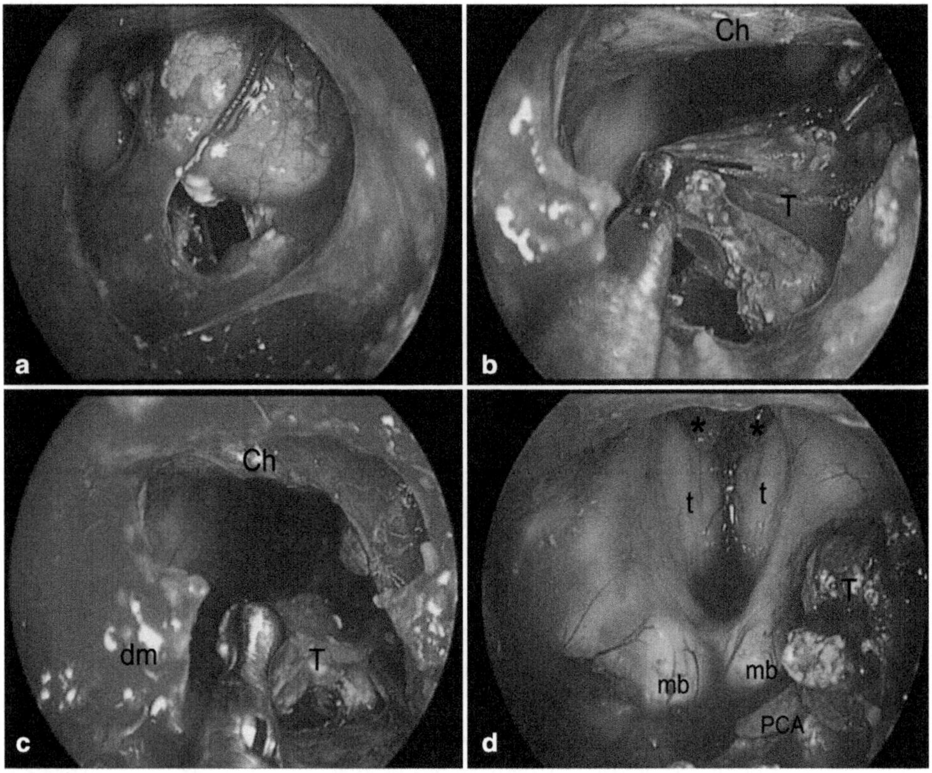


**Fig. 18.** Intraoperative pictures of the suprasellar craniopharyngioma showed in Fig. 17. a) initial visualization of the lesion after the dural opening. b, c) Piecemeal removal of the lesion. d) Endoscopic control after the removal. Note the presence of a calcified tumor remnant adherent to the left posterior communicating artery. *Ch* Chiasm; *T* tumor; *dm* dura mater; *t* thalamus; *mb* mammilary bodies; *PCA* posterior cerebral artery; * choroids plexus

the main landmarks within the sphenoid sinus are not easily recognizable, thus increasing the risk of injury to the intracavernous ICAs and the optic nerves. In cases of retrosellar extension of the lesion, the presence of a high dorsum can increase the difficulty of reaching and managing the tumor. The consistency, blood supply, and adherence to the surrounding neurovascular structures by the tumor can represent an obstacle to the approach. The narrow space for the instruments might create troubles in cases of hemorrhage. Other limitations are the steep learning curve before becoming confident with this peculiar view of the anatomical structures and the longer operative times at least initially when using a transcranial approach.

- *Tuberculum sellae meningiomas*

In the management of tuberculum sellae meningiomas (see Fig. 19a, b), tumor removal is preceded by the coagulation of the dural attachment,

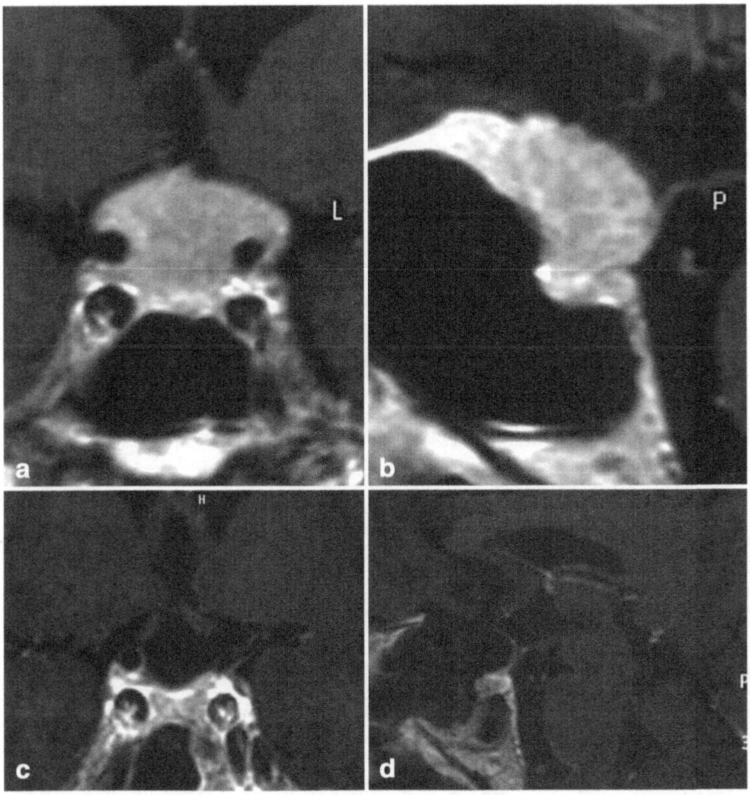


**Fig. 19.** a, b) Coronal and sagittal pre-operative MRI images showing a case of tuberculum sellae meningioma. c, d) Coronal and sagittal post-operative MRI images of the same patient confirming the total removal of the lesion

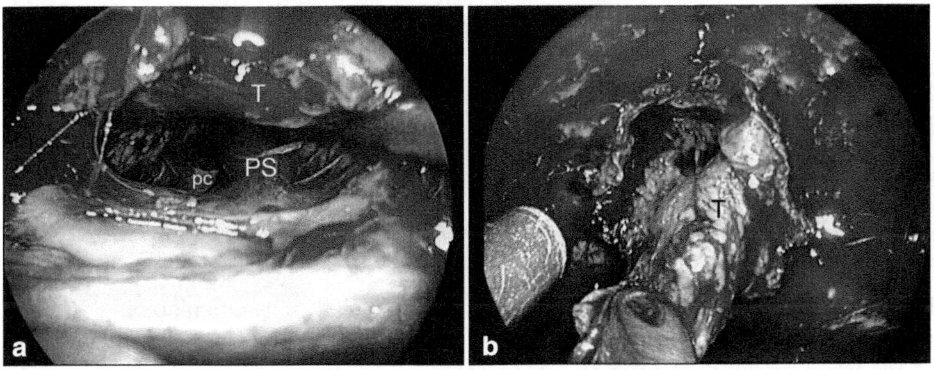


**Fig. 20.** Intraoperative pictures of the case of tuberculum sellae meningioma showed in Fig. 19. a) The mobilization of the inferior pole of the tumor permits to identify the pituitary stalk and the posterior clinoid process. b) Progressive internal debulking of the tumor mass. *T* Tumor; *Ps* pituitary stalk; *pc* posterior clinoid process

which permits an early tumor devascularization and offers an initial advantage. Then the dura and the underlying base of the meningioma is opened and the tumor is debulked with suction and radiofrequency cold bipolar coagulation (SurgiMax, Ellman Innovations, Oceanside, NY, U.S.A.). After the tumor is devascularized and debulked, the surrounding arachnoid is dissected away from the tumor's capsule. Usually the dissection starts from the inferior pole of the tumor which is elevated allowing the early identification of the pituitary stalk, of the optic nerves' inferior aspect and of the chiasm and both the superior hypophyseal arteries (see Fig. 20a, b). Gently blunt dissection of the tumor from the inferior surface of the optic nerves and chiasm is performed, with a meticulous identification and preservation of the vascular supply to the under face of the optic pathway. After the inferior aspect of the optic apparatus has been freed from the tumor, the

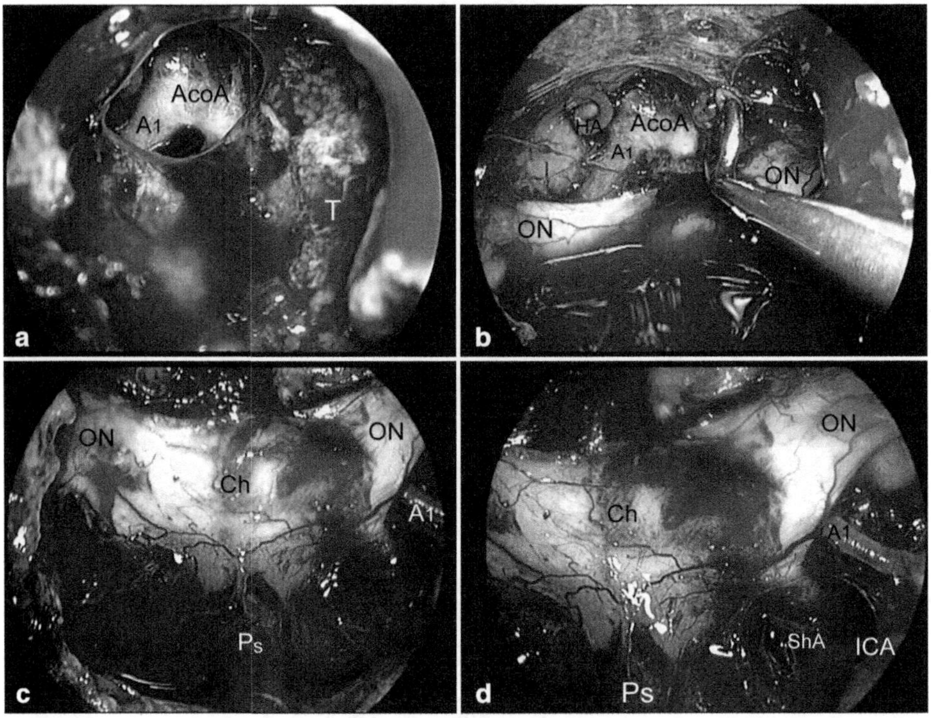


**Fig. 21.** Intraoperative pictures of the case of tuberculum sellae meningioma showed in Fig. 19. a, b) The superior aspect of the tumor was dissected from the anterior part of the Willis' circle. c, d) After the lesion removal, the panoramic endoscopic view of the surgical cavity shows the chiasm, the optic nerves and the A1 segment of the left anterior cerebral artery. *Ch* Chiasm; *ON* optic nerve; *A1* anterior cerebral artery; *A2* anterior cerebral artery; *AcoA* anterior communicating artery; *Ps* pituitary stalk; *ICA* internal carotid artery

lateral and the superior part of the tumor are dissected. Proceeding towards the lateral part of the meningioma, an arachnoidal plane is usually found against the internal carotid arteries. The safe removal of the upper pole of the tumor requires gentle pulling of the capsule from below, which brings into direct view the suprachiasmatic area, where there is the AComA complex. The arachnoidal layers are dissected and these arteries are freed (see Fig. 21a, b). Once the tumor has been freed from any adherence, it is removed. In the final step of the procedure the operative field is inspected and accurate hemostasis is checked (see Fig. 21c, d).

As for craniopharyngiomas, the transtuberculum/transplanum approach to tuberculum sellae meningiomas presents some disadvantages related to the approach and to the characteristic of the tumor itself. The degree of pneumatization of the sphenoid sinus is important for the recognization of the main landmarks within the sphenoid sinus and to guarantee safe bone removal; in the case of a small sella, the distance between the optic nerves and the ICAs is narrower and potentially more dangerous. Concerning the tumor-related limits, we consider as contraindication for the extended transsphenoidal approach either the involvement of the optic canal and the encasement of the 3rd cranial nerve. Finally a more anterior dural attachment requires a very large osteo-dural opening, thus increasing the difficulties of the skull base reconstruction.

## *Approach to the ethmoidal planum*

The introduction of functional endoscopic sinus surgery (FESS) in the early eighties allowed the ENT surgeons to approach chronic inflammatory pathologies of the nasal and paranasal sinuses [94, 112, 141–144]. Their experience has improved knowledge of the anatomy of this area and resulted in the evolution of the endoscopic approach to the anterior skull base. Due to its lesser surgical morbidity as compared to other techniques, the endoscopic endonasal technique for the management of lesions of spheno-ethmoidal region has become popular for CSF leaks, and subsequently for meningoencephaloceles (see Figs. 22, 23 and 24) and selected benign tumors of the anterior skull base [20, 70, 74, 108, 123, 147]. More recently the collaboration among ENT surgeons and neurosurgeons has brought advances in the use of the endoscopic endonasal technique in neurosurgery, thus permitting the pure endonasal treatment of intradural lesions, such as olfactory groove meningiomas or esthesioneuroblastomas [86]. The surgical approach to the ethmoid planum is tailored to the position and to the extension of the lesion. In this way it will be different for CSF leaks, meningoencephaloceles and tumors located on the cribiform plate. While approaching this region it is important to exactly know the position of some relevant structures, such as the anterior

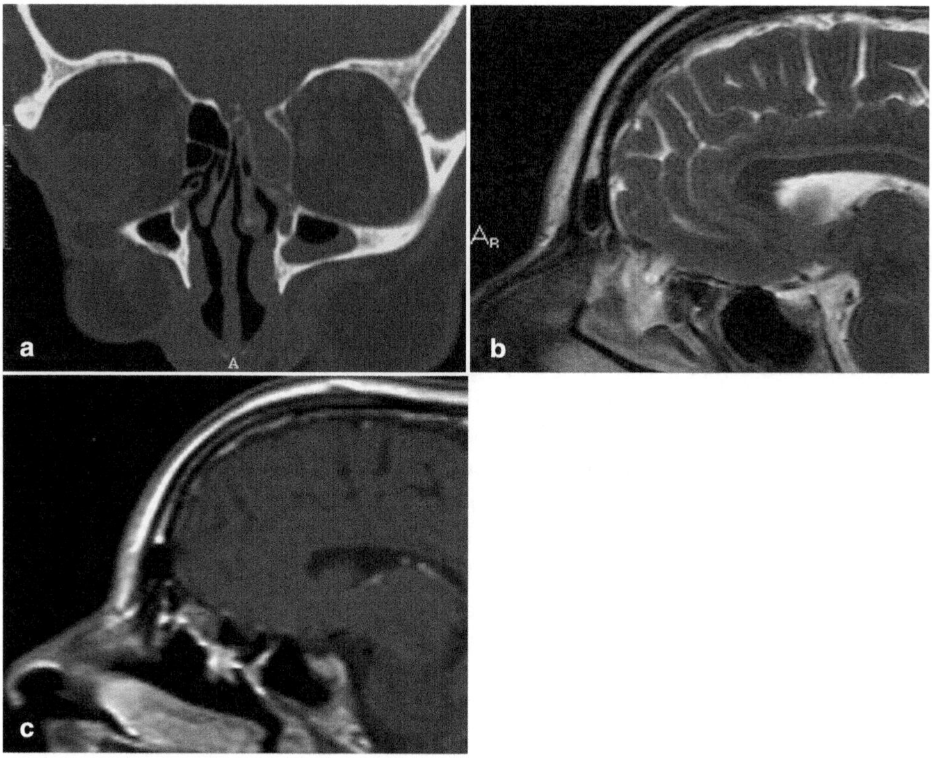


**Fig. 22.** Pre-operative neuroradiological studies showing a left ethmoidal meningoencephalocele. a) Coronal CT scan and b) sagittal MRI. c) Post-operative sagittal MRI, showing the complete removal of the meningoencephalocele and presence of reconstruction material in the anterior ethmoid

and posterior ethmoidal arteries or the papyracea, to avoid complications especially to the orbit.

## *Approaches to the cavernous sinus and lateral recess of the sphenoid sinus (LRSS)*

Different types of transcranial approaches have been adopted and popularized for the treatment of the cavernous sinus pathologies [44, 119, 135]. However these approaches require neuro-vascular manipulation and are related to a significant rate of morbidity and mortality. In order to reduce the risk of cranial nerves damage, a variety of transsphenoidal, transmaxillary, transmaxillosphenoidal, transethmoidal and transsphenoethmoidal microsurgical approaches have been proposed over the past two decades to remove lesions involving the anterior portion of the cavernous sinus [32, 37, 50, 54, 71, 75, 96, 99, 126]. These extradural approaches offer direct access to the anterior portion of the

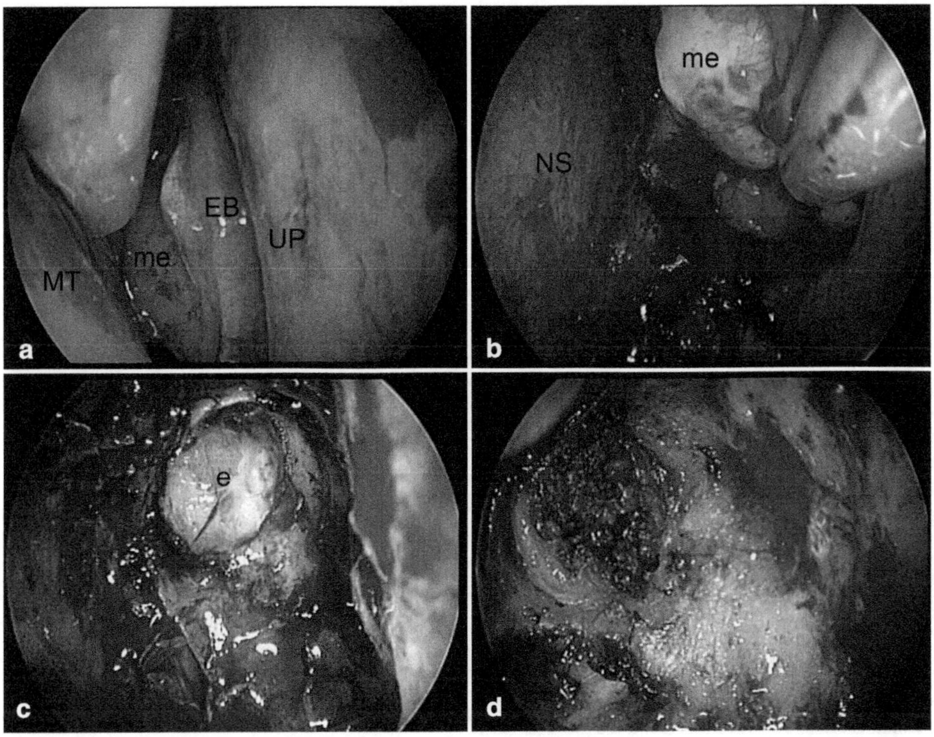


**Fig. 23.** Endoscopic endonasal removal of the meningoencephalocele showed in Fig. 22. a) Passing laterally to the middle turbinate, the meningoencephalocele becomes immediately visible. b) After removal of the middle turbinate, the sac of the meningoencephalocele is better identificated. c) After the removal of the meningeal layer, the encephalocele is identificated. d) The encephalocele is coagulated. *e* Encephalocele; *NS* nasal septum; *MT* middle turbinate; *EB* ethmoid bulla; *UP* uncinate process; *me* meningoencephalocele

cavernous sinus, but are limited by a deep, narrow surgical corridor that does not allow either an adequate exposure of the surgical field, specially of the lateral compartment of the cavernous sinus. The increasing use of the endoscope in transsphenoidal pituitary surgery has led some authors to consider the feasibility of the endoscopic transsphenoidal approach in the treatment of selected lesions arising from or involving this area, such as pituitary adenomas and chordomas [55, 83].

Different endoscopic endonasal surgical corridors have been described to gain access to different areas of the cavernous sinus [2, 55]. These corridors have been related to the position of the intracavernous carotid artery (ICA). The first approach permits access to a compartment of the cavernous sinus medial to the ICA, while a second approach allows access to a compartment lateral to the ICA.

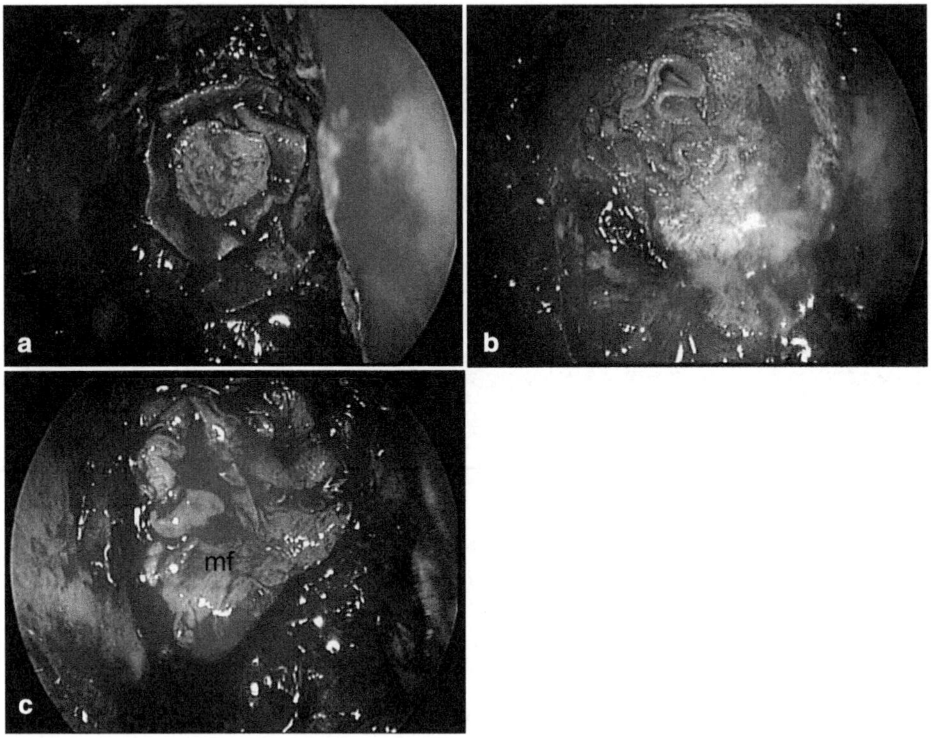


**Fig. 24.** Endoscopic endonasal removal of the meningoencephalocele showed in Fig. 22. Reconstruction of the bone and dural defects a, b) a single layer of dural substitute (bovine pericardium) and a sized piece of LactoSorb® have been positioned extradurally on the bone-dural defect and pushed intradurally. c) The reconstruction is completed with the positioning of the muchoperichondrium harvested from the middle turbinate. *mf* Mucosal flap

- *Approach to the medial compartment of the cavernous sinus*

The approach to the medial compartment is indicated for lesions arising from the sella and projecting through the medial wall of the cavernous sinus, without extension into the lateral compartment. Actually it is mainly indicated in cases of pituitary adenomas. The procedure begins with the introduction of the endoscope through the nostril controlateral to the parasellar extension of the lesion. This because the endoscopic approach is paramedian and the view provided by the endoscope is much wider on the contralateral side. After the sphenoidotomy and the accurate identification of all the bony landmarks on the sphenoid sinus posterior wall, the sellar floor and the dura are widely opened on the same side of the parasellar extension of the lesion. After the removal of the intra-suprasellar portion of pituitary adenoma, the intracavernous portion of the lesion is faced. The tumor itself enlarges the C-shaped parasellar carotid artery, thus making easier the suctioning and the curettage through this corridor. The completeness of the lesion removal is confirmed by the venous bleeding, easily controlled with irrigation and temporary sellar packing with haemostatic agents and/or cottonoids.

- *Approach to the lateral compartment of the cavernous sinus and to the lateral recess of the sphenoid sinus (LRSS)*

  The approach to the lateral compartment is indicated in the case of tumors involving the entire cavernous sinus and arising from the sella, such as pituitary adenomas, or lesions coming from surrounding areas (middle cranial fossa, clivus, pterygopalatine fossa), such as chordomas and chondrosarcomas. This approach is ipsilateral to the parasellar extension of the lesion. In the nasal phase of the approach, the surgical corridor is created by the removal of the middle turbinate, the lateralization of the middle turbinate in the other nostril and the removal of the posterior part of the nasal septum. The anterior wall of the sphenoid sinus and its septa are then widely removed in order to expose all the landmarks on the posterior wall of the sphenoid sinus. The bulla ethmoidalis and the anterior and posterior ethmoid cells are removed on the same side of the parasellar extension of the lesion, to create a wide surgical corridor between the nasal septum and the lamina papiracea. In order to preserve the medial wall of the orbit and the anterior and posterior ethmoidal arteries, an extensive lateral and superior surgical exposure has to be avoided while anterior and posterior ethmoid cells are opened.

  The nasal mucosa covering the vertical process of the palatine bone is dissected around the tail of the middle turbinate and carried upwards to identify the spheno-palatine foramen. The orbital process of the palatine bone and part of the posterior wall of the maxillary sinus are removed. The spheno-palatine artery is then isolated with bipolar coagulation or the use of haemoclip, if necessary At this point the medial pterygoid process is removed, with the microdrill providing a direct access to the lateral recess of the sphenoid sinus (LRSS) and thus to the lateral compartment of the cavernous sinus.

  Once the anterior face of the lesion has been exposed, before opening the dura, the use of Neuronavigation and the micro-Doppler is mandatory in identifying the exact position of the ICA. The tumor removal proceeds from the extracavernous to the intracavernous portion. In the case of tumours occupying mainly the lateral compartment of the cavernous sinus, the growth of the lesion usually displaces the ICA medially and pushies the cranial nerves laterally. The dura is then opened as far as possible from the ICA, which, in case of pituitary adenomas, allows the lesion to emerge under pressure. Delicate manouveres of curettage and suction usually allow the removal of the parasellar portion of the lesion, in the same fashion as for the intrasellar portion. Only after the removal has been completed will some bleeding begin, which is usually easily controlled with the use of hemostatic agents.

### *Approach to the clivus, cranio-vertebral junction and anterior portion of the foramen magnum*

The retroclival area and the cranio-vertebral junction can be involved in numerous and different disorders: intradural and extradural tumors, bone malformations, inflammatory diseases and trauma. Several approaches to these regions have been developed through anterior, antero-lateral and postero-lateral routes [6, 34, 36, 67, 93, 104, 111, 118, 128]. The most physiological and shortest route to the clival area and the anterior aspect of the cranio-vertebral junction is represented by an anterior approach through the pharynx. The transoral approach has been mainly used for treatment of extradural lesions and craniovertebral junction decompression and some authors have reported the treatment of intradural lesions [35, 72, 116]. The endoscope through the nose has been used for the management of clival lesions and more recently also for lesions located at the CVJ, either extradural [59, 84, 87, 89, 90] or intradural

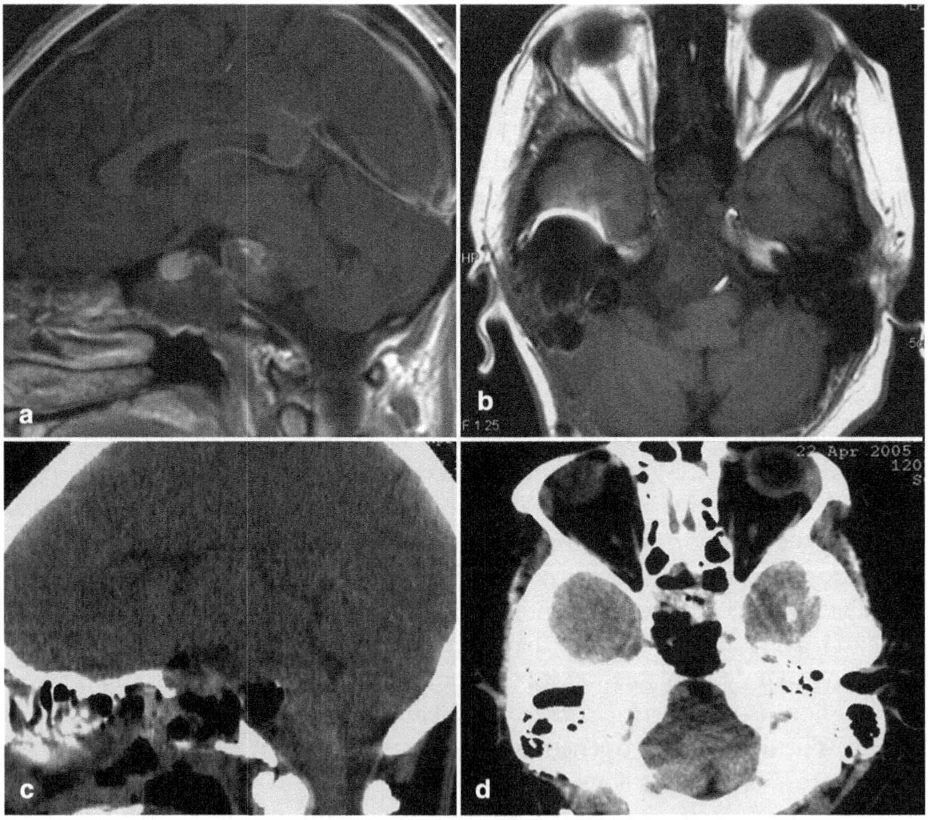


**Fig. 25.** a, b) Sagittal and coronal pre-operative MRI images showing a case of clival chordoma. c, d) Sagittal and coronal post-operative CT images of the same patient showing the subtotal removal of the lesion

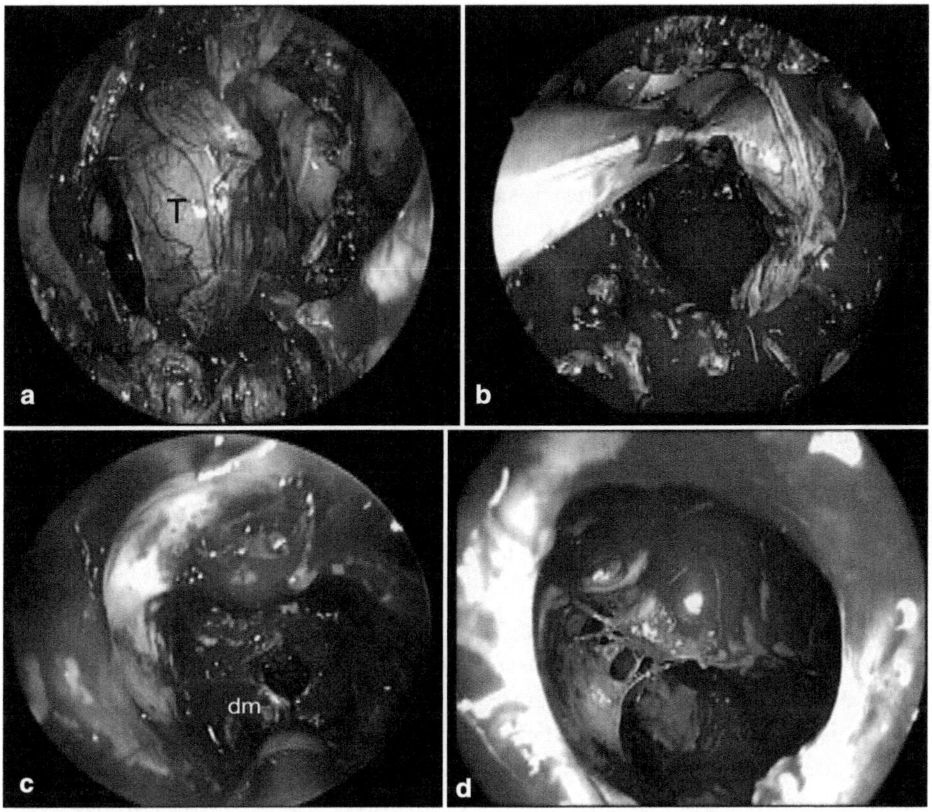


**Fig. 26.** Intraoperative pictures of the case of clival cordoma showed in Fig. 25. a) After performing the anterior sphenoidotomy, the tumor becomes immediately visible. b) The tumor has completely eroded the clival bone and is removed in piecemeal fashion after central debulking. c) After removal of the extradural portion of the tumor, a dural defect was identificated. d) Close up view through the dural defect during the intradural removal of the tumor mass

[89, 139] (see Figs. 25 and 26). The endoscopic endonasal approach provides the same advantages of direct route and minimal neurovascular manipulation offered by the transoral approach, but with a wider and closer view. Furthermore it avoids some of the disadvantages related to the transoral approach, such as the need for mouth retractors and splitting of the soft palate. However these approaches actually share some limits, that are the inadequate exposure of the lateral aspects of large tumors and the risk of meningitis and cerebrospinal fluid (CSF) leak, specially in case of intradural extension of the lesion.

- *Surgical procedure*

The access to the clivus needs a lower trajectory in respect to that necessary for the sellar region. After the preliminary steps (middle turbinectomy, removal of the posterior par of the nasal septum, wide sphenoidotomy) the procedure goes on with the removal of the inferior wall of the sphenoid sinus up to identify the Vidian nerves, that represent the lateral limits of the surgical corridor. The vomer and the inferior wall of the sphenoid sinus are completely removed, preserving the mucosa covering these structures, in order to create an useful mucosal flap for the closure of the surgical field. The bone of the clivus, according with the surgical necessity, is drilled and removed. At the level of the sphenoidal portion of the clivus the approach is limited laterally by the bony protuberances of intracavernous carotid artery. Furthermore it is important to highlight that the abducens nerve enters the cavernous sinus by passing through the basilar sinus medially than the paraclival tract of the intracavernous carotid artery; therefore particular attention should be paid during bone removal in this area in order to avoid damage to this nerve. In case of lower extension of the lesion, it is possible to extend downward the bone removal up to the C2 vertebral body.

## *Reconstruction techniques*

Reconstruction of the sella is a fundamental step of the procedure, either in microsurgical and endoscopic transsphenoidal surgery [13, 21, 137]. During an extended endoscopic endonasal approach, especially to the suprasellar area or to the clivus, a large osteo-dural opening is usually necessary and the subarachnoid space is often deliberatively entered. As a matter of facts, the creation of an intraoperative CSF leakage could be considered part of the surgical technique in extended transsphenoidal approach. Thus, the presence of a conspicuous intraoperative CSF leakage requires effective closures techniques to successfully avoid postoperative CSF leaks and the related undesirable complications (namely, meningitis and hypertensive pneumocephalus). Such complications are directly related with the failure of the skull base reconstruction at the end of the operation and the consequent postoperative CSF leak, which has been reported to as high as 65% of cases; however, it ranges from 9 to 21% [45, 49, 60, 61, 85, 91, 138]. Bacterial meningitis has been reported ranging from 0.5 to 14% [10, 30, 49, 51, 85] while tension pneoumocephalus occurs in fewer than 0.5% of cases and can be precipitated by lumbar CSF diversion in presence of an inadequate cranial base reconstruction [7, 49, 131, 132].

The presence of large osteo-dural defects makes inadequate the use of the conventional sellar floor reconstruction techniques, even though the criteria remain the same. During these extended approaches, the brain pulsation exerts high pressures over the wide skull base defect. For this reason a hard but easy to shape material is needed to create an initial barrier against the cranial pressure. In the majority of cases a synthetic copolymer of 82% polylactic acid and 18% polyglycolic acid (LactoSorb, Walter Lorenz Surgical, Inc., Jacksonville, FL) has been used. It becomes malleable at a temperature of 70°, making it easy to be shaped according to the defects, and becomes rigid in few seconds of cooling at room temperature. It is completely reabsorbed within 1 year, decreasing the risk of foreign body reaction. As a dural substitute, that has to be combined with the bone substitute, the human pericardium is used (Tutoplast®). This material is very malleable, easy to cut with scissors and also simple to distend over the skull base defect.

In our experience [26], we have adopted three different reconstruction techniques, according with the different surgical conditions.

1. Intradural reconstruction (so-called inlay). This type of reconstruction is easily performed when the size of the bony and dural openings coincide. A large fragment of dehydrated human pericardium is positioned to cover the entire dural and bony defect. Then, a piece of Lactosorb®, that has been previously cut slightly larger than the dural opening, is gently pushed against the dural substitute through the dural edges. In this way the dural substitute is transposed intradurally, as well as the fragment of Lactosorb®, remaining extradural the exceeding borders of the pericardium (see Fig. 27).
2. Intra-extradural reconstruction (inlay-overlay). This technique can be realized only when the dural window is smaller than the bony defect. A fragment of pericardium is fashioned and cut to a size a little bit larger than that of the dural window. The soft consistence of this material permits its easy insertion in an underlay position. A piece of Lactosorb® is then embedded extradurally, in a manner such that it is supported by at least two opposed edges of the bony defect, thus totally covering the dural defect beneath (see Fig. 28).

**Fig. 27.** Schematic drawings showing the so-called intradural (inlay) technique

**Fig. 28.** Schematic drawings showing the intra-extradural (inlay-overlay) technique

3. Extradural reconstruction (overlay). A large piece of human pericardium is placed over the bony defect, but the fragment of Lactosorb® is embedded in the extradural space dragging the dural substitute in overlay position. This kind of reconstruction seems to provide the most effective watertight barrier against CSF (see Fig. 29).

**Fig. 29.** Schematic drawings showing the extradural (overlay) technique

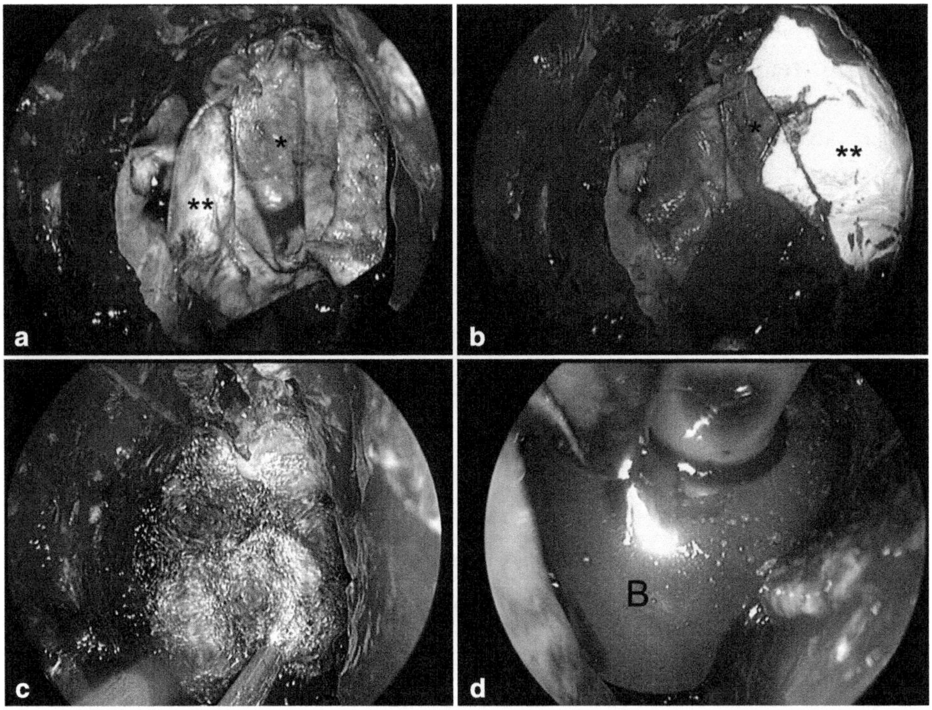


**Fig. 30.** Intraoperative image of the extradural (overlay) technique. a) The fragments of Tutoplast® and Lactosorb® are in the extradural space and the exceeding borders of the dural substitute cover the surrounding bone. b) A multilayer apposition of dural substitute was performed. c) Packing of the sphenoid sinus was performed with surgicel and fibrin glue. d) A 12-French Foley catheter inflated with 8 cc of saline solution was positioned in front of the sphenoid sinus to hold the reconstruction materials. * Lactosorb®; ** Tutoplast®; *B* balloon

After the osteo-dural defect has been sealed, the reconstruction continues with the packing of the sphenoid sinus.

Fragments of dural substitute are placed in multilayer fashion on the posterior wall of the sphenoid sinus, covering the skull base defect and the surrounding bone, where the mucosa has been stripped to favor adherence. The remaining sphenoid cavity is filled with surgicel and fibrin glue. The vascularized mucoperichondral septal flap, prepared at the beginning of the operation, as previously described, is then used to cover the skull base defect and the entire posterior wall of the sphenoid sinus [66]. An inflated Foley catheter (12–14 French), filled with 7–8 cc of physiologic solution, is placed in front of the sphenoid sinus cavity, to support the reconstruction (see Fig. 30). The Foley catheter is usually removed five days after the operation. After its removal an endoscopic inspection of the nasal cavities is performed, to check the correct positioning of the reconstruction materials and the eventual presence of CSF leak. Postoperative lumbar CSF drainage is not usually used.

## Results and complications

Between January 2004 and April 2006 we performed 33 extended endonasal transsphenoidal approaches for lesions arising from or involving the sellar region and the surrounding areas. The most representative pathologies of this series were the ten craniopharyngiomas, the six giant adenomas and the five meningiomas; we also used this procedure in three cases of chordomas, three of Rathke's cleft cysts and three of meningo-encephaloceles, one case of optic nerve glioma, one olfactory groove neuroendocrine tumor and one case of fibro-osseous dysplasia. Twenty patients were females and thirteen were males (mean age 47, 3 years) (see Table 1).

**Table 1.** *Patient series*

| Disease | No. of cases |
|---|---|
| Tuberculum sellae meningiomas | 4 |
| Clival meningioma | 1 |
| Craniopahryngiomas | 10 |
| Rathke's cleft cysts | 3 |
| Giant pituitary adenomas | 6 |
| Meningo-encephaloceles | 3 |
| Clival chordomas | 3 |
| Optic nerve glioma | 1 |
| Olphactory groove neuroendocrine tumor | 1 |
| Fibro-osseous displasia | 1 |
| Total | 33 |

**Table 2.** *Craniopharyngiomas' series*

| Age/sex | Tumor location | Tumor charac-teristics | Pre-operative signs | Pre-operative visual symptoms | Previous surgical procedures | Tumor removal | Complications | Postoperative endocrinol outcome | Post-operative visual outcome |
|---|---|---|---|---|---|---|---|---|---|
| 70, F | Infrasellar Suprasellar | Cystic | – | BT hemianopia | Transcranial approach | Total | – | – | Improved |
| 58, M | Infrasellar Suprasellar | Solid | Pan HP DI | BT hemianopia AD (R 1/200; L 1/20) | Trans-sphenoidal approach | Subtotal | CSF leak | Unchanged | Improved |
| 68, M | Intra-extraventricular | Solid | – | SBT quadrantopia | – | Total | – | Pan-HP | Improved |
| 63, M | Suprasellar | Cystic + Solid | – | BT hemianopia AD (R 1/30) | Transcranial approach | Subtotal | – | – | Improved |
| 58, M | Intra-extraventricular | Cystic + Solid | Pan HP DI | – | Transcranial approach | Total | – | Unchanged | – |
| 57, M | Intraventricular | Solid | Pan HP | BT hemianopia AD (L 1/30) | – | Total | CSF leak DI | Unchanged | Improved |
| 47, F | Intra-extraventricular | Cystic + Solid | DI | AD (R 1/30; L 2/10) | – | Partial | – | Unchanged | Improved R Worsening L |
| 57, F | Intra-extraventricular + Hydrocephalus | Cystic + Solid | Progressive neurological deterioration | – | – | Total | Brainstem hemorrhage | – | – |
| 68, M | Intra-extraventricular | Cystic + Solid | Pan HP | BT hemianopia AD (R 6/10; L 3/10) | – | – | DI CSDH | Unchanged | Improved |
| 26, F | Intra-extraventricular | Cystic + Solid | Hyperprolact | – | – | Total | DI | Unchanged | – |

*N* Normal size; *Pan HP* panhypopituitarism; *DI* diabetes insipidus; *BT* bitemporal; *SBT* superior bitemporal; *VA* visual acuity; *CSDH* chronic subdural hematoma.

Tumor removal, as assessed by post-operative MRI, revealed complete removal of the lesion in 2/6 pituitary adenomas, 7/10 craniopharyngiomas (see Table 2), 4/5 meningiomas, 3/3 Rathke's cleft cyst, 3/3 meningo-encephalocele. Subtotal removal (>80% based on the three-month post-operative 1.5 Tesla sellar MRI) was obtained in the four giant pituitary adenomas (3 non-functioning and 1 PRL-secreting) because of the extensive involvement of one or both the cavernous sinuses, in 3 craniopharyngiomas, in one clival meningioma, in one chordoma, and either in the case of optic nerve glioma and olphactory groove neuroendocrine tumor. Finally only partial removal was possible for one craniopharyngioma and two chordomas and biopsy only was performed in the case of fibro-osseous dysplasia.

In two cases of craniopharyngiomas, the incomplete removal was due to the partial calcification of the lesion, firmly adherent to the left posterior cerebral artery in the first one, and of a portion of capsule to the right optic nerve in the other. One patient underwent a partial removal because the pituitary stalk and the infundibular recess of the third ventricle were diffusely involved by the lesion and some remnants were intentionally left to avoid making pituitary function worse in the young patient.

Of 13 subjects with pre-operative visual function defects, three patients with meningioma had a complete recovery and six, who had a craniopharyngioma, improved; in one patient with a giant non-functioning pituitary macroadenoma, a preoperative severe bitemporal haemianopia occurred postoperatively further worsening vision in the left eye, with the only persistence of the light perception. We observed worsening of visual acuity in one eye and improvement in the other in three cases; the first one was a patient with craniopharyngioma, the second was the patient with the optic nerve glioma and the third was a patient with an infra-extraventricular craniopharyngioma.

Concerning surgical complications, 3 patients, two with a craniopharyngioma, one with a clival meningioma and one with a recurrent giant pituitary macroadenoma involving the entire left cavernous sinus, developed a CSF leak and a second operation was necessary in order to review the cranial base reconstruction and seal the leak. One of them (the patient with the giant Knosp grade 4 pituitary adenoma) developed a bacterial meningitis, which resolved after a cycle of intravenous antibiotic therapy with no permanent neurological deficits. One patient with an intra-suprasellar non-functioning adenoma presented with a generalized epileptic seizure a few hours after the surgical procedure, due to the intraoperative massive CSF loss and consequent presence of intracranial air. In one case of craniopharyngioma immediately after the procedure we observed rapid worsening of the level of consciousness and bilateral midriasis. CT scan showed a brain stem haemorrhage. The patient died few days later.

Pituitary dysfunction did not improve in any patient who already had some degree of pituitary hypofunction; however only one postoperative additional hypopituitarism was reported. In three cases of craniopharyngioma and in one case of meningioma a new permanent diabetes insipidus was observed. One patient developed a sphenoid sinus mycosis, cured with antimycotic therapy. Epistaxis and airway difficulties were never observed.

## Conclusions

The endoscope, after Gerard Guiot's first attempt to explore the sellar cavity following the lesion removal [65] and, then, after the endonasal experience of the ENT surgeons in Functional Endoscopic Sinus Surgery (FESS) [94, 141, 142, 145], has gained a stable position in transsphenoidal surgery, due to its vision inside the anatomy that offers wider view of the target area and permits to perform less invasive approaches.

The experience in surgery of the sellar region, the wide area of vision of the endoscope and the attainment of a specific endoscopic skill have gradually permitted to extend the area of the approach to the suprasellar, parasellar and infrasellar regions. The target of the surgical deed in transnasal surgery can be directed towards pathologies once approachable only with the more invasive transcranial surgery [8, 14, 15, 19, 39, 81]. Indeed, such extended endoscopic approaches, although at a first glance might be considered something that everyone can do, require an advanced and specialized training, either in the lab, with *ad hoc* anatomical dissections, and in the operating room, after having performed a sufficient number of standard sellar operations and having become familiar with the endoscopic skill, endoscopic anatomy and complication avoidance and management.

It is difficult today to define the boundaries and the future limits of the transsphenoidal extended approaches because the work is still in progress, but the train has moved and is bringing with it technical advances of which we think that patients and young generations will benefit.

## Acknowledgements

To Manfred Tschabitscher, MD, Professor of Anatomy at the University of Wien, who has guided our group along these last ten years of endoscopic transsphenoidal surgery.

## References

1. Al-Mefty O, Ayoubi S, Smith RR (1991) The petrosal approach: indications, technique, and results. Acta Neurochir Suppl 53: 166–170
2. Alfieri A, Jho HD (2001) Endoscopic endonasal approaches to the cavernous sinus: surgical approaches. Neurosurgery 49: 354–362

3. Alfieri A, Jho HD (2001) Endoscopic endonasal cavernous sinus surgery: an anatomic study. Neurosurgery 48: 827–837
4. Arita K, Kurisu K, Tominaga A, Kawamoto H, Iida K, Mizoue T, Pant B, Uozumi T (1998) Trans-sellar color Doppler ultrasonography during transsphenoidal surgery. Neurosurgery 42: 81–85; discussion 86
5. Baskin DS, Wilson CB (1986) Surgical management of craniopharyngiomas. A review of 74 cases. J Neurosurg 65: 22–27
6. Bertalanffy H, Seeger W (1991) The dorsolateral, suboccipital, transcondylar approach to the lower clivus and anterior portion of the craniocervical junction. Neurosurgery 29: 815–821
7. Candrina R, Galli G, Rossi M, Bollati A (1989) Tension pneumocephalus after transsphenoidal surgery for acromegaly. J Neurosurg Sci 33: 311–315
8. Cappabianca P, Alfieri A, de Divitiis E (1998) Endoscopic endonasal transsphenoidal approach to the sella: towards functional endoscopic pituitary surgery (FEPS). Minim Invasive Neurosurg 41: 66–73
9. Cappabianca P, Alfieri A, Thermes S, Buonamassa S, de Divitiis E (1999) Instruments for endoscopic endonasal transsphenoidal surgery. Neurosurgery 45: 392–395; discussion 395–396
10. Cappabianca P, Cavallo LM, Colao A, de Divitiis E (2002) Surgical complications associated with the endoscopic endonasal transsphenoidal approach for pituitary adenomas. J Neurosurg 97: 293–298
11. Cappabianca P, Cavallo LM, de Divitiis E (2004) Endoscopic endonasal transsphenoidal surgery. Neurosurgery 55: 933–940; discussion 940–931
12. Cappabianca P, Cavallo LM, Esposito F, de Divitiis E (2004) Endoscopic endonasal transsphenoidal surgery: procedure, endoscopic equipment and instrumentation. Childs Nerv Syst 20: 796–801
13. Cappabianca P, Cavallo LM, Esposito F, Valente V, De Divitiis E (2002) Sellar repair in endoscopic endonasal transsphenoidal surgery: results of 170 cases. Neurosurgery 51: 1365–1371; discussion 1371–1362
14. Cappabianca P, de Divitiis E (2007) Back to the Egyptians: neurosurgery via the nose. A five-thousand year history and the recent contribution of the endoscope. Neurosurg Rev 30: 1–7; discussion 7
15. Cappabianca P, de Divitiis E (2004) Endoscopy and transsphenoidal surgery. Neurosurgery 54: 1043–1048; discussions 1048–1050
16. Cappabianca P, de Divitiis O, Maiuri F (2003) Evolution of transsphenoidal surgery. In: de Divitiis E, Cappabianca P (eds) Endoscopic endonasal transsphenoidal surgery. Springer, Wien New York, pp 1–7
17. Cappabianca P, Frank G, Pasquini E, de Divitiis O, Calbucci F (2003) Extended endoscopic endonasal transsphenoidal approaches to the suprasellar region, planum sphenoidale & clivus. In: de Divitiis E, Cappabianca P (eds) Endoscopic endonasal transsphenoidal surgery. Springer, Wien New York, pp 176–187
18. Carmel P (1993) Craniopharyngioma: transcranial approaches. In: Apuzzo ML (ed) Brain surgery: complication avoidance and management. Churchill Livingstone, New York, pp 339–356
19. Carrau RL, Jho HD, Ko Y (1996) Transnasal-transsphenoidal endoscopic surgery of the pituitary gland. Laryngoscope 106: 914–918

20. Carrau RL, Snyderman CH, Kassam AB, Jungreis CA (2001) Endoscopic and endoscopic-assisted surgery for juvenile angiofibroma. Laryngoscope 111: 483–487
21. Castelnuovo P, Locatelli D, Mauri S (2003) Extended endoscopic approaches to the skull base. Anterior cranial base CSF leaks. In: de Divitiis E, Cappabianca P (eds) Endoscopic endonasal transsphenoidal surgery. Springer, Wien New York, pp 137–158
22. Castelnuovo P, Pistochini A, Locatelli D (2006) Different surgical approaches to the sellar region: focusing on the "two nostrils four hands technique". Rhinology 44: 2–7
23. Cavallo LM, Cappabianca P, Galzio R, Iaconetta G, de Divitiis E, Tschabitscher M (2005) Endoscopic transnasal approach to the cavernous sinus versus transcranial route: anatomic study. Neurosurgery 56: 379–389
24. Cavallo LM, de Divitiis O, Aydin S, Messina A, Esposito F, Iaconetta G, Talat K, Cappabianca P, Tschabitscher M (2007) Extended endoscopic endonasal transsphenoidal approach to the suprasellar area. Anatomic considerations: Part 1. Neurosurgery (in press)
25. Cavallo LM, Messina A, Cappabianca P, Esposito F, de Divitiis E, Gardner P, Tschabitscher M (2005) Endoscopic endonasal surgery of the midline skull base: anatomical study and clinical considerations. Neurosurg Focus 19: E2
26. Cavallo LM, Messina A, Esposito F, de Divitiis O, Dal Fabbro M, de Divitiis E, Cappabianca P (2007) Skull base reconstruction in extended endoscopic transsphenoidal approach for supra-sellar lesions. J Neurosurg (in press)
27. Chanda A, Nanda A (2002) Partial labyrinthectomy petrous apicectomy approach to the petroclival region: an anatomic and technical study. Neurosurgery 51: 147–159; discussion 159–160
28. Cho CW, Al-Mefty O (2002) Combined petrosal approach to petroclival meningiomas. Neurosurgery 51: 708–716; discussion 716–708
29. Cinalli G, Cappabianca P, de Falco R, Spennato P, Cianciulli E, Cavallo LM, Esposito F, Ruggiero C, Maggi G, de Divitiis E (2005) Current state and future development of intracranial neuroendoscopic surgery. Expert Rev Med Devices 2: 351–373
30. Ciric I, Ragin A, Baumgartner C, Pierce D (1997) Complications of transsphenoidal surgery: results of a national survey, review of the literature, and personal experience. Neurosurgery 40: 225–236; discussion 236–227
31. Cook SW, Smith Z, Kelly DF (2004) Endonasal transsphenoidal removal of tuberculum sellae meningiomas: technical note. Neurosurgery 55: 239–244; discussion 244–236
32. Couldwell WT, Sabit I, Weiss MH, Giannotta SL, Rice D (1997) Transmaxillary approach to the anterior cavernous sinus: a microanatomic study. Neurosurgery 40: 1307–1311
33. Couldwell WT, Weiss MH, Rabb C, Liu JK, Apfelbaum RI, Fukushima T (2004) Variations on the standard transsphenoidal approach to the sellar region, with emphasis on the extended approaches and parasellar approaches: surgical experience in 105 cases. Neurosurgery 55: 539–547; discussion 547–550
34. Crockard HA, Pozo JL, Ransford AO, Stevens JM, Kendall BE, Essigman WK (1986) Transoral decompression and posterior fusion for rheumatoid atlanto-axial subluxation. J Bone Joint Surg Br 68: 350–356
35. Crockard HA, Sen CN (1991) The transoral approach for the management of intradural lesions at the craniovertebral junction: review of 7 cases. Neurosurgery 28: 88–97; discussion 97–88
36. Crumley RL, Gutin PH (1989) Surgical access for clivus chordoma. The University of California, San Francisco, experience. Arch Otolaryngol Head Neck Surg 115: 295–300

37. Das K, Spencer W, Nwagwu CI, Schaeffer S, Wenk E, Weiss MH, Couldwell WT (2001) Approaches to the sellar and parasellar region: anatomic comparison of endonasal-transsphenoidal, sublabial-transsphenoidal, and transethmoidal approaches. Neurol Res 23: 51–54
38. de Divitiis E (2006) Endoscopic transsphenoidal surgery: stone-in-the-pond effect. Neurosurgery 59: 512–520
39. de Divitiis E, Cappabianca P (2002) Endoscopic endonasal transsphenoidal surgery. In: Pickard JD (ed) Advances and technical standards in neurosurgery. Springer, Wien New York, pp 137–177
40. de Divitiis E, Cappabianca P, Cavallo LM (2002) Endoscopic transsphenoidal approach: adaptability of the procedure to different sellar lesions. Neurosurgery 51: 699–705; discussion 705–697
41. de Divitiis E, Cavallo LM, Cappabianca P, Esposito F (2007) Extended endoscopic endonasal transsphenoidal approach for the removal of suprasellar tumors: part 2. Neurosurgery 60: 46–58; discussion 58–49
42. Delashaw JB Jr, Tedeschi H, Rhoton AL (1992) Modified supraorbital craniotomy: technical note. Neurosurgery 30: 954–956
43. Doglietto F, Prevedello DM, Jane JA Jr, Han J, Laws ER Jr (2005) Brief history of endoscopic transsphenoidal surgery – from Philipp Bozzini to the First World Congress of Endoscopic Skull Base Surgery. Neurosurg Focus 19: E3
44. Dolenc VV, Lipovsek M, Slokan S (1999) Traumatic aneurysm and carotid-cavernous fistula following transsphenoidal approach to a pituitary adenoma: treatment by transcranial operation. Br J Neurosurg 13: 185–188
45. Dusick JR, Esposito F, Kelly DF, Cohan P, DeSalles A, Becker DP, Martin NA (2005) The extended direct endonasal transsphenoidal approach for nonadenomatous suprasellar tumors. J Neurosurg 102: 832–841
46. Elias WJ, Chadduck JB, Alden TD, Laws ER Jr (1999) Frameless stereotaxy for transsphenoidal surgery. Neurosurgery 45: 271–275; discussion 275–277
47. Erdogmus S, Govsa F (2006) The anatomic landmarks of ethmoidal arteries for the surgical approaches. J Craniofac Surg 17: 280–285
48. Esposito F, Becker DP, Villablanca JP, Kelly DF (2005) Endonasal transsphenoidal transclival removal of prepontine epidermoid tumors: technical note. Neurosurgery 56: E443
49. Esposito F, Dusick JR, Fatemi N, Kelly DF (2007) Graded repair of cranial base defects and cerebrospinal fluid leaks in transsphenoidal surgery. Neurosurgery 60: ONS1–ONS9
50. Fahlbusch R, Buchfelder M (1988) Transsphenoidal surgery of parasellar pituitary adenomas. Acta Neurochir (Wien) 92: 93–99
51. Fahlbusch R, Honegger J, Buchfelder M (1996) Clinical features and management of craniopharyngiomas in adults. In: Tindall GT, Cooper PR, Barrow DL (eds) The practice of neurosurgery. Williams & Wilkins, Baltimore, pp 1159–1173
52. Fahlbusch R, Honegger J, Paulus W, Huk W, Buchfelder M (1999) Surgical treatment of craniopharyngiomas: experience with 168 patients. J Neurosurg 90: 237–250
53. Fahlbusch R, Schott W (2002) Pterional surgery of meningiomas of the tuberculum sellae and planum sphenoidale: surgical results with special consideration of ophthalmological and endocrinological outcomes. J Neurosurg 96: 235–243
54. Fraioli B, Esposito V, Santoro A, Iannetti G, Giuffre R, Cantore G (1995) Transmaxillosphenoidal approach to tumors invading the medial compartment of the cavernous sinus. J Neurosurg 82: 63–69

55. Frank G, Pasquini E (2003) Approach to the cavernous sinus. In: de Divitiis E, Cappabianca P (eds) Endoscopic endonasal transsphenoidal surgery. Springer, Wien New York, pp 159–175
56. Frank G, Pasquini E (2002) Endoscopic endonasal approaches to the cavernous sinus: surgical approaches. Neurosurgery 50: 675
57. Frank G, Pasquini E, Doglietto F, Mazzatenta D, Sciarretta V, Farneti G, Calbucci F (2006) The endoscopic extended transsphenoidal approach for craniopharyngiomas. Neurosurgery 59: ONS75–ONS83
58. Frank G, Pasquini E, Mazzatenta D (2001) Extended transsphenoidal approach. J Neurosurg 95: 917–918
59. Frank G, Sciarretta V, Calbucci F, Farneti G, Mazzatenta D, Pasquini E (2006) The endoscopic transnasal transsphenoidal approach for the treatment of cranial base chordomas and chondrosarcomas. Neurosurgery 59: ONS50–ONS57; discussion ONS50–ONS57
60. Gardner PA, Kassam AB, Snyderman CH, Carrau RL, Minz A (2006) Outcomes following purely endoscopic endonasal resection of anterior skull base meningiomas. 17th Annual Meeting North American Skull Base Society, p S12
61. Gardner PA, Kassam AB, Snyderman CH, Carrau RL, Minz A (2006) Outcomes following purely endoscopic endonasal resection of suprasellar craniopharingiomas. 17th Annual Meeting North American Skull Base Society, pp S19–S20
62. Goel A, Desai K, Muzumdar D (2001) Surgery on anterior foramen magnum meningiomas using a conventional posterior suboccipital approach: a report on an experience with 17 cases. Neurosurgery 49: 102–106; discussion 106–107
63. Goel A, Muzumdar D, Desai KI (2002) Tuberculum sellae meningioma: a report on management on the basis of a surgical experience with 70 patients. Neurosurgery 51: 1358–1364
64. Grisoli F, Diaz-Vasquez P, Riss M, Vincentelli F, Leclercq TA, Hassoun J, Salamon G (1986) Microsurgical management of tuberculum sellae meningiomas. Results in 28 consecutive cases. Surg Neurol 26: 37–44
65. Guiot G (1973) Transsphenoidal approach in surgical treatment of pituitary adenomas: general principles and indications in non-functioning adenomas. In: Kohler PO, Ross GT (eds) Diagnosis and treatment of pituitary adenomas. Excerpta Medica, Amsterdam, pp 159–178
66. Hadad G, Bassagasteguy L, Carrau RL, Mataza JC, Kassam A, Snyderman CH, Mintz A (2006) A novel reconstructive technique after endoscopic expanded endonasal approaches: vascular pedicle nasoseptal flap. Laryngoscope 116: 1882–1886
67. Hadley MN, Spetzler RF, Sonntag VK (1989) The transoral approach to the superior cervical spine. A review of 53 cases of extradural cervicomedullary compression. J Neurosurg 71: 16–23
68. Hakuba A, Liu S, Nishimura S (1986) The orbitozygomatic infratemporal approach: a new surgical technique. Surg Neurol 26: 271–276
69. Hakuba A, Tanaka K, Suzuki T, Nishimura S (1989) A combined orbitozygomatic infratemporal epidural and subdural approach for lesions involving the entire cavernous sinus. J Neurosurg 71: 699–704
70. Hao SP, Wang HS, Lui TN (1995) Transnasal endoscopic management of basal encephalocele – craniotomy is no longer mandatory. Am J Otolaryngol 16: 196–199

71. Hashimoto N, Kikuchi H (1990) Transsphenoidal approach to infrasellar tumors involving the cavernous sinus. J Neurosurg 73: 513–517
72. Hayakawa T, Kamikawa K, Ohnishi T, Yoshimine T (1981) Prevention of postoperative complications after a transoral transclival approach to basilar aneurysms: technical note. J Neurosurg 54: 699–703
73. Honegger J, Buchfelder M, Fahlbusch R, Daubler B, Dorr HG (1992) Transsphenoidal microsurgery for craniopharyngioma. Surg Neurol 37: 189–196
74. Hosemann W, Nitsche N, Rettinger G, Wigand ME (1991) [Endonasal, endoscopically controlled repair of dura defects of the anterior skull base]. Laryngorhinootologie 70: 115–119
75. Inoue T, Rhoton AL Jr, Theele D, Barry ME (1990) Surgical approaches to the cavernous sinus: a microsurgical study. Neurosurgery 26: 903–932
76. Jallo GI, Benjamin V (2002) Tuberculum sellae meningiomas: microsurgical anatomy and surgical technique. Neurosurgery 51: 1432–1440
77. James D, Crockard HA (1991) Surgical access to the base of skull and upper cervical spine by extended maxillotomy. Neurosurgery 29: 411–416
78. Jane JA Jr, Han J, Prevedello DM, Jagannathan J, Dumont AS, Laws ER Jr (2005) Perspectives on endoscopic transsphenoidal surgery. Neurosurg Focus 19: E2
79. Javed T, Sekhar LN (1991) Surgical management of clival meningiomas. Acta Neurochir Suppl 53: 171–182
80. Jho HD (1999) Endoscopic pituitary surgery. Pituitary 2: 139–154
81. Jho HD, Carrau RL, Ko Y (1996) Endoscopic pituitary surgery. In: Wilkins H, Rengachary S (eds) Neurosurgical operative atlas. American Association of Neurological Surgeons, Park Ridge, pp 1–12
82. Jho HD, Ha HG (2004) Endoscopic endonasal skull base surgery: part 1. The midline anterior fossa skull base. Minim Invasive Neurosurg 47: 1–8
83. Jho HD, Ha HG (2004) Endoscopic endonasal skull base surgery: part 2. The cavernous sinus. Minim Invasive Neurosurg 47: 9–15
84. Jho HD, Ha HG (2004) Endoscopic endonasal skull base surgery: part 3. The clivus and posterior fossa. Minim Invasive Neurosurg 47: 16–23
85. Kaptain GJ, Vincent DA, Sheehan JP, Laws ER Jr (2001) Transsphenoidal approaches for the extracapsular resection of midline suprasellar and anterior cranial base lesions. Neurosurgery 49: 94–100; discussion 100–101
86. Kassam A, Snyderman CH, Mintz A, Gardner P, Carrau RL (2005) Expanded endonasal approach: the rostrocaudal axis: part I. Crista galli to the sella turcica. Neurosurg Focus 19: E3
87. Kassam A, Snyderman CH, Mintz A, Gardner P, Carrau RL (2005) Expanded endonasal approach: the rostrocaudal axis: part II. Posterior clinoids to the foramen magnum. Neurosurg Focus 19: E4
88. Kassam AB, Gardner P, Snyderman C, Mintz A, Carrau R (2005) Expanded endonasal approach: fully endoscopic, completely transnasal approach to the middle third of the clivus, petrous bone, middle cranial fossa, and infratemporal fossa. Neurosurg Focus 19: E6
89. Kassam AB, Mintz AH, Gardner PA, Horowitz MB, Carrau RL, Snyderman CH (2006) The expanded endonasal approach for an endoscopic transnasal clipping and aneurysmorrhaphy of a large vertebral artery aneurysm: technical case report. Neurosurgery 59: ONSE162–ONSE165

90. Kassam AB, Snyderman C, Gardner P, Carrau R, Spiro R (2005) The expanded endonasal approach: a fully endoscopic transnasal approach and resection of the odontoid process: technical case report. Neurosurgery 57: E213
91. Kato T, Sawamura Y, Abe H, Nagashima M (1998) Transsphenoidal-transtuberculum sellae approach for supradiaphragmatic tumours: technical note. Acta Neurochir (Wien) 140: 715–718; discussion 719
92. Kawase T, Shiobara R, Toya S (1991) Anterior transpetrosal-transtentorial approach for sphenopetroclival meningiomas: surgical method and results in 10 patients. Neurosurgery 28: 869–875; discussion 875–866
93. Kawashima M, Tanriover N, Rhoton AL Jr, Ulm AJ, Matsushima T (2003) Comparison of the far lateral and extreme lateral variants of the atlanto-occipital transarticular approach to anterior extradural lesions of the craniovertebral junction. Neurosurgery 53: 662–674; discussion 674–665
94. Kennedy DW (1985) Functional endoscopic sinus surgery. Technique. Arch Otolaryngol 111: 643–649
95. Kim J, Choe I, Bak K, Kim C, Kim N, Jang Y (2000) Transsphenoidal supradiaphragmatic intradural approach: technical note. Minim Invasive Neurosurg 43: 33–37
96. Kitano M, Taneda M (2001) Extended transsphenoidal approach with submucosal posterior ethmoidectomy for parasellar tumors. Technical note. J Neurosurg 94: 999–1004
97. Kouri JG, Chen MY, Watson JC, Oldfield EH (2000) Resection of suprasellar tumors by using a modified transsphenoidal approach. Report of four cases. J Neurosurg 92: 1028–1035
98. Lakhdar A, Sami A, Naja A, Achouri M, Ouboukhlik A, El Kamar A, El Azhari A (2003) Epidermoid cyst of the cerebellopontine angle. A surgical series of 10 cases and review of the literature. Neurochirurgie 49: 13–24
99. Lalwani AK, Kaplan MJ, Gutin PH (1992) The transsphenoethmoid approach to the sphenoid sinus and clivus. Neurosurgery 31: 1008–1014
100. Lang DA, Neil-Dwyer G, Iannotti F (1993) The suboccipital transcondylar approach to the clivus and cranio-cervical junction for ventrally placed pathology at and above the foramen magnum. Acta Neurochir (Wien) 125: 132–137
101. Lasio G, Ferroli P, Felisati G, Broggi G (2002) Image-guided endoscopic transnasal removal of recurrent pituitary adenomas. Neurosurgery 51: 132–136; discussion 136–137
102. Laufer I, Anand VK, Schwartz TH (2007) Endoscopic, endonasal extended transsphenoidal, transplanum transtuberculum approach for resection of suprasellar lesions. J Neurosurg 106: 400–406
103. Laws ER (1980) Transsphenoidal microsurgery in the management of craniopharyngioma. J Neurosurg 52: 661–666
104. Laws ER Jr (1984) Transsphenoidal surgery for tumors of the clivus. Otolaryngol Head Neck Surg 92: 100–101
105. Laws ER, Kanter AS, Jane JA Jr, Dumont AS (2005) Extended transsphenoidal approach. J Neurosurg 102: 825–827; discussion 827–828
106. Liu JK, Decker D, Schaefer SD, Moscatello AL, Orlandi RR, Weiss MH, Couldwell WT (2003) Zones of approach for craniofacial resection: minimizing facial incisions for resection of anterior cranial base and paranasal sinus tumors. Neurosurgery 53: 1126–1135; discussion 1135–1127

107. Liu JK, Weiss MH, Couldwell WT (2003) Surgical approaches to pituitary tumors. Neurosurg Clin N Am 14: 93–107
108. Locatelli D, Rampa F, Acchiardi I, Bignami M, De Bernardi F, Castelnuovo P (2006) Endoscopic endonasal approaches for repair of cerebrospinal fluid leaks: nine-year experience. Neurosurgery 58: ONS246–ONS256; discussion ONS256–ONS247
109. MacDonald JD, Antonelli P, Day AL (1998) The anterior subtemporal, medial transpetrosal approach to the upper basilar artery and ponto-mesencephalic junction. Neurosurgery 43: 84–89
110. Mason RB, Nieman LK, Doppman JL, Oldfield EH (1997) Selective excision of adenomas originating in or extending into the pituitary stalk with preservation of pituitary function. J Neurosurg 87: 343–351
111. Menezes AH, VanGilder JC (1988) Transoral-transpharyngeal approach to the anterior craniocervical junction. Ten-year experience with 72 patients. J Neurosurg 69: 895–903
112. Messerklinger W (1987) Role of the lateral nasal wall in the pathogenesis, diagnosis and therapy of recurrent and chronic rhinosinusitis. Laryngol Rhinol Otol (Stuttg) 66: 293–299
113. Miller E, Crockard HA (1987) Transoral transclival removal of anteriorly placed meningiomas at the foramen magnum. Neurosurgery 20: 966–968
114. Moon HJ, Kim HU, Lee JG, Chung IH, Yoon JH (2001) Surgical anatomy of the anterior ethmoidal canal in ethmoid roof. Laryngoscope 111: 900–904
115. Nakamura M, Samii M (2003) Surgical management of a meningioma in the retrosellar region. Acta Neurochir (Wien) 145: 215–219; discussion 219–220
116. Nanda A, Vincent DA, Vannemreddy PS, Baskaya MK, Chanda A (2002) Far-lateral approach to intradural lesions of the foramen magnum without resection of the occipital condyle. J Neurosurg 96: 302–309
117. Ohhashi G, Kamio M, Abe T, Otori N, Haruna S (2002) Endoscopic transnasal approach to the pituitary lesions using a navigation system (InstaTrak system): technical note. Minim Invasive Neurosurg 45: 120–123
118. Pasztor E, Vajda J, Piffko P, Horvath M, Gador I (1984) Transoral surgery for craniocervical space-occupying processes. J Neurosurg 60: 276–281
119. Perneczky A, Knosp E, Matula C (1988) Cavernous sinus surgery. Approach through the lateral wall. Acta Neurochir (Wien) 92: 76–82
120. Perneczky A, Muller-Forell W, van Lindert E, Fries G (1999) Keyhole concept in neurosurgery. Thieme, Stuttgart New York
121. Puxeddu R, Lui MW, Chandrasekar K, Nicolai P, Sekhar LN (2002) Endoscopic-assisted transcolumellar approach to the clivus: an anatomical study. Laryngoscope 112: 1072–1078
122. Rabadan A, Conesa H (1992) Transmaxillary-transnasal approach to the anterior clivus: a microsurgical anatomical model. Neurosurgery 30: 473–481; discussion 482
123. Raftopoulos C, Baleriaux D, Hancq S, Closset J, David P, Brotchi J (1995) Evaluation of endoscopy in the treatment of rare meningoceles: preliminary results. Surg Neurol 44: 308–317; discussion 317–308
124. Reisch R, Bettag M, Perneczky A (2001) Transoral transclival removal of anteriorly placed cavernous malformations of the brainstem. Surg Neurol 56: 106–115; discussion 115–106
125. Reisch R, Perneczky A (2005) Ten-year experience with the supraorbital subfrontal approach through an eyebrow skin incision. Neurosurgery 57: 242–255; discussion 242–255

126. Sabit I, Schaefer SD, Couldwell WT (2000) Extradural extranasal combined transmaxillary transsphenoidal approach to the cavernous sinus: a minimally invasive microsurgical model. Laryngoscope 110: 286–291
127. Samii M, Ammirati M (1988) The combined supra-infratentorial pre-sigmoid sinus avenue to the petro-clival region. Surgical technique and clinical applications. Acta Neurochir (Wien) 95: 6–12
128. Samii M, Klekamp J, Carvalho G (1996) Surgical results for meningiomas of the craniocervical junction. Neurosurgery 39: 1086–1094; discussion 1094–1085
129. Sandeman D, Moufid A (1998) Interactive image-guided pituitary surgery. An experience of 101 procedures. Neurochirurgie 44: 331–338
130. Sano K (1980) Temporo-polar approach to aneurysms of the basilar artery at and around the distal bifurcation: technical note. Neurol Res 2: 361–367
131. Satyarthee GD, Mahapatra AK (2003) Tension pneumocephalus following transsphenoid surgery for pituitary adenoma – report of two cases. J Clin Neurosci 10: 495–497
132. Sawka AM, Aniszewski JP, Young WF Jr, Nippoldt TB, Yancz P, Ebersold MJ (1999) Tension pneumocranium, a rare complication of transsphenoidal pituitary surgery: Mayo Clinic experience 1976–1998. J Clin Endocrinol Metab 84: 4731–4734
133. Schwartz TH, Stieg PE, Anand VK (2006) Endoscopic transsphenoidal pituitary surgery with intraoperative magnetic resonance imaging. Neurosurgery 58: ONS44–ONS51; discussion ONS44–ONS51
134. Seifert V, Raabe A, Zimmermann M (2003) Conservative (labyrinth-preserving) transpetrosal approach to the clivus and petroclival region – indications, complications, results and lessons learned. Acta Neurochir (Wien) 145: 631–642; discussion 642
135. Sekhar LN, Ross DA, Sen CN (1993) Cavernous sinus and sphenocavernous neoplasms. Anatomy and surgery. In: Sekhar LN, Janecka IP (eds) Surgery of cranial base tumors. Raven Press, New York, pp 521–604
136. Sepehrnia A, Knopp U (2002) The combined subtemporal-suboccipital approach: a modified surgical access to the clivus and petrous apex. Minim Invasive Neurosurg 45: 102–104
137. Spaziante R, E. dD, Cappabianca P, Zona G (2006) Repair of the sella following transsphenoidal surgery. In: Schmidek HH, Roberts DW (eds) Chmidek and sweet operative neurosurgical techniques indications, methods and results. W. B. Saunders, Philadelphia, pp 390–408
138. Spencer WR, Levine JM, Couldwell WT, Brown-Wagner M, Moscatello A (2000) Approaches to the sellar and parasellar region: a retrospective comparison of the endonasal-transsphenoidal and sublabial-transsphenoidal approaches. Otolaryngol Head Neck Surg 122: 367–369
139. Stamm AC, Pignatari SS, Vellutini E (2006) Transnasal endoscopic surgical approaches to the clivus. Otolaryngol Clin North Am 39: 639–656, xi
140. Stamm AM (2006) Transnasal endoscopy-assisted skull base surgery. Ann Otol Rhinol Laryngol (Suppl) 196: 45–53
141. Stammberger H (1986) Endoscopic endonasal surgery – concepts in treatment of recurring rhinosinusitis: Part I. Anatomic and pathophysiologic considerations. Otolaryngol Head Neck Surg 94: 143–147
142. Stammberger H (1986) Endoscopic endonasal surgery – concepts in treatment of recurring rhinosinusitis: part II. Surgical technique. Otolaryngol Head Neck Surg 94: 147–156

143. Stammberger H, Hosemann W, Draf W (1997) Anatomic terminology and nomenclature for paranasal sinus surgery. Laryngorhinootologie 76: 435–449
144. Stammberger H, Posawetz W (1990) Functional endoscopic sinus surgery. Concept, indications and results of the Messerklinger technique. Eur Arch Otorhinolaryngol 247: 63–76
145. Stankiewicz JA (1989) The endoscopic approach to the sphenoid sinus. Laryngoscope 99: 218–221
146. Talacchi A, Sala F, Alessandrini F, Turazzi S, Bricolo A (1998) Assessment and surgical management of posterior fossa epidermoid tumors: report of 28 cases. Neurosurgery 42: 242–251; discussion 251–242
147. Tosun F, Carrau RL, Snyderman CH, Kassam A, Celin S, Schaitkin B (2003) Endonasal endoscopic repair of cerebrospinal fluid leaks of the sphenoid sinus. Arch Otolaryngol Head Neck Surg 129: 576–580
148. Tschabitscher M, Galzio RJ (2003) Endoscopic anatomy along the transnasal approach to the pituitary gland and the surrounding structures. In: Divitiis ED, Cappabianca P (eds) Endoscopic endonasal transsphenoidal surgery. Springer, Wien New York, pp 21–39
149. Weiss M (1987) The transnasal transsphenoidal approach. In: Apuzzo MLJ (ed) Surgery of the third ventricle. Williams & Wilkins, Baltimore, pp 476–494
150. White DV, Sincoff EH, Abdulrauf SI (2005) Anterior ethmoidal artery: microsurgical anatomy and technical considerations. Neurosurgery 56: 406–410; discussion 406–410
151. Yamasaki T, Moritake K, Hatta J, Nagai H (1996) Intraoperative monitoring with pulse Doppler ultrasonography in transsphenoidal surgery: technique application. Neurosurgery 38: 95–97; discussion 97–98

# Management of brachial plexus injuries

G. Blaauw[1], R. S. Muhlig[2], and J. W. Vredeveld[3]

[1] Department of Neurosurgery, University Hospital, Maastricht, The Netherlands
[2] Rehabilitation Out-Patient Clinic, S.G.L., Heerlen, The Netherlands
[3] Department of Neurophysiology, Atrium Medical Centre, Heerlen, The Netherlands

With 9 Figures

## Contents

## Abstract

Most brachial plexus lesions are traction injuries sustained during birth, but in adolescents and older people they are usually caused by traffic accidents or following a fall in the home. A minority are the result of penetrating injury after civilian assault or trauma encountered during wartime.

Birth palsy cases (obstetric brachial plexus palsy) and the remaining cases (traumatic brachial plexus palsy) are viewed differently with regard to treatment and outcome and so these two groups are usually discussed in separate chapters. In this paper we treat both groups in parallel because as far as primary (= nerve) surgery is concerned, many treatment problems and solutions are present in both groups and are therefore comparable.

*Keywords:* Brachial plexus injuries; birth palsy; obstetric brachial plexus palsy; traumatic brachial plexus palsy; management of brachial plexus injuries.

## Introduction

In the nineteen-sixties, there was a revival of primary (= nerve) surgery of brachial plexus injuries in some neurosurgical centres. The wide application of the surgical microscope, new techniques for nerve repair, innovative imaging techniques, etc. gave rise to a fresh interest in the surgical treatment of brachial plexus palsy cases, because there was an expectation that the results of surgery could now be rewarding. But surgery was prolonged, results were modest and interest soon waned in most centres. In a few centres, however, the realization of a functional concept governing surgical treatment gave a new impetus to continue, because the value of the outcome was taken into account. As a logical consequence, secondary surgery, such as osteotomy, tendon- or muscle transfer, was included in the total treatment policy as soon as the results of the nerve surgery had become clear. The introduction of treatment of birth palsy cases gave an extra incentive, because results were often much more rewarding in these children.

In this paper we shall discuss indications and surgical techniques for brachial plexus injuries from a functional point of view. In addition to this overview, the reader is referred to the extensive literature for further information. Although both obstetric and non-obstetric brachial plexus palsy are traumatic in origin (mostly traction injuries), it is quite normal for clinical features and surgical approach to be discussed separately.

## Epidemiology

The incidence of obstetric brachial plexus injury is better documented than that of traumatic, non-obstetric injury. Official registration institutions in The Netherlands (SIG) quoted an incidence of 1.02‰ in 1995, 1.34‰ in 1996, and 0.90‰ in 1997 [11]. The reported incidence from other countries in the last three decades of the twentieth century varies considerably from 0.42 [24] to 2.5 per 1000 births [4, 31, 33, 62, 65]. Risk factors are breech presentation, macrosomia and shoulder dystocia [43].

| |
|---|
| The reported incidence of obstetric brachial plexus injury in different countries varies from 0.42 to 2.5 per 1000 births. |

The incidence of traumatic, adult lesions is difficult to evaluate. In The Netherlands, numbers ranging from 82 (1992) to 119 cases (1994) have been reported, constituting complete or partial supraclavicular lesions or infraclavicular lesions; sometimes double lesions are present. Most adult lesions are the result of motorcycle accidents, but the number of open lesions due to shotgun- or stabbing injuries is increasing. About 30% of the patients have concomitant injuries of the head, thorax or internal organs, and fracture of the humeral shaft or injury to the glenohumeral joint is usually present. The subclavian artery is torn in 15% of supraclavicular and in 30% of infraclavicular lesions; damage to the spinal cord is found in 5% of complete lesions [8].

According to Bonnard *et al.* [15], the palsy is complete in 60%, nearly complete in 20% and partial in 20% of cases.

## Anatomical features

Although significant intra- and interindividual variability exists, the basic feature is that the brachial plexus is formed by the anterior spinal nerves from the four lowest cervical roots and the first thoracic root (Fig. 1). The spinal nerves result from a fusion of multiple small spinal rootlets originating from the anterior and posterior horns. The rootlets leading to the posterior horn have all passed through the cells in the spinal ganglion. The rootlets emanating from the anterior horn are axons emerging from cells in the grey matter of the anterior horn. Berthold *et al.* [6] described the junction between roots and spinal cord, identifying a central-peripheral transition zone lying outside the spinal cord at varying levels along the roots. The zone demarcates clear histological differences and is relevant to the level of intradural injury. This and the possibility of selective avulsion of either ventral or dorsal rootlets, makes it clear that different types of intradural lesion of the spinal roots may be present (Table 1). This accounts for the varying rates of recovery illustrating the terms partial and total avulsion [55].

On emerging from the foramen, the spinal nerves undergo a complicated process of joining and dividing of nerve elements to form the brachial plexus. The nerves unite to form three trunks: upper (C5 and C6), middle (C7), and lower (C8 and T1). Each trunk divides into two branches: anterior and posterior. The anterior branches (divisions) join to form the two anterior cords, lateral and medial. The musculocutaneous nerve and the lateral root of the median nerve stem from the lateral cord. The medial cord gives rise to the

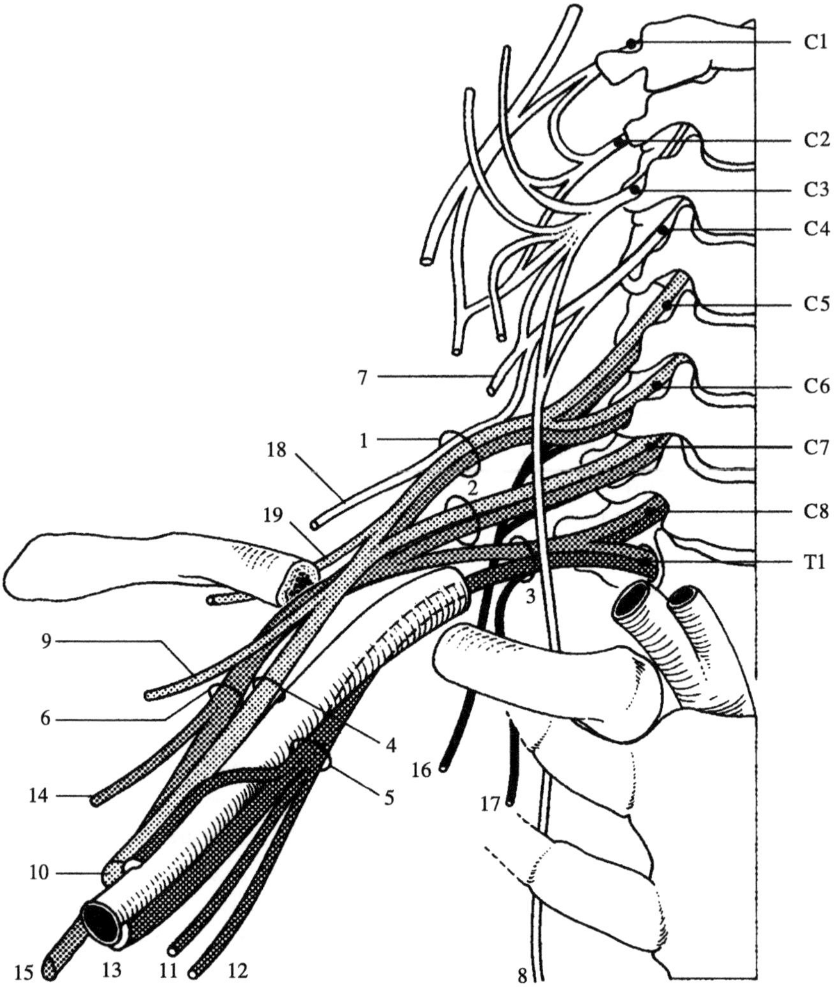


**Fig. 1.** Anatomical diagram of the brachial plexus and significant nerve branches (from Blaauw and Pons, 1999; by courtesy of De Tijdstroom). ▫ Lateral cord, ▪ posterior cord, ■ medial cord, *1* upper trunk (from C5 and C6), *2* middle trunk (from C7), *3* lower trunk (from C8 and D1), *4* lateral cord (from anterior divisions of upper and middle trunk), *5* medial cord (from anterior division of lower trunk), *6* posterior cord (from posterior divisions of all three trunks), *7* supraclavicular nerve, *8* phrenic nerve, *9* musculocutaneous nerve, *10* median nerve, *11* medial cutaneous antebrachial nerve, *12* medial cutaneous brachial nerve, *13* ulnar nerve, *14* axillary nerve, *15* radial nerve, *16* long thoracic nerve, *17* medial pectoral nerve, *18* dorsal scapular nerve, *19* suprascapular nerve

medial root of the median nerve, the ulnar nerve, the medial cutaneous nerve, and the medial antebrachial cutaneous nerve. The lateral and medial roots of the median nerve unite to form the median nerve. The three posterior divisions unite to form the posterior cord, which gives rise to the axillary and radial

**Table 1.** *Classification of preganglionic injury shows the types graphically [55]. For example myelographic figure 3 is illustrative of type B4*

| Type | | |
|---|---|---|
| A | | Roots torn central to transitional zone. True avulsion |
| B | | Roots torn distal to transitional zone |
| | Type 1 | Dura torn within spinal canal, DRG displaced in neck |
| | Type 2 | Dura torn at mouth of foramen: DRG more or less displaced |
| | Type 3 | Dura not torn. DRG not displaced |
| | Type 4 | Dura not torn. DRG not displaced, either ventral or dorsal roots intact |

*DRG* Dorsal root ganglion.

nerves. For detailed information of anatomical features the reader is referred to the exemplary book by Kline *et al.* [37].

A lesion to the brachial plexus can be situated at any level from the origin of the nerve root to the division in the axillary region. The most common lesion is caused by traction and usually results in a combination of rupture of upper plexus elements and avulsion of one or several lower roots supplying the brachial plexus. Extraforaminal lesions are as a rule postganglionic lesions and are referred to as nerve ruptures.

Microscopic neuroanatomical examination of the posterior horns initially only defined a few well delimited regions, such as the substantia gelatinosa and Lissauer's zone. The unique pattern of spinal grey organization in the cat consisted of juxtaposed cell layers, as specified in the original description by Rexed [54]. The second layer corresponded exactly to the earlier description of the substantia gelatinosa Rolandi. Later, physiological experiments on the Rexed layers of the dorsal horn revealed their importance as specific regions for the modulation of sensory information from all regions of the body. Six Rexed layers are recognized, each with its particular cytological feature and typical cellular organization. The neurochemical features of each layer are also different. Afferent and specific nociceptive fibres take care of the input and modulate the neurochemical processes. Damage to the posterior horn deregulates the systems in the layers, causing the typical pain in non-obstetric brachial plexus injury.

## Clinical features

### *Obstetric palsy*

Clinical examination usually allows a diagnosis of the extent and level of the injury. In obstetric injury, the birth weight of the neonates born after breech delivery contrasts with that of the cases of brachial plexus palsy following vertex presentation [69], the latter cases being almost invariably macrosomic neonates.

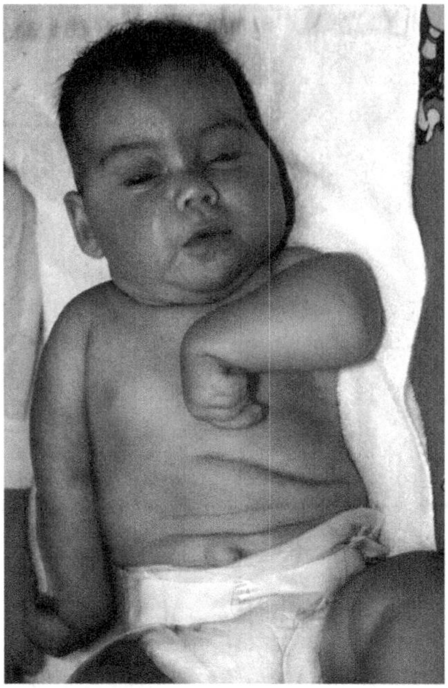

**Fig. 2.** Boy with a bilateral upper palsy following breech delivery. On the left side the lesion shows early proximal recovery. On the same side he has a Horner's syndrome and a phrenic palsy, which required plication of the diaphragm

In most children, a functional disturbance of the arm is noted directly after birth, although in some the cause is initially suspected to be a fracture. A local haematoma may point to the site of the trauma. A fractured clavicle is more frequent than a fractured humerus. Dislocations and/or fractures of the cervical spine emphasize the traumatic birth. Sometimes there are also fractures of the lower limbs. Hemiphrenic nerve palsy may be present. Bilateral lesions mainly occur following breech delivery (Fig. 2): phrenic nerve lesions and especially bilateral brachial plexus lesions are typical of a breech delivery [13].

On the whole the cases can be divided into Narakas' classification system [46]. This classification is based on an examination 2–3 weeks of age and on the clinical course of children during the first 8 weeks after birth. These observations were correlated with nerve injuries classified in five degrees following Sunderland [64], and they are depicted in Table 2.

In a later publication Narakas classified the patients in four groups, because previously group IV was divided into two groups, but Narakas' experience showed that there were no significant differences between them regarding late sequelae [47]. Narakas' classification assesses the future of the palsy and excludes many mild cases, which recover full function in a matter of days.

**Table 2.** *Narakas classification of obstetric brachial plexus palsy*

| | Clinical picture | Pathology grades (Sunderland's degrees [64]) | Recovery |
|---|---|---|---|
| Type I | C5–C6 | 1 and 2 | Complete or almost in 1–8 wks |
| Type II | C5–C6 | Mixed 2 and 3 | Elbow flexion: 1–4 wks<br>Elbow extension: 1–8 wks |
| | C7 | Mixed 1 and 2 | Limited shoulder: 6–30 wks |
| Type III | C5–C6 | 4 or 5 | Poor shoulder: 10–40 wks<br>Elbow flexion: 16–40 wks |
| | C7 | 2 or 3 | Elbow extension: 16–20 wks<br>Wrist: 40–60 wks |
| | C8–T1 (no Horner's sign) | 1 | Hand complete: 1–3 wks |
| Type IV | C5–C7 | 4 and/or 5 | Poor shoulder: 10–40 wks<br>Elbow flexion: 16–40 wks |
| | C8 | Mixed 2–3 | Elbow extension: incomplete, poor: 20–60 wks or nil |
| | T1 (temporary Horner's sign) | 1 and 2 | Wrist: 40–60 wks<br>Hand complete: 20–60 wks |
| Type V | C5–C7 | 5 | Shoulder and elbow as above |
| | C7 | or avulsed | |
| | C8 | 3 or avulsed | Wrist poor or only extension; poor flexion or none |
| | T1 | 2 and 3 | |
| | C8–T1 (Horner's sign usually present) | avulsed | Very poor hand with no or weak flexors and extensors; no intrinsics |

*From* Narakas AO (1986) Injuries to the brachial plexus. In: Bora FW Jr (ed) The pediatric upper extremity: diagnosis and management. WB Saunders, Philadelphia, p 247.

*Group I*: This includes paralysis of shoulder abduction and external rotation, of elbow flexion and of supination of the forearm resulting in adduction-endorotation posture of the shoulder, extension of the elbow and fixed pronation of the forearm. It is caused by a lesion to roots C5 and C6, or upper trunk, and is often called Duchenne's or Erb's paralysis (Fig. 3).

*Group II*: This is an extended Duchenne's/Erb's palsy: spinal nerve C7 is involved, as indicated by a palsy of the elbow, wrist and finger extensors and paralysis of the latissimus dorsi. The elbow may lie slightly flexed and waiter's tip position of the hand is pronounced (Fig. 4). In groups I and II pectoralis major, finger and thumb flexors are usually active, but muscle atrophy often

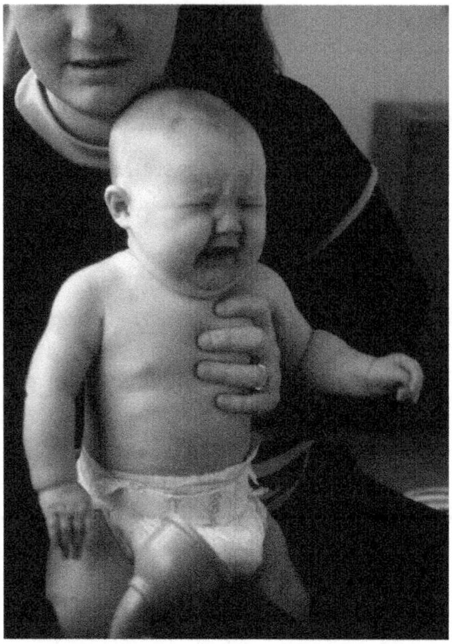

**Fig. 3.** A child with a C5–C6 lesion

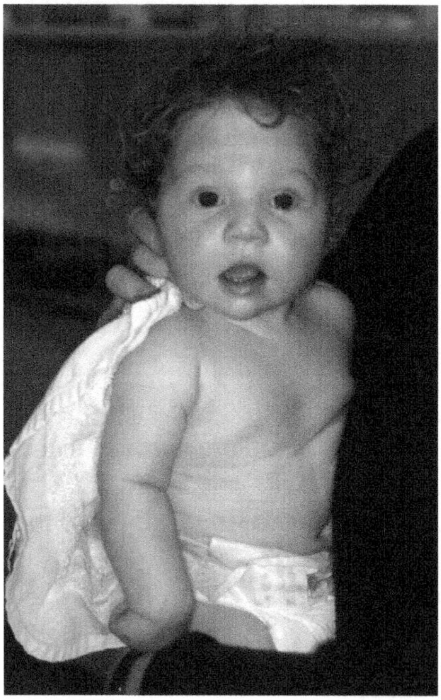

**Fig. 4.** A child with a C5–C6–C7 lesion. Note waiter's tip position of hand

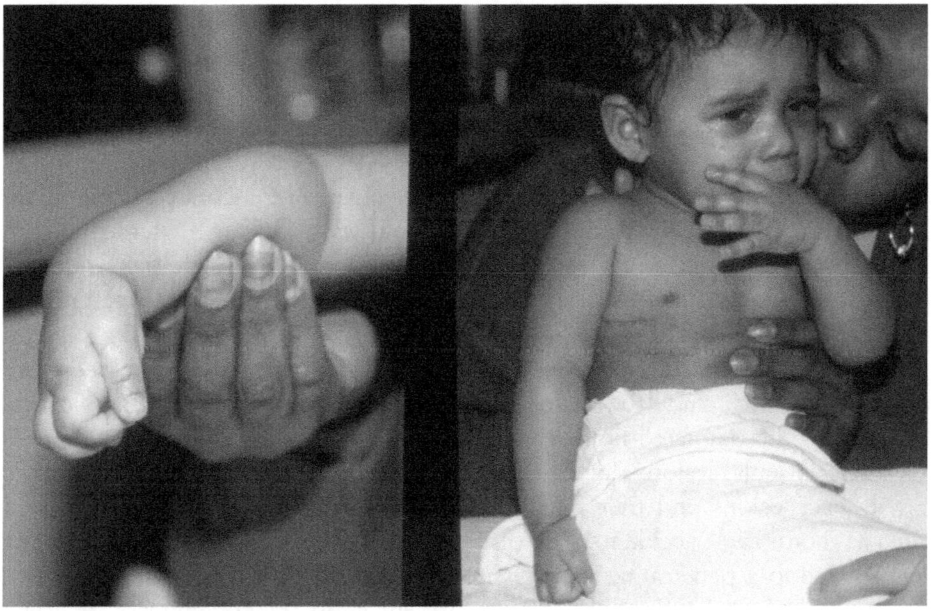

**Fig. 5.** A child with a total lesion

develops early. Distal sensation and vasomotor control are usually unaffected. In the majority of obstetric lesions there is paralysis of the upper roots only, of C5 and C6, or of C5, C6 and C7.

*Group III*: The injury has extended to spinal nerves C8 and T1. There is no Horner's syndrome. In some cases where the injury to the lower nerves of the brachial plexus is of a lesser degree, partial recovery of the hand function usually takes place and serious deficit of the muscles to shoulder and elbow persists. Sometimes the opposite is true and recovery of function is more pronounced proximally than distally. This is referred to as lower brachial plexus or Klumpke's palsy.

*Group IV*: There is (almost) complete motor and sensory deficit of the arm. A Horner's syndrome is present (Fig. 5).

## Non-obstetric, traumatic palsy

In non-obstetric palsy we must take into account:

1. *The type of lesion*: is there a stretch and/or avulsion injury or is there a focal penetration or laceration involving the plexus as in gunshot wounds and a variety of mechanisms of injury such as those resulting from iatrogenic causes.

2. *Age*: although we obtained some surprising successes in older patients, recovery patterns after nerve surgery in children revealed a degree of recovery which was superior to that observed after nerve repair in adults. Sunderland reported on this issue in 1968 [64].

3. *Level of lesion*: the attitude to a total lesion is different from that to an upper plexus lesion; the latter is usually surgically treated at an early stage with the aim of controlling shoulder function and elbow flexion; infraclavicular lesions are more amenable to reconstructive surgery and thus seem to have a better prognosis.

4. *Time of surgery*: early repair has a greater chance of success, preferably no later than 2 months post-injury for blunt injuries and immediately for open injuries; repair carried out after more than 6 months is regarded as useless.

5. *Pain*: which is always present in preganglionic lesions, can sometimes be relieved by nerve transfers.

In traumatic brachial plexus palsy, important features to be obtained from the case history include the violence of the injury and the mode of application of force to the damaged limb.

Infraclavicular lesions due to shoulder dislocation or to humeral fracture are low impact lesions and they have a better prognosis than high impact lesions such as motor cycle accidents. The distinction between supra- and infraclavicular lesions due to a penetrating injury is not difficult but it is sometimes less clear, especially when a longitudinal force is present as in traction injuries. In these cases, double lesions may be present. There are usually special features which make it easier to distinguish between supra- and infraclavicular lesions.

The findings of sensory examination are very important. Partial or full sensory function in the presence of motor paralysis clearly points to good prognosis: neurapraxia is considered to be present. This may be found in skin areas supplied by one or several nerves or roots.

| |
|---|
| Partial or full sensory function in the presence of motor paralysis is indicative of a good prognosis. |

Lesions in each group can be complete or partial and are often a combination of preganglionic (damaged roots) and postganglionic lesions. The latter can be supra- and retroclavicular lesions, in which case trunks are involved. Infraclavicular lesions involve damage to cords and/or nerves.

## Special investigations

These include neurophysiological and image producing techniques, such as CT-myelography, MRI and sonography.

### *Neurophysiology*

In *adult lesions*, the EMG can help in the analysis of the severity and extent of the lesion. For this purpose, the EMG investigation has to be based upon a

**Table 3.** *Neurophysiological protocol*

*Sensory nerve action potentials (SNAPs)*
- Radial nerve to first digit (C6, upper trunk)
- Median nerve to first and third digit (C6, C7 upper and middle trunk)
- Ulnar nerve to fifth digit (C8, lower trunk)
- Medial (C8/T1, lower trunk) and lateral (C6, upper trunk) cutaneous nerves to forearm (not routinely in neonates)

*Needle EMG*

| Muscle examined | Root | Trunk | Cord | Nerve(s) |
|---|---|---|---|---|
| Abductor pollicis brevis | (C7), C8, **T1** | (middle), **lower** | medial | median |
| First dorsal interosseus | C8, **T1** | **lower** | medial | ulnar |
| Flexor carpi radialis | (C6), **C7**, (C8) | **upper**, **middle**, (lower) | **lateral**, medial | median |
| Flexor carpi ulnaris | **C8**, **T1** | **lower** | lateral, **medial** | ulnar |
| Extensor digitorum communis | (C6), **C7**, C8 | (upper), **middle**, lower | posterior | radial |
| Brachioradialis | (C5), **C6** | **upper** | posterior | radial |
| Biceps brachii | **C5**, **C6** | **upper** | lateral | musculocutaneus |
| Triceps brachii | (C6), **C7**, **C8** | (upper), **middle**, lower | posterior | radial |
| Deltoid | **C5**, C6 | **upper** | posterior | axillary (circumflex) |
| Pectoralis major | C5, **C6**, **C7**, **C8**, T1 | **upper**, middle, **lower** | lateral, medial | lateral and medial pectoral |
| Infraspinatus | (C5), C6 | **upper** | | suprascapular |
| Trapezius | | | | accessory |
| Rhomboids | C4, **C5** | | | dorsal scapular |
| Serratus anterior | **C5**, **C6**, C7 | | | long thoracic |

The main innervation is indicated in normal and bold, bold indicating the most important; innervation sporadically found is shown between brackets.

combination of measuring the sensory nerve action potentials (SNAPs) for finding extraforaminal lesions and the needle-EMG for finding lesions of the motor fibres in a myotome (Table 3). If the lesion is complete, all muscles innervated by this root (normal SNAP), trunk or cord (both absent SNAP) will show pathological spontaneous muscle fibre activity. In the first case the sensory ganglion is positioned extramedullary and the lesion is preganglionic, thus the SNAP is normal. When the lesion is in the trunk or cord it is distal to the ganglion and SNAP is thus absent. Bonney and Gilliatt have as early as 1958 shown that in a preganglionic lesion there is evidence of conductivity in the intact sensory axons (no Wallerian degeneration), but this may not have contact with the central nervous system [16]. Basically from each root, trunk or cord, at least 2 muscles innervated by different nerves should be sampled in order to pinpoint the exact location. Problems appear when there are multiple lesions, the most important of which is root avulsion. Root avulsion can be missed when there is also a more peripheral lesion in the same myotome. Using these basic principles, however, we were able to analyze correctly more than 80% of the adult traumatic brachial plexus lesions; sometimes we also found more distal lesions, information which proved important for the surgeon when deciding what to do during the operation [74].

In *obstetric lesions*, EMG can make an important contribution to the solution of the lesion's aetiology and the likely prognosis [51]. Generally, the neurophysiological data at 3–4 months of age seem to indicate a much smaller lesion than found during operation if interpreted in the same way as in adults. This stimulated an investigation into these differences. It was found that there are many differences between adults and neonates quite apart from the size:

1. The pathological spontaneous muscle fibre activity, sometimes also called denervation activity, appeared much earlier than in adults: in neonates as early as days 4–5, and also disappeared much sooner when collateral innervation was possible [19]. This means that for the EMG-analysis of a lesion, the search for reinnervation is even more important than just looking for pathological spontaneous muscle fibre activity.

2. Focusing on the biceps brachii muscle, innervation could be demonstrated from more roots than in adult patients. We called this "luxury innervation" [72]. In the biceps brachii muscle the C7 root appeared to be most important in neonates, whereas in adults innervation from this root of the biceps brachii muscle is only minimal or absent [73].

3. Also at the level of the muscle fibres, polyneural innervation could be demonstrated by the Groningen group of Gramsbergen *et al.* [32].

4. Using the somatosensory evoked potential technique (SEP), "luxury innervation" at the root level could also be demonstrated for the somatosensory pathways [20].

5. Smith [60] reported that mixed nerve action potentials (NAPs) of the median nerve appeared to offer prognostic information in obstetric lesions. She suggested an important role for electrodiagnosis in obstetric brachial palsy: firstly to determine the extent and level of involvement of individual components of the plexus; secondly to identify root avulsion; and thirdly, to identify the nature of the lesion in terms of neurapraxic, axonotmetic and neurotmetic injury, and thus to assist in making a prognosis [60].

These median nerve-NAPs give an estimation of the number of functioning nerve fibres, both sensory and motor. The fact that the median nerve contains many fibres from C7 also indicates the possibility of recovery of the biceps brachii in neonates, based upon possible spontaneous reinnervation by the "luxury innervation": a low amplitude of the median nerve-NAP means severe loss of C7 fibres, thereby loss of the "luxury innervation", and hence loss of possibility of spontaneous reinnervation.

6. We think that central factors also play an important role in obstetric brachial palsy. Although innervation of muscles may exist – e.g. in root avulsions of both C5 and C6, the EMG may show considerable innervation of the biceps brachii in neonates, but not in adults; in most cases, this innervation cannot be used by the infant at the age of 4 months. Using magnetic cortical stimulation (Magstim) and measuring the motor evoked potentials (MEPs) from the biceps brachii muscle, we could demonstrate the existence of corticospinal connections to the "luxury innervation", although the infant could not use these voluntarily. This indicates that cortical plasticity may be responsible for the, sometimes limited, spontaneous recovery seen in many of these infants.

Van Dijk *et al.* [70] also reported from their patient material, that EMG performed close to the time of possible intervention (3 months) usually reveals a discrepancy: motor unit potentials are seen in clinically paralyzed muscles. They explained this in five ways: an overly pessimistic clinical examination; overestimation of EMG recruitment due to small muscle fibres; persistent fetal innervation; developmental apraxia; or misdirection, in which axons reach inappropriate muscles.

Bisinella *et al.* [10] reported results of neurophysiological prediction of outcome in 73 children who showed slow recovery (biceps function returning after 3 months of age) and whose results of neurophysiological investigations were relatively favourable. Following the protocol defined by Smith in the London Peripheral Nerve Injury and Congenital Hand Unit, the cases were regarded as favourable on the basis of their NAP and EMG findings. These cases did not, therefore, undergo nerve surgery but later showed recovery of muscular function. A number did, however, require surgery for medial rotation contracture (11 cases) or posterior dislocation (21 cases) of the shoulder.

*In summary*: the EMG in neonates must be interpreted differently from that in adults, but the EMG can make important contributions to the likely prognosis [51]; also the search for reinnervation is very important. In case of doubt, the median nerve-NAP can provide prognostic information indicating the possibility of spontaneous recovery, even at an early age. We also tried to use the MEP for this purpose, but this technique did not give reliable information about prognosis below the age of 3–4 months.

> Pathological spontaneous muscle fibre activity appears in neonates as early as 4–5 days following brachial plexus birth injury. Interpretation of electromyographic data in peripartal plexus lesions is quite different from the results gained from traumatic lesions.

## Myelography, CT-myelography, MRI and ultrasonography

Since the accidental demonstration of a traumatic meningocele in a patient who had sustained a brachial plexus injury [45], many radiological findings have been published. These were reviewed by Rankine [53]. CT-myelography remains useful for detecting intradural lesions i.e. total and/or partial avulsions (Figs. 6–8) particularly in obstetric cases. The accuracy of MRI for determining nerve root avulsion matches CT-myelography only in adults [22].

It remains to be seen whether ultrasonography can reliably identify postganglionic brachial plexus injuries, when significant soft-tissue disruption to the normal landmarks is expected. Another difficulty is that nerves may become

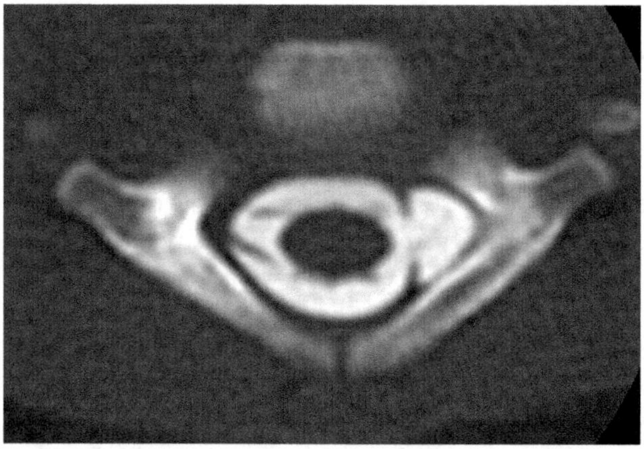

**Fig. 6.** At the left side dorsal and ventral rootlets are absent and a meningocele is present, illustrating the picture of complete root avulsion

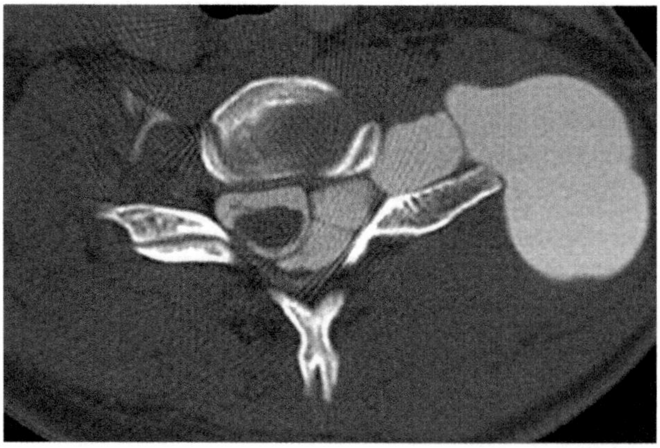

**Fig. 7.** Large traumatic meningocele in the presence of root avulsion extending into the soft tissues of the neck

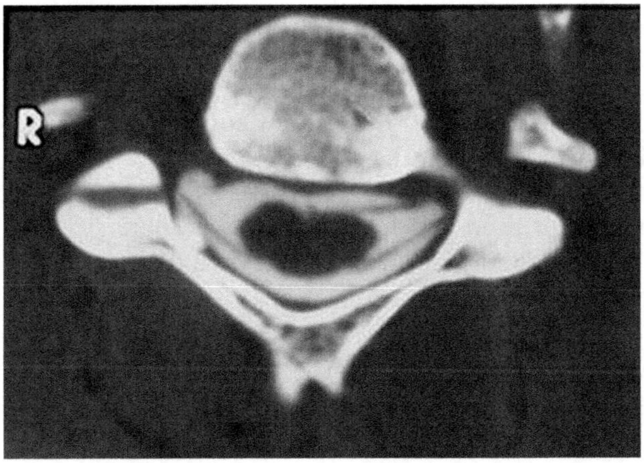


**Fig. 8.** Partial avulsion: at the right side the dorsal rootlet is normal, while the ventral rootlet is absent in the presence of a small traumatic meningocele

invisible when they are situated beneath bone such as the brachial plexus under the clavicle.

*Fluoroscopy* of the chest is necessary to confirm the absence of phrenic paralysis.

## Indication and surgical approach

### *Obstetric palsy*

When we advise surgery in a case of obstetric brachial plexus injury, it is important to operate at an age when there is no anaesthesia risk in a medical environment well suited to the care of the very young, because the risk of complication is high [38]. It is important to realise that obstetric brachial plexus injuries are mainly supraclavicular lesions. This means that we cope in general with two types of injury: upper and total lesions of roots and/or trunks.

In a recent extensive review on the natural history of obstetric brachial plexus palsy [52 ], no restriction for language was applied and articles published in medical periodicals not identified in the initial Medline query were added if these had appeared after 1965; a total of 1020 articles was found. Criteria for inclusion were as follows: the study had to be prospective; the study population had to be on a demographic basis; a follow-up of at least three years; and assessment of end-result preferably using a pre-defined assessment protocol. It was concluded that no study had the width of scope necessary to answer the expected natural course of obstetric brachial plexus palsy. Two studies which came closest to these strict criteria showed that 20–30% residual deficits can be expected. The authors of the review concluded that the often-cited excellent prognosis for this type of birth injury could not be (considered to be) based on their criteria for scientifically sound evidence.

The often-cited excellent prognosis following the natural course for brachial plexus birth injury is not based on scientifically sound evidence.

The difficulty is that at present there are no universally accepted criteria for the categorization of function for surgical or non-operative treatment. Bae *et al.* [3] determined the intraobserver and interobserver reliability of the modified Mallet Classification [40], Toronto Test Score [41], and Hospital for Sick Children Active Movement Scale [21] in the evaluation of patients with brachial plexus birth palsy. They concluded that these three systems are reliable instruments and can be used to assess functional outcomes. They stressed that reliability does not imply validity of these instruments as this was not tested.

The modified Mallet Classification, the Toronto Test Score and the Active Movement Scale are reliable methods of quantifying upper-extremity function in patients with brachial plexus birth palsy and may be used clinically and to assess functional outcomes.

At present, surgical exploration of the brachial plexus is considered to be indicated if spontaneous recovery is insufficient at a preset age. Absence of biceps function at 3 months of age is regarded by many as the key indicator for surgery in upper brachial plexus lesions [27], in persisting total lesions, surgery should be performed earlier. Others use a combined score of different movements to decide whether nerve surgery may be performed at a later date but not later than 9 months [18].

Which methods of nerve surgery are available? These consist of nerve repairs and nerve transfers. Nerve repairs are possible when adequate proximal and distal stumps are available following resection of neuromas, but interposition of sural or other grafts is usually necessary to cover the gap. Nerve transfers are an adjunct if nerve repair is only partially possible (Tables 4 and 5). The transfer of an uninjured nerve to the distal stump of an injured nerve can be very successful. Favourable transfers are: accessory to suprascapular nerve for recovery of shoulder functions and medial pectoral branches to musculo-cutaneous nerve if the pectoralis muscle is contracting [12] or intercostals to musculo-cutaneous nerve if the pectoralis nerve is not working. Several other transfers are available, but these are not as widely used [8]. We do not believe that the sacrifice of such an important function as exerted by the hypoglossal nerve is balanced by the gain demonstrated in our series [14].

If an upper brachial plexus palsy is present, we often find a neuroma of the upper trunk, sometimes also of the middle trunk; the neuroma is resected until a healthy zone is reached. When avulsion is present this is recognized and it

**Table 4.** *Nerve transfers which are frequently used (Narakas [48])*

| Nerve | Introduced by | Remarks |
|---|---|---|
| Spinal accessory nerve (No. XI) | Mentioned by Tuttle (U.S.A) in 1913. Reintroduced by Kotani (Japan) 1963 | Frequently applied for the shoulder (spinati and deltoid) and for elbow flexors |
| Pectoral nerve | Stoffel (Germany) 1920, Lurje 1948 | Particularly for elbow flexors |
| Intercostal nerves | Ciasserini (Italy), Yeoman and Seddon (1963), Kotani, Tsuyama, Hara perfected this method (1972) | Particularly for the musculocutaneous nerve but also for the median nerve and other nerves |
| Healthy parts of the brachial plexus itself or proximal roots (intraplexal neurotization) for elbow flexors | Harris en Low (U.K.) 1903, Narakas (1972) | This may cause synkineses |

**Table 5.** *Infrequent transfers*

| Nerve | Introduced by | Remarks |
|---|---|---|
| Hypoglossal nerve (No. XII) | Narakas (Switzerland) 1980, Slooff (Netherlands) 1992 | Used for shoulder and elbow function. Serious clinical morbidity, poor results and abandoned (Blaauw *et al.* 2006) |
| Phrenic nerve | Gu (China) 1983 | Not routinely used in Western countries. In OBPP now abandoned by Chen |
| Long thoracic nerve | Förster (Germany) 1928, Lurje (Russia) 1948, Narakas (Switzerland) 1972 | Causes scapula alata and instability of the shoulder |
| Contralateral pectoral nerve or brachial plexus parts (particularly part of medial trunk) | Gilbert (France) 1984, Gu (China) 1989 | Long transplants are necessary; associated movements |

means that reconstruction to the proximal root is impossible. Fortunately C5 usually withstands avulsion and may thus be used for reinnervation.

In complete lesions the principle of repair is that everything should be done to improve hand function. As the lower roots are avulsed in most of these cases, it will be necessary to use upper roots for reinnervation of distal arm muscles by connecting upper roots to the lower trunk.

> In obstetric lesions the principle of repair is that everything should be done to improve hand function: hand function is more important than proximal extremity function.

## *Non-obstetric, traumatic brachial palsy*

Emergency surgery is indicated in the case of life-endangering concomitant lesions, such as vascular trauma. At the time of repair of vascular and bone lesions the extent of the nerve lesion can be estimated and nerve surgery need not be delayed. If deemed necessary following initial surgery, the patient should be referred as quickly as possible to a centre capable of handling brachial plexus surgery. Penetrating injuries must also be surgically explored as soon as possible. Figure 9a and b are graphical representations of the management in

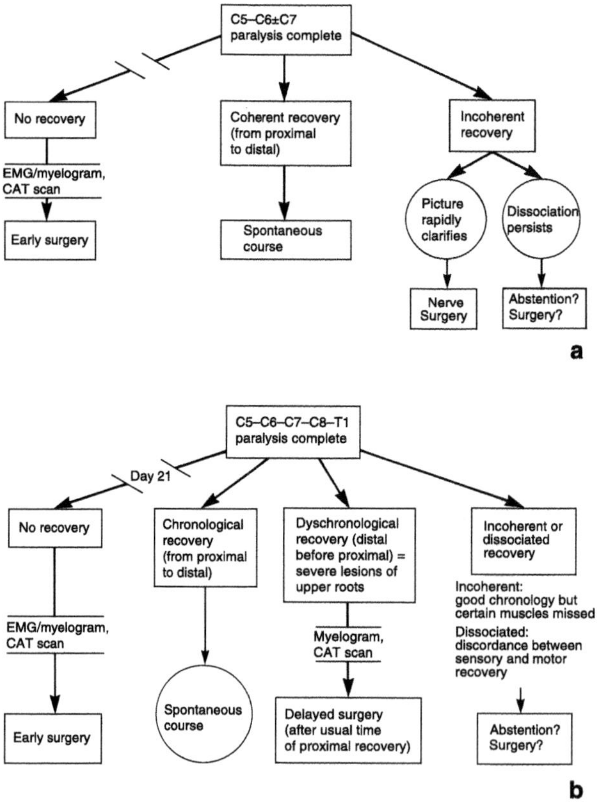


**Fig. 9(a and b).** Alnot's algorithms for the care of upper and total lesions

total and upper supraclavicular lesions [2]. Kline digresses extensively upon the significance of other injury categories [36].

Which techniques are currently used for reinnervation? This depends largely on the extent of the brachial plexus injury. Millesi has provided detailed graphic instructions concerning the surgical techniques [42]. In his book he shows the technique of nerve repair and the details of individual nerves and their significance.

Are root avulsions present and how many? Does the injury consist of rupture of nerve elements? Are they supra- and/or infraclavicular? It is important to realise that one is not dealing with a uniform type of plexus injury in all the patients. The brachial plexus injury is not a lesion in one nerve element but in a complex nerve structure. Thus the surgical treatment in an individual patient is a combination of the surgical possibilities and the functional goals to be achieved. We must accept that in the case of total lesions, which usually include multiple avulsions especially of the lower roots, manual function is seldom achieved following surgery.

Associated vascular lesions must be repaired immediately. Fractures and dislocations should be dealt with at the same time. Further treatment consists of the prevention of trophic changes and joint stiffness. Active mobilization is started as soon as possible, as is passive mobilization. The palsy is assessed by repeated motor and sensory examinations and by progression of Tinel's sign. If there are no signs of recovery from injury after a short period of time (±3 weeks), cervical CT-myelography, MRI and neurophysiological studies are performed, because there is an indication for surgery.

Surgical treatment of brachial plexus injury patients was performed a few decades ago by Seddon and his co-worker Brooks and they demonstrated the efficacy of transfer of intercostal nerves to the musculocutaneous nerve, but the rationale and techniques of surgery in brachial plexus injuries may still be difficult to comprehend. Several surgical techniques are available but their application depends on functional goals and not on reinnervation of individual muscles. More vigorous attempts are made to achieve recovery of motor function than recovery of sensation. This is assumed to occur more or less simultaneously. Thus, following the evaluation of the patient's functional status, goals are formulated and means are sought.

| Early surgery is essential; surgical treatment after 6 months is useless. |
|---|

In cases with total paralysis, management depends on the presence of root avulsion. Myelography often shows traumatic meningoceles at C8 and T1, and often at C7; C6 may have an abnormal aspect, and C5 is usually normal. In these cases at surgery, the one or two normal roots are used to obtain proximal reinnervation. If only one root is to be grafted, repair of the suprascapular nerve and the lateral cord or the anterior division of the upper trunk is performed. The goal is to obtain stabilization of the shoulder, an active pectoralis major muscle for thoraco-humeral grip, flexion of the elbow, and some palmar sensibility. Motor recovery of the hand will not be achieved. If two roots are available it is sometimes possible to graft parts of the posterior cord to improve radial nerve or axillary nerve function. If surgery reveals meningoceles on all roots, one will find total avulsion of C5–T1. In these cases neurotizations are performed using intercostal nerves, the spinal accessory nerve, or superficial cervical plexus in order to obtain some shoulder control and elbow flexion. In Table 3 a summary of nerve transfers is shown. Reimplantation of avulsed nerve roots may be useful for selected cases [17].

When spontaneous recovery takes place in the first month from proximal to distal, this may indicate that we have a case which can achieve significant recovery. This occurs especially in patients with shoulder dislocation. Early recovery from distal to proximal may indicate the presence of a repairable supraclavicular lesion which will often be operated on at an early stage. This management is graphically represented in Fig. 9a and b (from Alnot [2]).

> In closed adult traumatic brachial plexus palsy, nerve surgery is usually postponed, but not for too long; early exploration is preferable when there is doubt about prognosis.

In cases of paralysis of C5, C6 $\pm$ C7, the prognosis is dominated by the fact that the hand is normal or only partially involved but can still be used. Surgery must be performed at an early stage and a satisfactory functional result is achieved by nerve repair or graft and/or nerve transfer. The results of direct reinnervation are better than those of (later) secondary surgery.

In infraclavicular lesions distal to the level of the terminal branches of the plexus, such as the axillary nerve, the musculocutaneous nerve, and the radial nerve, a sensory and motor paralysis implies a complete rupture, and it is necessary to operate before the third month. In lesions at the level of the cords, diagnosis and indication for surgery may be difficult.

> In adult complete traumatic brachial plexus palsy, the treatment goal is to obtain stabilization of the shoulder, an active pectoralis major for thoraco-humeral grip, active flexion of the elbow, and some palmar sensibility.

## Secondary surgical techniques

Primary (nerve) surgery is followed by careful observation of functional recovery. At least two years must elapse before the results of brachial plexus repair can be properly analyzed, because reinnervation after grafting or following nerve transfer is always a long process. Amongst other things it depends on the age of the patient, the time between injury and surgical repair, the type of injury and the distance between graft and end-organ.

When the results of reinnervation are clear, the requirement to improve shoulder-, elbow-, wrist- and hand function is evaluated. What are the options for improving these functions?

## *Obstetric lesions*

It was expected that primary surgery would diminish the sequelae of obstetric birth palsy. Although primary surgery achieved greater functionality, a number of joint problems persisted due to imbalance of muscular function which may cause serious malformations during growth, in particular gleno-humeral deformities.

Upper brachial plexus lesion (Erb's palsy) is the most common type. An isolated lower lesion (so-called Klumpke's palsy, although she did not in fact describe this) is extremely rare (if at all present [1]); it may be the clinical presentation of a total lesion with significant recovery of the upper part of the brachial plexus and persisting palsy of the lower plexus parts. Thus we are left with upper lesions and total lesions with lesion of upper plexus elements as the common denominator; hence it is understandable that impairments and disabilities by glenohumeral deformities are most common, although they are less frequent in patients who had early nerve surgery. It is, therefore, important to offer nerve reconstruction when the prognosis is known.

At the beginning of the last century, when nerve reconstruction was not yet widely practiced, the occurrence of a fixed internal rotation contracture of the shoulder in 40–60% of cases was described [35, 57, 67, 68, 75]. In 1934, L'Episcopo [39] concluded that the disability resulting from upper obstetrical palsy is in fact often due to a severe internal contracture of the shoulder and this opinion is still valid.

> In obstetric birth palsy, prevention of internal rotation contracture of the shoulder is very important because the contracture may give rise to a number of serious gleno-humeral deformities.

From these experiences we are familiar with many aspects of the shoulder problems and some surgical solutions. Neurosurgeons are usually not trained to offer these surgical solutions, and so hand-, plastic- or orthopaedic surgeons are often called in to assist. A number of deformities may also develop secondarily, such as:

1. Posterior subluxation of the humeral head: passive lateral rotation of the arm in the shoulder is restricted. There is no secondary deformity of acromion, coracoid or glenoid.

2. Posterior dislocation; the humeral head can be seen and palpated behind the glenoid. Reposition of the humeral head is possible causing a "click". Passive lateral rotation is more restricted.

3. Complex subluxation/dislocation of the humeral head: at this stage marked skeletal deformities are present such as elongated coracoid, elongated and downward hooked acromion, bifacetal glenoid, retroversion of the glenoid, torsion deformity of the humerus. Passive external rotation is usually impossible [8].

It is clear that prevention of internal rotation deformity of the shoulder is necessary in obstetric brachial plexus palsy. Thus the parents are instructed to exercise the arm. Sometimes this is not sufficient to prevent contracture, necessitating surgical measures. First of all, persisting shoulder impairment due to internal rotation contracture and concomitant external rotation weakness around the shoulder needs attention. Subscapular release or subscapular tendon lengthening is sometimes required at an early stage when contracture is evident. Then patients with rotator cuff muscle imbalance, minimal joint contracture and no glenohumeral deformity are treated with latissimus dorsi transfer, sometimes with additional teres major tendon transfer or humeral derotation osteotomy. Patients with a glenohumeral deformity or dislocation are treated with some form of surgical reduction supplemented by tendon transfers and musculocutaneous lengthenings.

In the elbow, insufficient flexion, extension or pro- and supination may be present. For elbow flexion a flexor-pronator plasty (Steindler's operation [63]) may be indicated. Our group reported results in 26 patients, showing a good result in 23 cases [71]. To improve pronation, especially in supination contracture, osteotomy of the radius is undertaken, forcing the hand in pronation, eventually supplemented with biceps rerouting transfer. Elbow extension is usually sufficiently enhanced by the force of gravity.

Weakness of wrist and/or finger extension is a recurring problem both in upper brachial plexus lesions and in total lesions following initial nerve surgery. If strong wrist and finger flexors are present, it is possible to deal with this problem using tendon transfer. The results of hand function following nerve reconstruction in total lesions are often modest but are greatly appreciated by the patients and their environment and are useful [34]. Secondary surgery is not standardized for these patients, but is tailored to the functional result in the individual patient.

## *Non-obstetric lesions*

Secondary surgery in patients with brachial plexus palsy who underwent primary surgery is intended to achieve greater functional results; only in obstetric palsy is it also performed to redress malfunction due to growth disturbances.

Thus growth does not cause a problem in the non-obstetric palsy group and as the results of primary surgery are not as good as in obstetric cases, the role of secondary surgery is not equal in the treatment procedure.

If sufficient shoulder function is not regained following nerve surgery, arthrodesis of the shoulder is a useful alternative. Normal function of the trapezius and serratus muscles is required. The strength of the arthrodesed shoulder is better than that obtained by muscular transfers. The procedure is indicated when at least some recovery of elbow function is achieved.

Elbow flexion plays a key role in the global function of the upper extremity. If, following primary surgery, elbow flexion is not regained, surgery is mandatory. In upper palsies a flexor-pronator plasty (Steindler's operation) is indicated and is usually successful, when active wrist extension is adequate. If this operation is not possible, bipolar latissimus dorsi transfer or triceps-to-biceps transfer may be considered.

Especially for the distal motor functions of the paralyzed arm, free muscle transfers may be undertaken. In special cases wrist and finger flexion and extension may be regained [22].

It is our contention that amputation is very seldom indicated and should not be undertaken because of pain. Functional braces are rarely utilized, and cosmetic prostheses for social use are always less satisfactory than the paralyzed arm.

## Results of both primary and secondary surgery

The results of brachial plexus reconstruction in adults are generally modest, especially in cases of total lesions. Although the same techniques are used in neonates the results are far better, because of shorter regeneration distances, stronger potential for regeneration, and the greater capacity for brain adaptation.

### *Obstetric lesions*

One of the biggest problems is being able to compare the results of the different treatment policies because of lack of consensus about the method of assessment and how to use the various scoring systems. This of course makes it complicated to compare, for example, the results of a more conservative attitude in treating obstetric palsy with a more aggressive surgical approach. The Brachial Plexus Group in Heerlen uses several assessment methods [44]. Bae *et al.* [3] have demonstrated that the modified Mallet Classification [40], the Toronto Test Score [41] and the Active Movement Scale [21] are reliable methods of quantifying upper-extremity function in patients with brachial plexus birth palsy and may be used clinically and to assess functional outcomes.

Using the Mallet scale, Gilbert [29] reviewed 237 patients who had undergone brachial plexus reconstruction before 1996. Of these, 103 patients were operated for C5–C6 lesions. Including those patients (one-third) who had required secondary surgery, he concluded that 80% had a good or excellent result (grades IV–V) and 20% were average (grade III). In 61 patients who had C5–C6–C7 defects (7 patients had subscapularis release and 25 had tendon transfers for the shoulder following primary surgery), the results were excellent or good (grade IV–V) in 61%, average (grade III) in 29%.

Complete paralysis and associated root ruptures and avulsions are severe, and the results cannot be evaluated before completion of growth. From Gilbert's patient group, a series of 73 patients with complete paralysis operated on from 1978 to 1994 were followed with a mean follow-up of 6.4 years [34]. Secondary operations (mainly on the shoulders) were necessary on 123 occasions. Although the results show that the shoulders and elbows did not do as well as in upper-type lesions, because in these cases upper roots were used to reinnervate lower roots, the results at the level of the hand were encouraging, showing 75% useful results after 8 years, even in patients with avulsion injuries of the lower roots. In this paper, scoring scales for elbow and hand function were used.

In our series of more than 500 neurosurgical obstetric cases, we examined functional results of 171 cases who had undergone accessory nerve transfer to the suprascapular nerve with at least a 2-year follow-up. We evaluated active external glenohumeral rotation, because this is particularly exerted by the infraspinatus muscle which is innervated by the suprascapular nerve and thus reflects specifically the result of the transfer. Results were evaluated in patients who had had the transfer more than 24 months earlier using the Mallet scale. In 4 cases, data were lost and 14 cases, which had required a latissimus dorsi transfer to improve external rotation, had to be excluded. Thus, we could evaluate 153 cases. Results were not good in 47 cases (Mallet scale 2 in 38 cases (22%) and Mallet scale 3 in 9 cases (5%)), but in 106 cases (62%) the Mallet scale was 4. Possible reasons for the failures could be technical, lack of neurotization of the infraspinatus muscle for unknown reason, or lack of central learning.

## *Non-obstetric lesions*

As mentioned earlier and supported by international colleagues the results in severely injured patients are modest [15], partly because surgery is often performed late and now we know that timing is everything. In these cases we aim to achieve some recovery of shoulder and elbow function, in particular elbow flexion, and in a few cases – especially in adolescents – some strength is regained in wrist flexors and extensors. A certain degree of protective sensibility in the hand may also be regained but the distal muscles remain paralysed.

Particularly in upper (partial) palsies the ability to actively move the shoulder and elbow so that the good and functionally not injured wrist and hand may be used, is important. Thus surgical measures to induce key functions in the shoulder and elbow either by nerve surgery sometimes followed by secondary surgery or by secondary surgery alone, are essential.

## Summary of management of patients with brachial plexus lesions

In *obstetric lesions* Gilbert's biceps rule in upper lesions is applied, while total lesions can be operated earlier. Thus we recommend that surgery should take place before three months of age for global palsy cases and at three months in upper (Erb's type) lesions, for best functional results. Even in complete lesions the end results at the level of the hand are encouraging [29]. When spontaneous recovery takes place in the first month from proximal to distal this may indicate that we have a case which can achieve significant recovery. In partial lesions operation is advised when paralysis of abduction of the shoulder and of flexion of the elbow persists after the age of three months and neurophysiological investigations predict a poor prognosis. Operation is carried out earlier in complete lesions showing no sign of clinical recovery [9].

In *non-obstetric* lesions, associated vascular lesions must be repaired immediately at the same time as the nerves [8]. In closed lesions without a vascular rupture, nerve surgery is usually postponed, but not too long and early exploration is preferable when there is doubt concerning prognosis. Fractures and dislocations should also be dealt with early. Further treatment consists of the prevention of trophic changes and joint stiffness. Active mobilization is started as soon as possible, as is passive mobilization. The palsy is assessed by repeated motor and sensory examinations, and by progression of Tinel's sign. Tinel's sign on day 1 is an early indication of the presence of nerve rupture.

If recovery does not take place during the first weeks following the injury, this may be an urgent indication to operate, because otherwise it may be too late to achieve good results. When there is a surgical indication, cervical CT-myelography and neurophysiological studies are performed.

## Pain following traumatic brachial plexus injury

Pain is common after non-obstetric traction lesions of the brachial plexus. Also postganglionic lesions are not associated with pain. Pain almost exclusively can create a serious problem in patients with avulsion of the lower roots supplying the brachial plexus. It seems reasonable to suppose that the more violence exerted on the spinal cord, the greater the deafferentation and the greater the change in abnormal circuits after sprouting, with a larger number of cells firing spontaneously and upsetting some of the Rexed layers in the posterior horn.

In 1911, Frazier and Skillern [26] set out to perform dorsal rhizotomy in a patient, a physician, with intractable pain from closed traction lesion of the brachial plexus. They exposed the cervical cord by laminectomy and found the anterior and posterior rootlets of C6, C7 and C8 to be absent: "the roots evidently had been torn completely from the cord".

The patient's description of the pain was characteristic: "the pain is continuous; it does not stop a minute either day or night. It is either burning or compressing.... In addition, there is, every five minutes, a jerking sensation similar to that obtained by touching ... a Leyden jar. It is like a zigzag made in the sky by a stroke of lightning. The upper part of the arm is mostly free of pain; the lower part from a little above the elbow to the tip of the fingers, never."

It is all there, the characteristic pain in extensive traumatic brachial plexus palsy. The pain is severe, there are two parts to it (one constant, the other intermittent and unpredictable), and it is worst in the hand and forearm. The typical pain following brachial plexus injury often develops very quickly, within hours, but in some cases not until several weeks after the accident. It is not clear whether the neurochemical mechanisms underlying these pain sensations are the same in all these conditions.

Treatment with tegretol, tryptizol, peripheral analgesics or opiates frequently only has limited success. Cannabis seems to be more effective. Alcohol is helpful, probably because it relaxes the patient and helps to induce sleep. A fairly characteristic feature is that a really good night's sleep can often give marked relief of pain. None of our patients have become alcoholics or drug addicts because they soon learned that apart from other social and psychological mechanisms, work is the best method of pain relief, and they cannot therefore risk being drowsy.

An expectative management is adopted in all these cases because the majority of the patients will be able to cope with the situation with acceptable remaining pain one year after the injury, only for it to return in situations of stress, underlying illness, or marked changes in the weather. Surgical repairs and reconstructions are regarded as playing a role in the diminution of pain. About 10% of the patients request further measures one year or more after the injury because of intractable pain. According to Wynn Parry [76], the most useful modality for the management of avulsion pain was regarded to be prolonged transcutaneous electrical stimulation, but we now doubt this. Berman *et al.* [5] concluded that nerve repair can reduce pain from spinal root avulsions and that the mechanism may involve successful regeneration, and/or restoration of peripheral connections prior to their function, possibly in muscle.

Sadly, there is a significant number of patients who do not respond to nerve reconstruction, electrical stimulation, drugs, or distraction by work and hobbies and who do not lose their pain over a period of time.

The hypothesis that abnormal electrophysiological phenomena in the posterior horn are responsible for the pain syndromes, has led to the introduction of neuromodulation on the one hand, and on the other to surgical destruction of circumscribed areas in the posterior horn by a so-called DREZ-lesion (Dorsal Root Entry Zone-lesion).

We have used neuromodulation in a certain number of cases with only modest success. An important condition for optimal pain diminution is a complete overlap of the pain area and the area in which paraesthesias are achieved by stimulation. This congruence is rarely reached, and so in almost all cases insufficient pain diminution occurred. This is probably caused by the deafferentation which arises following avulsion of multiple roots causing atrophy of the posterior horn. Although in some cases the patients achieved pain diminution of more than 70%, they became dissatisfied with this result in the course of their ailment, making them less motivated to continue neuromodulation treatment.

In 1974, Sindou *et al.* [58] described the neuroanatomical basis for DREZ lesioning as well as certain clinical indications for the procedure. Nashold and Ostdahl indicated the possibility that thermal destruction of the denervated neurones in the posterior horn could be a solution for persisting pain in brachial plexus lesions [49]. Thomas and Kitchen [66] concluded from their follow-up study that DREZ thermocoagulation is an effective procedure for relieving deafferentation pain. Sindou thinks that the long-term efficacy of this procedure strongly indicates that pain after brachial plexus avulsion originates from the deafferented (and gliotic) dorsal horn [59].

> Dorsal root entry zone thermocoagulation is an effective procedure for relieving deafferentation pain following brachial plexus injury.

We agree that long-term pain relief is good or complete in a high percentage of these patients. However, DREZ lesioning is an invasive procedure and we have found persistent, albeit mild, neurological deficits at the time of follow-up. The side-effects are rarely severe or functionally significant, but a few patients who are suffering permanent side-effects – locomotor deficits, in particular, impotence and proprioceptive loss – have doubts as to whether they were right in choosing the operation, because patients soon forget having had pain. It is useful to make a recording of the patient's feelings about his pain before the operation so that, if necessary, he can be reminded of his once desperate state.

## Acknowledgements

We are grateful to Professor Rolfe Birch, London, UK, for his helpful discussions. Mr Koen Koenders, Oud-Turnhout, Belgium, assisted in the preparation of the illustrations.

## References

1. Al-Qattan MM, Clarke HM, Curtis CG (1995) Klumpke's birth palsy: does it really exist? J Hand Surg (Br) 20: 19–23
2. Alnot J-Y (1988) Traumatic brachial plexus palsy in adults. In: Raoul Tubiana (ed) The hand, vol. III. WB Saunders, Philadelphia, pp 607–644
3. Bae DS, Waters PM, Zurakowski D (2003) Reliability of three classification systems measuring active motion in brachial plexus birth palsy. J Bone Joint Surg 85: 1733–1738
4. Bager B (1997) Perinatally acquired brachial plexus palsy – a persisting challenge. Acta Paediatr 86: 1214–1219
5. Berman JS, Birch R, Anand P (1998) Pain following human brachial plexus injury with spinal cord avulsion and the effect of surgery. Pain 75: 199–207
6. Berthold CH, Carlstedt T, Corneliuson O (1993) Anatomy of the mature transitional zone. In: Dyck PJ, Thomas PK, Griffin JW, Low PA, Poduslo JF (eds) Peripheral neuropathy, 3rd edn. WB Saunders, Philadelphia, pp 75–80
7. Birch R (1996) Brachial plexus injuries. J Bone Joint Surg 78-B: 986–992
8. Birch R, Bonney G, Wynn Parry CB (1998) Surgical disorders of the peripheral nerves. Churchill Livingstone, Edinburgh, pp 398–404
9. Birch R, Ahad N, Kono H, Smith (2005) Repair of obstetric brachial plexus palsy. Results in 100 children. J Bone Joint Surg (Br) 87-B: 1089–1095
10. Bisinella GL, Birch R, Smith SJM (2003) Neurophysiological prediction of outcome in obstetric lesions of the brachial plexus. J Hand Surg 28B: 148–152
11. Blaauw G, Pons C (1999) Letsels van de plexus brachialis. Elsevier/Bunge, Maarssen, pp 36–38
12. Blaauw G, Slooff ACJ (2003) Transfer of pectoral nerves to the musculocutaneous nerve in obstetric upper brachial plexus palsy. Neurosurgery 53: 338–341
13. Blaauw G, Muhlig RS, Kortleve JW, Tonino AJ (2004) Obstetric brachial plexus injuries following breech delivery: an adverse experience in The Netherlands. Semin Plast Surg 18: 301–307
14. Blaauw G, Sauter Y, Lacroix CLE, Slooff ACJ (2006) Hypoglossal nerve transfer in obstetric brachial plexus palsy. J Plast Reconstr Aesthetic Surg 59: 474–478
15. Bonnard C, Allieu Y, Alnot J-Y, Brunelli G, Merle M, Santos-Palazzi A, Sedel L, Raimondi PL, Narakas A (1996) Complete palsies and supraclavicular lesions. In: Alnot J-Y, Narakas A (eds) Traumatic brachial plexus injuries, Monographie de la Societé Française de Chirurgie de la Main (GAM). Expansion Scientifique Française, Paris, pp 126–155
16. Bonney G, Gilliatt RW (1958) Sensory nerve conduction after traction lesion of the brachial plexus. Proc R Soc Med 51: 365–367
17. Carlstedt T, Anand P, Hallin R, Misra PV, Norén G, Seferlis T (2000) Spinal nerve root repair and reimplantation of avulsed ventral roots into the spinal cord after brachial plexus injury. J Neurosurg Spine 93: 237–247

18. Clarke HM, Curtis CG (1995) An approach to obstetrical brachial plexus injuries. Hand Clin 11: 563–581
19. Colon AJ, Vredeveld JW, Blaauw G, Zandvoort JA (2003) Spontaneous muscle fiber activity appears early in cases of obstetric brachial plexopathy. Muscle Nerve 28: 515–516
20. Colon AJA, Vredeveld JW, Blaauw G, Slooff ACJ, Richards R (2003) Extensive somatosensory innervation in infants with obstetric brachial palsy. Clin Anat 16: 25–29
21. Curtis C, Stephens D, Clarke HM, Andrews D (2002) The active movement scale: an evaluative tool for infants with obstetrical brachial plexus palsy. J Hand Surg 27A: 470–478
22. Doi K (2001) Palliative surgery: free muscle transfers. In: Gilbert A (ed) Brachial plexus injuries. Martin Dunitz, London, pp 137–147
23. Doi K, Otsuka K, Okamoto Y, Fujii H, Hattori Y, Baliarsing AS (2002) Cervical nerve root avulsion in brachial plexus injuries: magnetic resonance imaging classification and comparison with myelography and computerized tomography myelography. J Neurosurg 96 Suppl 3: 277–284
24. Evans-Jones G, Kay SPJ, Weindling AM, Cranny G, Ward A, Bradshaw A, Hernon C (2003) Congenital brachial palsy: incidence, causes, and outcome in the United Kingdom and republic of Ireland. Arch Dis Child Fetal Neonatal Ed 88: F185–F189
25. Fairbank HAT (1913) Birth palsy: subluxation of the shoulder-joint in infants and young children. Lancet 1: 1217–1223
26. Frazier CH, Skillern PF (1911) Supraclavicular subcutaneous lesions of the brachial plexus not asociated with skeletal injuries. J Am Med Ass 57: 1957–1963
27. Gilbert A, Tassin JL (1984) Réparation chirurgicale du plexus brachial dans la paralysie obstétricale. Chirurgie 110: 70–75
28. Gilbert A (1995) Long-term evaluation of brachial plexus surgery in obstetrical palsy. Hand Clin 11: 583–594
29. Gilbert A (2001) Results of repair to the brachial plexus. In: Gilbert A (ed) Brachial plexus injuries. Martin Dunitz, London, pp 211–215
30. Gilbert A, Pivato G, Kheiralla T (2006) Long-term results of primary repair of brachial plexus lesions in children. Microsurgery 26: 334–342
31. Gordon M, Rich H, Deutschberger JD, Green M (1973) The immediate and long-term outcome of obstetric birth trauma. Am J Obstet Gynecol 117: 51–56
32. Gramsbergen A, IJkema-Paassen J, Nikkels PGJ, Hadders-Algra M (1997) Regression of polyneural innervation in the human psoas muscle. Early Hum Dev 49: 49–61
33. Greenwald AG, Schute PC, Shively JL (1984) Brachial plexus birth palsy: a 10-year report on the incidence and prognosis. J Pediatr Orthop 4: 689–692
34. Haerle M, Gilbert A (2004) Management of complete obstetric brachial plexus lesions. J Pediatr Orthop 24: 194–200
35. Hoffer MM, Phipps GJ (1998) Closed reduction and tendon transfer for treatment of dislocation of the glenohumeral joint secondary to brachial plexus birth palsy. J Bone Joint Surg 80A: 997–1001
36. Kline DG, Hudson AR (1995) Nerve injuries. Operative results for major nerve injuries, entrapments, and tumors. W.B. Saunders, Philadelpphia, pp 345–471
37. Kline DG, Hudson AR, Kim DH (2001) Atlas of peripheral nerve surgery. W.B. Saunders, Philadelphia, pp 1–75
38. La Scala GC, Rice SB, Clarke HM (2003) Complications of microsurgical reconstruction of obstetrical brachial plexus palsy. Plast Reconstruct Surg 111: 1383–1390

39. L'Episcopo JB (1934) Tendon transplantation in obstetrical paralysis. Am J Surg 25: 122
40. Mallet J (1972) Paralysie obstetricale du plexus brachial: traitement des sequelles. Primauté du traitement de l'épaule – Méthode d'expression des résultats. Rev Chir Orthop Reparatrice Appar Mot 58 Suppl 1: 166–168
41. Michelow BJ, Clarke HM, Curtis CG, Zuker RM, Seifu Y, Andrews DF (1994) The natural history of obstetrical brachial plexus palsy. Plast Reconstruct Surg 93: 675–681
42. Millesi H (1992) Chirurgie der peripheren Nerven. Urban & Schwarzenberg, München, pp 79–120
43. Mollberg M, Hagberg H, Bager B, Lilja H, Ladfors L (2005) Risk factors for obstetric brachial plexus palsy among neonates delivered by vacuum extraction. Obstetric Gynecol 106: 913–918
44. Muhlig RS, Blaauw G, Slooff ACJ, Kortleve JW, Tonino AJ (2001) Conservative treatment of obstetrical brachial plexus palsy (obpp) and rehabilitation. In: Gilbert A (ed) Brachial plexus injuries. Martin Dunitz, London, pp 173–187
45. Murphey F, Hartung W, Kirklin JW (1947) Myelographic demonstration of avulsing injury of the brachial plexus. Am J Roentgenol 58: 102–105
46. Narakas AO (1986) Injuries to the brachial plexus. In: Bore FW (ed) The pediatric upper extremity. Diagnosis and management. W. B. Saunders Company, Philadelphia, pp 247–258
47. Narakas AO (1987) Obstetrical brachial plexus injuries. In: Lamb DW (ed) The paralysed hand. (The hand and upper limb, vol. 2). Churchill Livingstone, Edinburgh, pp 116–135
48. Narakas AO (1991) Neurotization in the treatment of brachial plexus injuries. In: Gelberman RH (ed) Operative nerve repair and reconstruction. JB Lippincott Company, Philadelphia, pp 1329–1358
49. Nashold BS Jr, Ostdahl RH (1979) Dosal root entry zone lesions for pain relief. J Neurosurg 51: 59–69
50. Ostdahl RH (1996) DREZ surgery for brachial plexus avulsion pain. In: Nashold BS, Pearlstein RD (eds) The DREZ operation. The American Association for Neurological Surgeons, Illinois, pp 105–124
51. Pitt M, Vredeveld JW (2005) The role of electromyography in the management of the brachial plexus palsy of the newborn. Clin Neurophysiol 116: 1756–1761
52. Pondaag W, Malessy MJA, Van Dijk JG, Thomeer RTWM (2004) Natural history of obstetric brachial plexus palsy: a systematic review. Dev Med Child Neurol 46: 138–144
53. Rankine JJ (2004) Adult traumatic brachial plexus injury. Clin Radiol 59: 767–774
54. Rexed D (1952) The cytoarchitectonic organization of the spinal cord in the cat. J Comp Neurol 96: 414–495
55. Schenker M, Birch R (2001) Diagnosis of the level of intradural rupture of the rootlets in traction lesions of the brachial plexus. J Bone Joint Surg 83-B: 916–920
56. Seddon H (1972) Surgical disorders of the peripheral nerves. Churchill Livingstone, Edinburgh London, pp 32–36, 174–198
57. Sever JW (1918) The results of a new operation for obstetrical paralysis. Am J Orthop Surg 16: 248–257
58. Sindou MP, Fischer G, Goutelle A, Mansuy L (1974) La radicellotomie posterieure selective. Premiers resultats dans la chirurgie de la douleur. Neurochirurgie 20: 391–408
59. Sindou MP, Blondet E, Emery E, Mertens P (2005) Microsurgical lesioning in the dorsal root entry zone for pain due to brachial plexus avulsion: a prospective series of 55 patients. J Neurosurg 102: 1018–1028

60. Smith SJM (1996) The role of neurophysiological investigation in traumatic brachial plexus lesions in adults and children. J Hand Surg 21: 145–148
61. Smith SJM (1998) Electrodiagnosis. In: Birch R, Bonney G, Wynn Parry CB (eds) Surgical disorders of the peripheral nerves. Churchill Livingstone, Edinburgh, pp 482–487
62. Specht EE (1975) Brachial plexus palsy in the newborn. Incidence and prognosis. Clin Orthop 110: 32–34
63. Steindler A (1918) A muscle plasty for the relief of flail elbow in infantile paralysis. Inter Med J 35: 235–241
64. Sunderland S (1968) Nerves and nerve injuries. Churchill Livingstone, Edinburgh London, 633 pp
65. Tan KL (1973) Brachial palsy. J Obstet Gynaecol Br Commonw 80: 60–62
66. Thomas DGT, Kitchen ND (1994) Long term follow up of dorsal root entry zone lesions in brachial plexus avulsion. J Neurol Neurosurg Psychiatr 57: 737–738
67. Torode I, Donnan L (1998) Posterior dislocation of the humeral head in association with obstetrical paralysis. J Pediatr Orthop 18: 611–615
68. Troum S, Floyd WED, Waters PM (1993) Posterior dislocation of the humeral head in infancy associated with obstetrical paralysis. A case report. J Bone Joint Surg 75-A: 1370–1375
69. Ubachs JHM, Slooff ACJ, Peeters LLM (1995) Obstetric antecedents of surgical treated obstetric brachial plexus injuries. Br J Obstet Gynaecol 102: 813–817
70. Van Dijk JG, Pondaag W, Malessy MJ (2001) Obstetric lesions of the brachial plexus. Muscle Nerve 24: 1451–1461
71. Van Egmond C, Tonino A, Kortleve JW (2001) Steindler flexorplasty of the elbow in obstetric brachial plexus injuries. J Pediatr Orthop 21: 169–173
72. Vredeveld JW, Blaauw G, Slooff ACJ, Richards R (1997) "Luxury innervation": does it exist and play a role at the time of birth? Electroencephalogr Clin Neurophysiol 107: 1P
73. Vredeveld JW, Blaauw G, Slooff ACJ, Richards R, Rozeman CAM (2000) The findings in paediatric obstetric brachial palsy differ from those in older patients: a suggested axplanation. Dev Med Child Neurol 42: 158–161
74. Vredeveld JW, Slooff BCJ, Blaauw G, Richards R (2001) Validation of an electromyography and nerve conduction study protocol for the analysis of brachial plexus lesions in 184 consecutive patients with traumatic lesions. J Clin Neuromusc Dis 2: 123–128
75. Wickstrom J, Haslam ET, Hutchinson RH (1955) The surgical management of residual deformities of the shoulder following birth injuries of the brachial plexus. J Bone Joint Surg 27A: 27–36
76. Wynn Parry CB (1984) Pain in avulsion of the brachial plexus. Neurosurgery 15: 960–965

# Surgical anatomy of the jugular foramen

P.-H. Roche[1], P. Mercier[2], T. Sameshima[3], and H.-D. Fournier[2]

[1] Service de Neurochirurgie, Hôpital Sainte Marguerite, CHU de Marseille, Marseille, France
[2] Service de Neurochirurgie et Laboratoire d'anatomie de la faculté de Médecine d'Angers, France
[3] Carolina Neuroscience Institute, Raleigh, NC, USA

With 20 Figures

## Contents

## Abstract

The jugular foramen (JF) is a canal that makes communication between the posterior cranial fossa and the upper neck for one third of the cranial nerves and for the main venous channel of the brain. From a lateral view, the JF is protected by multiple layers of muscles and by the outer surface of the petrous bone. Surgical exposure of the JF is usually justified by the removal of benign tumors that grow in this region.

In the first part of the present study we describe the surgical anatomy of the JF. Then, we detail the relevant points of a stepwise surgical progression of three lateral skull base approaches with a gradual level of exposure and invasiveness. The infralabyrinthine transsigmoid transjugular-high cervical approach is a conservative procedure that associates a retrolabyrinthine approach to a lateral dissection of the upper neck, exposing the sinojugular axis without mobilization of the facial nerve. In the second step, the external auditory canal is transsected and the intrapetrous facial nerve is mobilized, giving more exposure of the carotid canal and middle ear cavity. In the third step, a total petrosectomy is achieved with sacrifice of the cochlea, giving access to the petrous apex and to the whole course of the intrapetrous carotid artery.

Using the same dissection of the soft tissues from a lateral trajectory, these three approaches bring solutions to the radical removal of distinct tumor extensions. While the first step preserves the facial nerve and intrapetrous neuro-otologic structures, the third one offers a wide but more aggressive exposure of the JF and related structures.

*Keywords:* Glomus tumor; jugular foramen; lower cranial nerves; meningioma; skull base surgery.

## Introduction

The jugular foramen (JF) is a deeply located region that makes a communication between the posterior fossa and the superior latero-cervical area. The JF is a complex area of the skull base through which important cranial nerves and vessels course in variable anatomic patterns [2, 23, 26, 28]. The pathology that involves the JF is mainly of tumoral origin. Tumors may affect the JF primarily (e.g., schwannomas, glomus tumors, meningiomas) or secondarily (e.g., posterior fossa meningiomas, chondrosarcomas, metastasis). Surgical resection is the treatment of choice in the majority of cases. Radical resection exposes the patient to lower cranial nerves (LCNs) deficits, which is the most important source of morbidity after these operations. However, recent advances in radiation therapy techniques like radiosurgery may be proposed as first stair treatment for small tumors or by second intention for larger ones, allowing a less invasive surgical management [15, 18].

The exposure of the internal porus of the JF is well standardized, coming from a regular retrosigmoid intradural neurosurgical route. Likewise, it remains usual to control the outside aperture of the JF by exposing the upper neck. However, exposure of the whole length of the JF with preservation of the LCNs and using a single approach is challenging and necessitates an expertise in the field of skull base surgery.

The aim of this study is to provide the comprehensive anatomy of the main skull base approaches that give access within and around the JF. In the second part of the paper, a selection of these approaches will be presented in a stepwise manner.

## Microanatomy of the jugular foramen region

Because of the locoregional extension of the disease that usually involve the JF and the complexity of the elements that are necessarily exposed by its surgical approaches, it is preferable to detail the regional anatomy rather than the foramen itself spoken.

### *General consideration*

The JF is located in the cranial base in the posterior aspect of the petrooccipital fissure. It is bounded anterolaterally by the petrous bone and posteromedially by the basioccipital bone. The long axis of the foramen is directed from posterolateral to anteromedial. The right foramen is usually larger than the left (Fig. 1). Like some other foramina of the skull base, the JF does not correspond to a simple hole but is a canal that displays horizontal portion lying over the jugular process of the occipital bone and a vertical portion covered by the jugular fossa of the temporal bone. Viewed from the inside, its shape mimicks a tear drop with a narrow anteromedial part and an enlarged posterolateral margin. The structures that traverse the JF are the jugular bulb, the inferior petrosal sinus, meningeal branches of the ascending pharyngeal and occipital arteries and lower cranial nerves with their ganglia [12]. Hovelacque [11] is generally credited with classifying the JF into two compartments: an anteromedial containing the glossopharyngeal nerve (IX) and the inferior petrosal sinus (IPS) and a

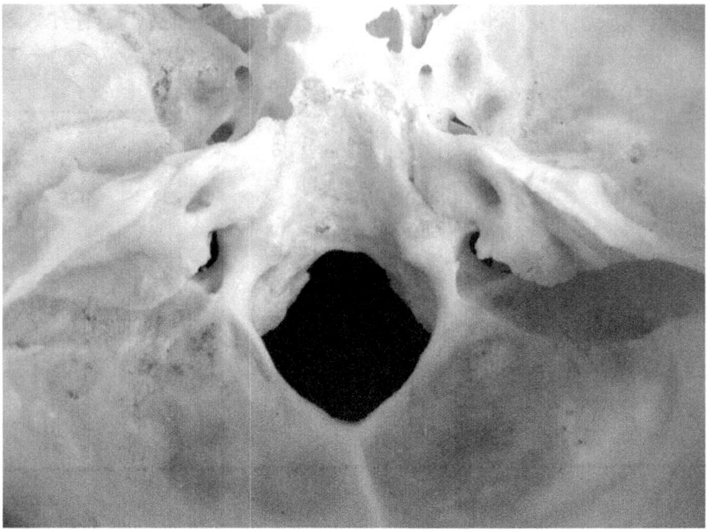

**Fig. 1.** Endocranial view of the bony anatomy of the JF showing the general configuration of the JF in the posterior fossa and the asymmetry of the right to left JF

posterolateral compartment containing the vagus (X), the spinal accessory nerve (XI), superior aspect of the jugular bulb and posterior meningeal artery.

A more recent description based on microsurgical anatomy from Katsuta *et al.* [12], has divided the JF into three compartments: A large posterolateral venous channel which receives the flow of the sigmoid sinus, a small anteromedial venous channel which receives the drainage of the inferior petrosal sinus, and an intermediary neural compartments which is located between the sigmoid and the petrosal parts. The neural part is an intrajugular part through which course the LCNs. The IX nerve is separated from X to XI nerves by the veinous channel that connect the petrosal part to the sigmoid part.

### *Bony limits of the JF and dura architecture*

The JF is delineated by bony boundaries that deserve a precise description.

Viewed from inside (Fig. 2), the superolateral limit of the JF is given by the inferior aspect of the posterior petrous bone. This upper border of the JF displays an anterior small excavation that is named pyramidal fossa in the apex of which opens the aperture of the cochlear acqueduct. The pyramidal fossa is an important landmark because it also houses the superior ganglion of the glossopharyngeal nerve, indicating the upper point of the LCNs. Backward, a posterior bony spine named the intrajugular process of the temporal bone is identified. This process constitutes the upper limit of the division between the petrosal and the sigmoid part of the JF. Behind this process, the petrous bone widen its circumference, and forms a large excavation that is named the jugular

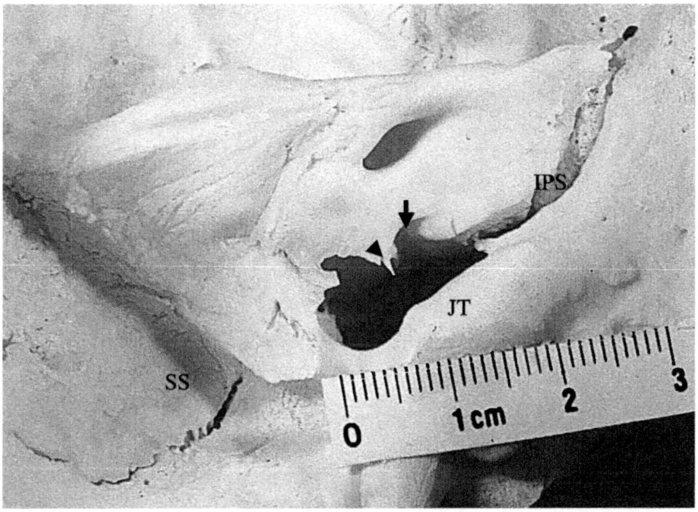


**Fig. 2.** Enlarged endocranial view of the left JF. Note the sharp bony boundaries of the JF. IPS indicates the groove of the inferior petrosal sinus. The black arrow shows the pyramidal fossa and the aperture of and endocochlear canal. The black arrowhead indicates the jugular spike of the temporal bone. *JT* Jugular tubercle of the occipital bone; *SS* groove of the sigmoid sinus

fossa. This excavation houses the jugular bulb (JB) and the jugular dome. The height of the dome is highly variable and a high jugular bulb (HJB) position may be an obstacle in some surgical procedures, as detailed previously [24]. At the posterior part of this excavation, lies a vertical bony ridge that is directed medially and named intrajugular ridge. This ridge makes a sharp division between the horizontal part of the sigmoid sinus and the jugular bulb. The inferomedial bony boundary of the JF is formed by the condylar part of the occipital bone and is also marked by a bony prominence that is named the intrajugular process of the occipital bone. This process constitutes the lower limit of the division between the petrosal and the sigmoid part of the JF. This bony anatomy is covered by the dura mater that completely hidden the jugular part of the JF. At the upper part of the JF, the dura thicken and makes a dural fold, which forms a roof to the glossopharyngeal meatus. The dura mater penetrates into the neural part of the JF and displays several fenestrations that give access to the LCNs; particularly there is a constant dural septum between the nerve IX and the nerve X. The dural guide plate that protects nerves IX–XI extends toward the exit of the JF where it joins to the pericranium on the inferior aspect of the outer skull base. The osteodural compartmentalization of the JF generally does not reach the outer skull base, as shown by the histological study conducted by Sen *et al.* [27].

Viewed from the outside (Fig. 3), the bony anatomy takes a circumferential shape due to the conformation of the jugular bulb and upper internal jugular

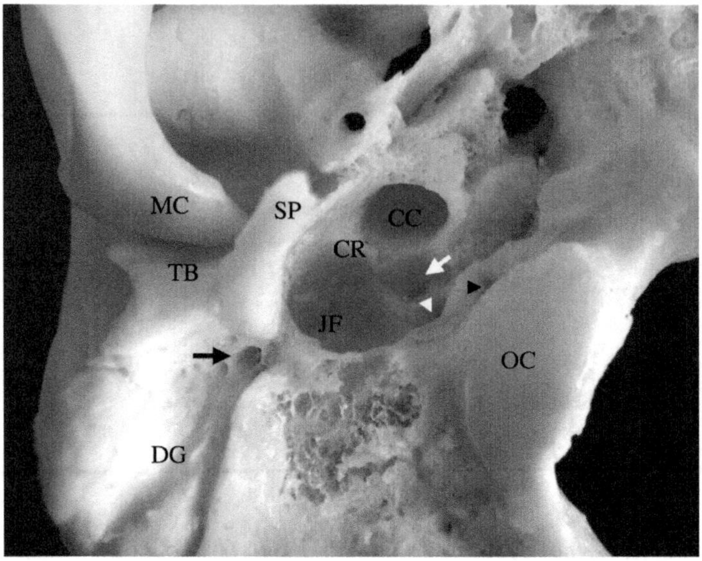


**Fig. 3.** Exocranial view of the right JF. *CC* Carotid canal, *CR* carotid ridge, *DG* digastric groove, *JF* jugular foramen, *MC* mandibular condyle, *OC* occipital condyle, *SP* styloid process, *TB* tympanic bone. The black arrow indicates the stylomastoid foramen, the black arrowhead indicates the external aperture of the hypoglossal canal, the white arrow shows the tympanicus canaliculus

vein. Anteriorly, the JF is limited by the carotid ridge, which is a transverse crest that separates the JF from the entry point of the carotid canal. Just anteromedial to this ridge a small hole is identified which is named the tympanic canaliculus and gives access to the tympanic nerve coursing toward the middle ear. The medial border of the JF is limited by the condylar part of the occipital bone and by the relief of the occipital condyle. The exit zone of the hypoglossal canal is identified at the anteromedial margin of the condyle. The posterior margin of the JF lies without special accident while its lateral margin is marked by several key landmarks in respect to surgical considerations: from the front to the back, just lateral to the carotid ridge is located the base of the styloid process. This process is attached to the vaginal part of the tympanic bone, which separates both the JF and the carotid canal from the glenoid fossa and temporomandibular join. The stylomastoid foramen is identified a few millimeters and lateral to the base of the styloid process. It is also located 5 mm lateral to the outer border of the JF. This foramen is just in front of the anterior edge of the digastric groove that is protected laterally by the mastoid tuberosity. These anatomic relationships clearly indicate that it is quite impossible to reach the depth of the JF and to control the LCNs inside the JF without mobilizing the third portion of the facial nerve. The same procedure is required if an access to the carotid canal is needed.

## *Neural contain of the jugular foramen*

During their course from the brain stem to the upper neck, the glossopharyngeal, vagus and accessory nerves, named lower cranial nerves (LCNs), run from a medial and horizontal trajectory to a lateral and vertical one. They also move from a craniocaudal distribution in their cisternal course to an anteroposterior one in the neck. These changing of trajectory from the brain stem to the neck, occur at the level of the JF where the LCNs converge. The shape of the jugular tubercle that represents the floor of the JF, allows these rerouting. The course of the LCNs can be subsequently classified in 3 segments: preforaminal or cisternal, intraforaminal, and extraforaminal or cervical.

### Intracisternal course (Fig. 4)

The glossopharyngeal nerve (CN IX) arises from the upper medulla dorsal to the olive. It consists of a dorsal root and most frequently of one small ventral root that is sometime difficult to identify. The nerve runs at the ventrocaudal aspect of the choroids plexus at the lateral recess of the fourth ventricule and courses anterolaterally in the cerebellomedullary cistern toward the antero-

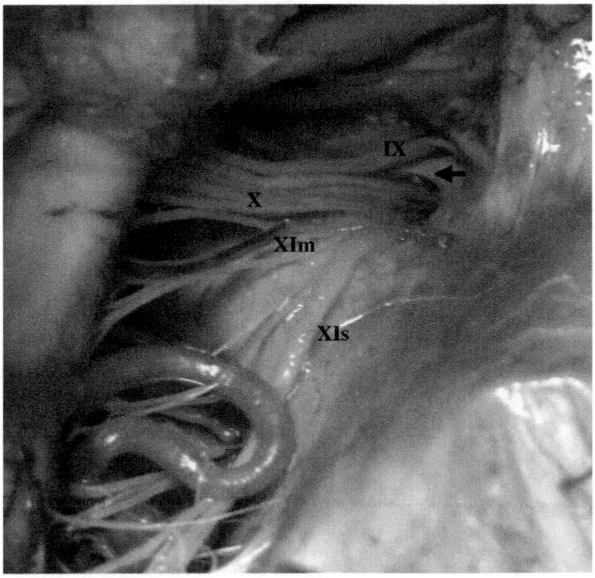


**Fig. 4.** Endocranial view of the right JF and lower cranial nerves after suboccipital exposure. The dura that covers the JF displays a septation (*black arrow*), which delineates two distinct apertures. The anterosuperior one contains the two bundles of the glossopharyngeal nerve (*IX*) while the posteroinferior one gives access to the vagus nerve (*X*), the medullary root of the spinal nerve (*XIm*) and the spinal root of the same nerve (*XIs*)

medial perforation of the dural covering of the jugular foramen. The nerve's intracisternal length between the brain stem and the dural porus is 15.65 mm (10–20 mm) [14]. The vagus nerve (CN X) consists of 8.6 (4–15) fiber bundles exiting from the retroolivary sulcus below the CN IX and following a cranio-caudal distribution. The intracisternal length of the fibers is equivalent to the CN IX. Both nerves are protected by the arachnoid membrane of the cerebellomedullary cistern and display close relationship with the first portion of the PICA.

The accessory nerve (CN XI) displays distinct cranial and spinal rootlets. A mean of 11 (6–16) cranial rootlets arise at the lower lever of the retroolivary sulcus while the spinal ones arise behind the first digitations of the dentate ligament, from the upper cervical cord. While approaching the inner dural orifice of the JF, cranial and spinal rootlets converge and most frequently penetrate the same dural hole then the vagus nerve.

## Intraforaminal course (Fig. 5)

Some amount of arachnoid membrane enters inside the foramen around a variable length of the nerve's course. While penetrating inside the JF via its

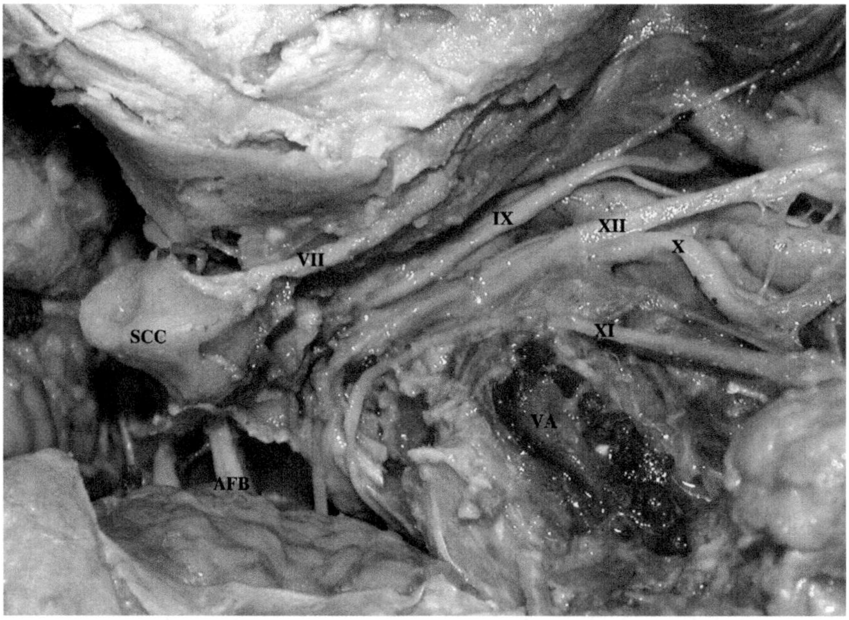


**Fig. 5.** Intraforaminal course of the lower cranial nerves on the right side. Note the change of direction and disposition of the nerves from their intracisternal portion to their extracranial course. *AFB* Acousticofacial bundle in the cerebellopontine angle, *SCC* superior semicircular canal, *VA* vertebral artery, *VII* facial nerve, *IX* glossopharyngeal nerve, *X* vagus nerve, *XI* spinal nerve, *XII* hypoglossal nerve

own dural porus the CN IX forms a superior and an inferior ganglion. The latter one is located just above or at the level of the external porus of the JF and gives off a branch, the tympanic branch (Jacobson's nerve) that enters the tympanic canaliculus to course in the middle ear at the surface of the promontory. The ganglion cells that belong to this nerve may give rise to glomus tumors (tympanic paragangliomas). The vagus nerve enters the JF behind the intrajugular process of the temporal bone. The dural bridge that separates the entry points of the IX and X nerves is not identified in the depth of the foramen. The rootlets of the CN X gather inside the foramen and form the superior ganglion of the vagus nerve. The average distance of the ganglion from the intracranial opening has been estimated to 2.6 mm, ranging from 2.2 to 3.0 mm [27]. This ganglion occupies the totality of the intraforaminal segment of the nerve and its average size was measured as 4.2 mm (range: 4.0–4.5 mm) in the same study [27]. At the level of the ganglion, there is a close relationship between the three LCNs which fibers establish connections. The superior vagal ganglion gives off an auricular branch (Arnold's nerve) that courses into the mastoid canaliculus toward the mastoid segment of the fallo-

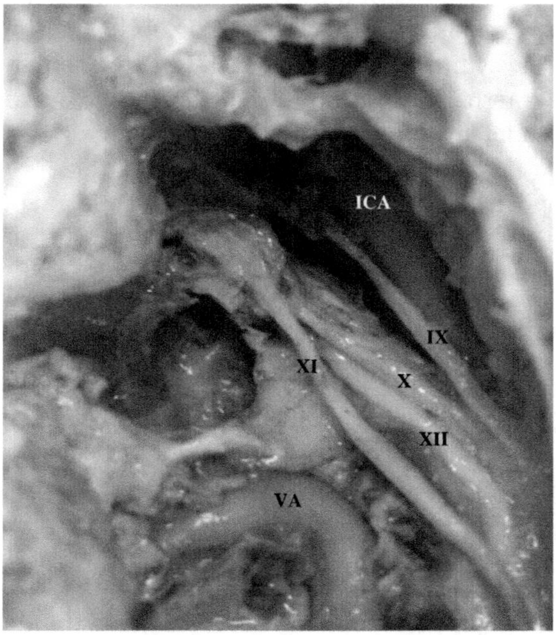


**Fig. 6.** Exocranial course of the lower cranial nerves on the right side. The jugular vein and jugular bulb have been resected. The internal carotid artery (*ICA*) is exposed in the carotid canal and the vertebral artery (*VA*) has been identified between the atlas and the axis. The hypoglossal nerve (*XII*) is identified just under and behind the vagus nerve (*X*)

pian canal and offers a branch to the facial nerve. This branch in its intrapetrous course may also give rise to glomus tumor. The cranial and spinal portions of the CN XI usually converge to enter the vagal meatus together. It is then difficult to separate the vagal from the accessory nerve inside the foramen because they display intimate interconnections at the level of the superior ganglion.

### Extraforaminal course (Fig. 6)

The exit of LCN from the JF can be visualized only by reflection of the internal jugular vein and microscopic dissection of the inner wall of the jugular bulb. The nerves exit anteromedial to the jugular bulb, separated from it by thin layers of connective tissue. At the caudal end of the JF, CN IX is anchored to the ICA and to the junction of the JB with the internal jugular vein by a dense connective tissue. The CN IX gives off its tympanic branch (see above) and runs inferoanteriorly, crossing the lateral wall of the internal carotid artery, medial to the styloid process at the level of which it divides into several branches. The vagus nerve exists the JF vertically, behind the CN IX and often joined with the accessory nerve. It forms the inferior vagal ganglion and courses posterior to the ICA. At the level of the lower ganglion, the vagus nerve gives off several branches that communicate with CNs IX, XI and XII. Another branch is connected to the sympathetic trunk which fibers penetrate the carotid canal and forms the internal carotid nerve. The accessory nerve separates from the vagal nerve under the JF and gradually crosses the outer surface of the jugular vein while descending and coursing backward. More rarely, the CN XI courses inferoposteriorly at the medial surface of the internal jugular vein.

## *Hypoglossal canal and nerve*

The hypoglossal canal does not belong to the JF, but takes place in its close vicinity. The CN XII leaves the medulla oblongata at the level of the preolivary sulcus and anterolaterally to enter the hypoglossal foramen. Then it courses through dense connective tissue in the hypoglossal canal, which is approximately 7.5 mm inferior to the FJ, under the jugular tubercle and at the top of the medial part of the occipital condyle. The exit point of the hypoglossal canal is just medial and under the outer margin of the JF. At this point, the CN XII passes adjacent to the vagus nerve at the level of the inferior ganglion of the vagus nerve and connects with it by several thin branches. Then the nerve runs anteromedial to the CN XI and crosses the posterior and lateral wall of the ICA under the nerve IX toward the tongue (Fig. 7). In the upper neck, the nerve is protected by the posterior belly of the digastric muscle.

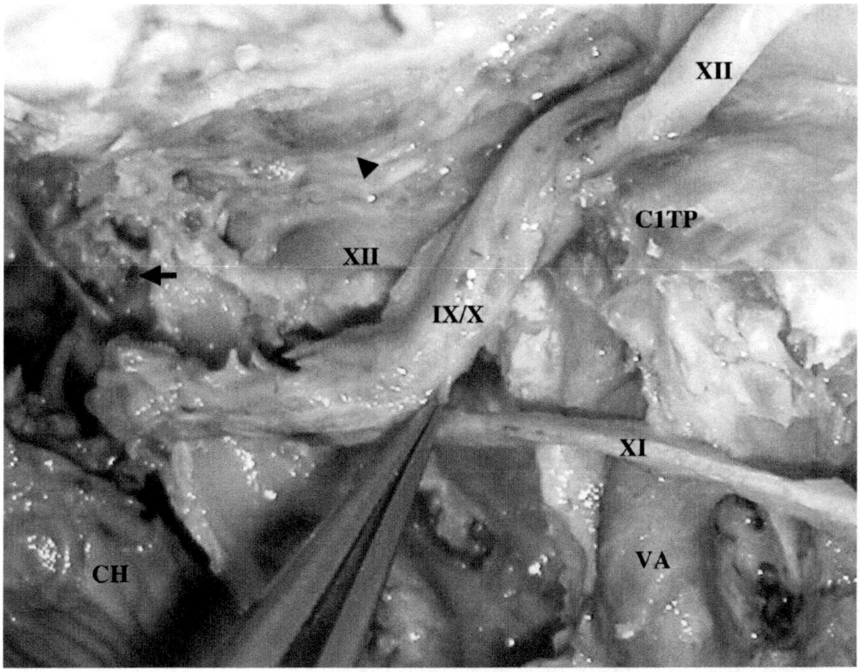


**Fig. 7.** Exocranial view of the lower cranial nerves (*IX*, *X* and *XI*) and hypoglossal nerve (*XII*) on the right side. The jugular vein and jugular bulb have been resected. The black arrowhead shows a branch of the ascending pharyngeal artery that feed the JF. Note the close relationship of the LCN in the upper neck with the transverse process of C1 (*C1TP*). The black arrow shows the opening of the inferior petrosal sinus. *CH* Cerebellar hemisphere

## *Venous relationships*

The sigmoid sinus drains into the posterior aspect of the jugular bulb (JB). The JB varies considerably in size and shape as described above. The dome of the JB can extend as high as the internal auditory canal or protrude in the mesotympanum. The JB lies beneath the floor of the middle ear cavity. This floor, which is usually formed by a compact bone, may be thin or dehiscent in cases with a HJB. The lateral wall of the JB is separated from the vertical segment (mastoid segment) of the facial nerve (Third portion) by the retrofacial and infralabyrinthine air cells. It is important to note that the wall of the jugular bulb is very thin and fragile because devoid of adventitia [13]. At its outside aperture, the JF is reinforced by a periosteal ring and acquires a normal venous structure while becoming the internal jugular vein.

The IPS (Fig. 8) is the major site of drainage for the cavernous sinus. There is usually one main sinus orifice located most frequently between the exit of IX and X. The IPS which has a variable course and drainage pattern, usually enters

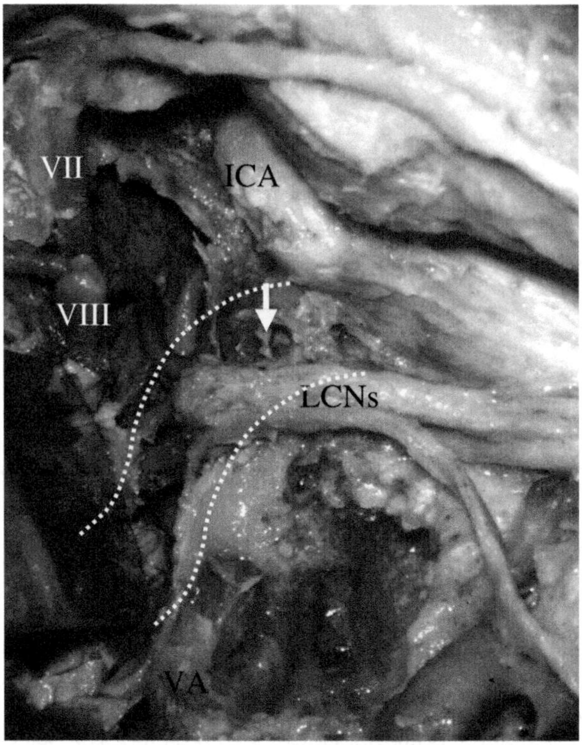


**Fig. 8.** Venous relationship of the jugular foramen region (*right side*). The sigmoid sinus, jugular bulb and internal jugular vein have been resected in order to expose the apertures of the inferior petrosal sinus. In this case, there are two channels that are divided by a fibrous septum (*white arrow*). Note that in this case, the CN IX is not separated from the CN X by the opening of the IPS. The double white dotted line indicates the position of the jugular bulb before transaction and removal

the anterior aspect of the jugular bulb in around 90% of cases; in other cases, the IPS shares its drainage into the JB and the internal jugular veins and more rarely exclusively into the internal jugular vein (10%). In other circumstances of poorly developed IPS, it drains into a deep cervical plexus of veins. In such cases, the IPS makes a plexiform confluens with the venous plexus of the hypoglossal canal, the inferior petroclival vein, and tributaries from the posterior condylar emissary vein. The posterior condylar emissary vein courses into the posterior condylar canal and enters the thicker inferior wall of the JF below the sigmoid sinus. This vein puts into communication the vertebral venous plexus to the jugular bulb. It usually opens into the posteromedial aspect of the junction between the SS and the JB. The venous plexus of the hypoglossal canal is also named anterior condylar vein. It communicates the marginal sinus of the foramen magnum with the jugular bulb (in 11.53% of cases [14]). It may do so directly or by the intermediary of a plexiform chamber located at the lower end of the IPS.

## *Arteries*

The region of the JF is mainly supplied by the occipital artery and the ascending pharyngeal artery. The occipital artery (OA) arises either the posterior or the lateral aspect of the external carotid artery (ECA), at a variable distance from the carotid bifurcation [1]. These authors have described three segments, the digastric segment, the suboccipital segment and the terminal segment. The digastric segment extends from the origin of the OA to the exit of the occipital groove. In its distal digastric segment, the OA runs medially to the posterior belly of the digastric muscle and the emergence of the facial nerve from the stylomastoid foramen. The OA gives off several muscular branches to the SCM, DM, and the group of muscles inserted on the transverse process of C1. The OA gives off meningeal branches from a "stylomastoid" trunk that enters the JF to reach the dura of the posterior fossa. The ascending pharyngeal artery (APA) belongs to the posterior group of the occipital artery's branches. In all specimens the APA gives off a posterior meningeal branch to the JF. This artery courses upward ventral to the ICA and IJV and enters the JF most often between CN X and XI. Several others meningeal branches from the APA pass through the foramen lacerum, JF and hypoglossal canal, to supply the surrounding dura of the posterior cranial fossa. The APA also gives rise to the inferior tympanic artery, which reaches the tympanic cavity by way of the tympanic canaliculus also shared by the Jacobson's nerve. An accessory supply is given by the posterior auricular artery, which arises above the posterior belly of the DM and courses between the parotid gland and the styloid process. It gives off a branch dedicated to the stylomastoid foramen that supply the facial nerve, and branches that may connect with the occipital artery to supply the JF. Muscular branches that come from the extracranial part of the vertebral artery (VA) may rarely feed the outside of the JF. While penetrating the dura mater in C1, the dural branches of the VA give supply to the dura of the craniocervical junction. In some cases, it can also provide feeders to the posterior part of the JF.

At the level of the skull base, the ICA courses just anterior to the jugular vein, being separated from it by the carotid ridge. At this level, both artery and vein are surrounded by the thick fibrous attachment of the carotid sheath to the periosteum of the skull base (Fig. 9). This periosteum is also in the continuum of the styloid ligaments. The ICA enters the carotid canal and describes a short vertical portion before turning at right angle and taking a horizontal course. While it changes of direction, the ICA is located just below the promontory that corresponds to the basal turn of the cochlea at the inner surface of the middle ear. Into the carotid canal, the ICA is surrounded by a loose venous plexus and by the carotid sympathetic nerves. It gives rise to a small branch

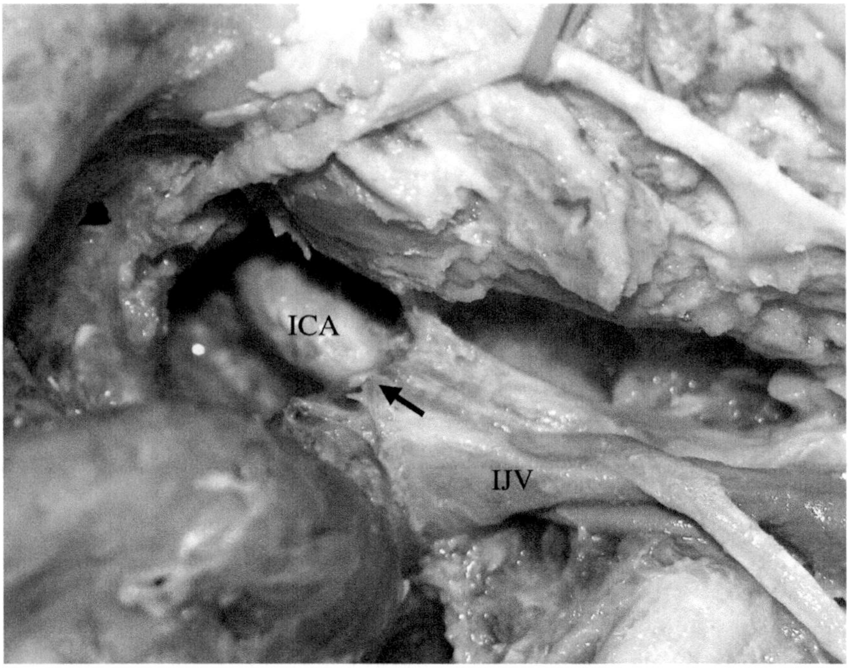


**Fig. 9.** General anatomy of the outer surface of the JF (*right side*). The bone has been resected and the upper neck has been dissected following a widened transcochlear technique. The close relationship between the carotid artery and the internal jugular vein are shown. The *black arrow* indicates the periosteal ring that ensheath both vessels at inferior margin of the JF. *ICA* Ascending portion of the intrapetrous internal carotid artery, *IJV* Internal jugular vein

named the caroticotympanic artery that reaches the tympanic cavity laterally through a small aperture.

## *Muscular environment*

We focus here on the muscles that cover the lateral area of the JF and that are exposed during the lateral approaches (Fig. 10).

The first group of muscles are inserted in the proximity of the mastoid process. The most superficial is the sternocleidomastoid muscle (SCM). It attaches above the mastoid process and the lateral border of the superior nuchal line. It runs obliquely downward and forward. Just under the SCM, the splenius capitus attaches at the mastoid tip and runs downward and backward. Deeper and medial to the mastoid tip, the posterior belly of the digastric muscle arises in the digastric groove and runs anteroinferiorly to reach the hyoid bone. This muscle is innervated by the facial nerve.

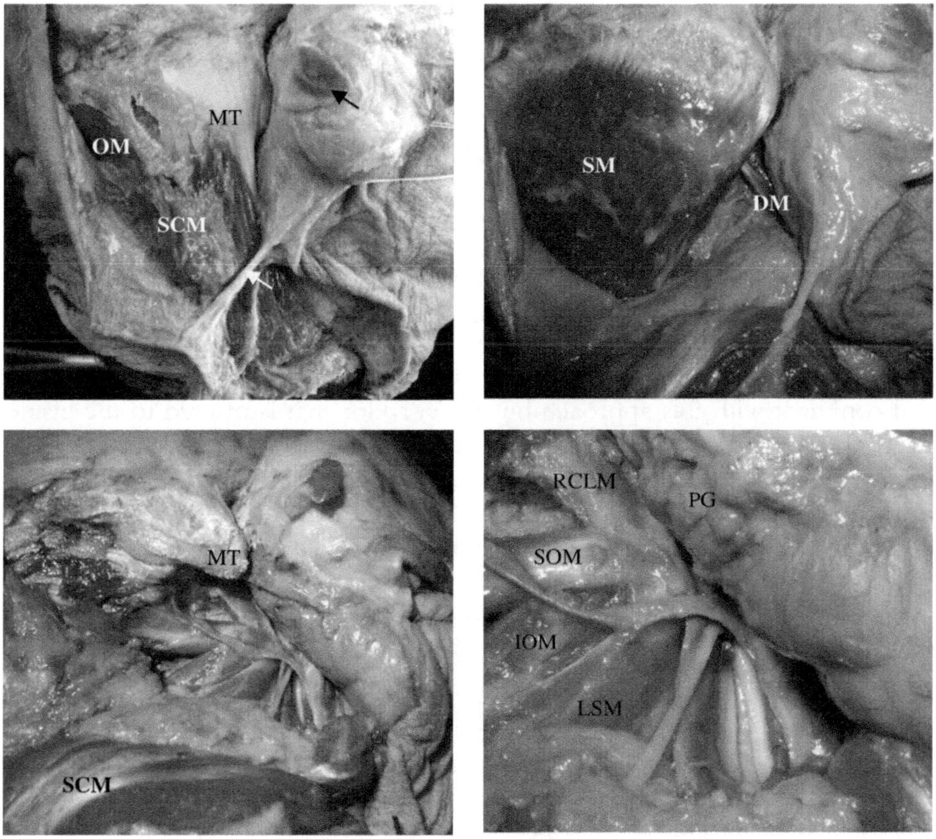


**Fig. 10.** Lateral view of the muscles that cover the region of the JF. The skin and galea have been elevated forward. The external auditory meatus has been preserved. The black arrow indicates the posterior auricular muscle. The white arrow indicates a branch of the superficial cervical plexus. The mastoid tip (*MT*) and the parotid gland (*PG*) are important landmarks. The superficial layers are shown at the top right and left of the figure. *OM* Occipital muscles, *SCM* sternocleidomastoid muscle, *DM* digastric muscle, *SM* splenius capitis muscle. The muscles that are inserted on the lateral process of C1 constitute the deep layer. *IOM* Inferior oblique muscle, *LSM* levator scapulae muscle, *RCLM* rectus capitis lateral muscle, *SOM* superior oblique muscle

The second group consists in the muscles that are attached to the styloid process. They are deeply seated just lateral and anterior to the JF. The styloglossus muscle is attached anteriorly, the stylohyoid laterally and the stylopharyngeal posteromedially.

The third group of muscle are mainly attached to the transverse process of the atlas. In this group, two muscles run upward: The rectus capitis lateral muscle is short and vertical, running toward the medial and anterior border of the digastric groove. The superior oblique muscle runs upward and backward toward the condylar part of the occipital bone. Two other muscles run posteroinferiorly, the inferior oblique muscle and the levator scapulae muscle.

## The approaches to the region of the jugular foramen

### *Classification and selection of the approach* (Fig. 11)

The number and complexity of the approaches that have been proposed for the control of the lesions involving the JF illustrates the lack of ideal procedure. As mentioned above, the inner portion of the JF is usually properly reached using a suboccipital retrosigmoid approach [25]. All neurosurgeons are familiar and confident with this approach but the corridor that is offered to the inside of the JF is limited and blind. It is generally reserved to control the cisternal extension of the disease (case illustration 1). Excepting this regular cisternal route, the other ones belong to the field of skull base procedures and can be classified following the target that is aimed.

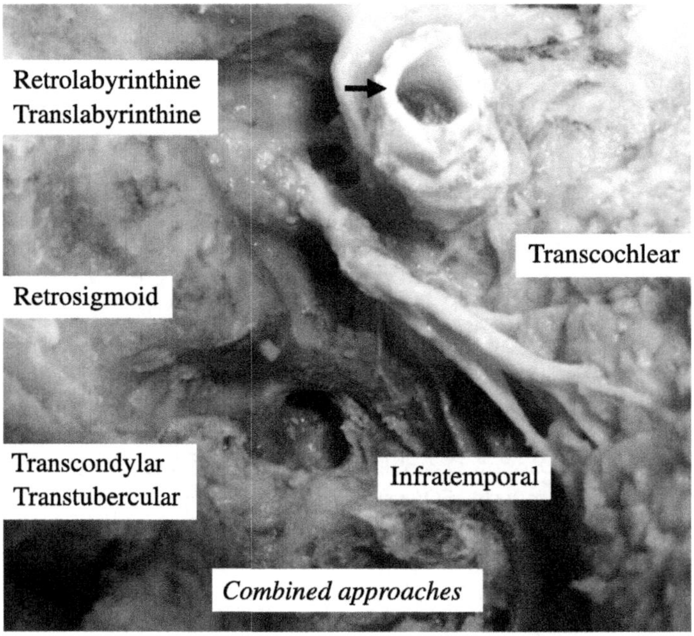


**Fig. 11.** Summary of the main surgical approaches to the region of the JF. The present dissection represents the final step of the infralabyrinthine transigmoid transjugular-high cervical approach. Several of these approaches can be used in a combined manner (*combined approaches*), depending on the extension of the disease and clinical condition. The black arrow indicates the cartilaginous wall of the outer meatus that has been cut

The inferolateral approaches are represented by transcondylar [3], juxta condylar [8], far lateral or extreme lateral approaches [29]. They target the posterolateral part of the JF and craniocervical junction.

The posterolateral approach is illustrated by the infralabyrinthine transigmoid transjugular-high cervical approach, as described below.

The superolateral approaches are the retrolabyrinthine and the translabyrinthine approaches. Both of them expose the jugular dome and bulb from above and do not control the lower cranial nerves in their intra and extraforaminal portion.

The anterolateral approaches associate a transpetrous and an upper neck exposure: The Fisch infratemporal fossa [4] approach and the widened transcochlear approach [19] belong to this group. In an attempt to obtain a similar exposure with a less invasive technique, it is possible to combine a retrolabyrinthine exposure with an upper neck dissection as we will detail below.

Selection of the approach depends on the tumor characteristics, patient examination, and expertise of the team.

The nature, the origin and the extension of the tumor are crucial points, obtained from high-resolution preoperative imaging. As stated by Lustig and Jackler [16], tumors located lateral to the cranial nerves are favourable for cranial nerve preservation during surgical excision. Recently, Ramina *et al.* [22], reviewed their experience about 106 consecutive tumors of the jugular foramen. Most of them were paragangliomas (57%) while schwannomas and meningiomas represented respectively 16 and 10% of cases. Excepting rare cases of primary cervical location [17], meningiomas usually grow up from the intradural compartment of the JF and shift the nerves that remain protected by arachnoid at the early stage of tumor development. They modify the adjacent petrooccipital bone and secondarily involve the inside of the foramen. Schwannomas are relatively uncommon in this location, representing less than 3% of intracranial schwannomas. They involve one or several rootlets of the LCNs from the beginning [25]. The early symptoms of presentation depend on the nerve of origin; however, this may not be true in cases of jugular foramen tumors, because the compartment is so narrow that all LCNs may be involved at the same time. Although these tumors can adopt various location in the foramen as described in published classifications [7], the dumbbell shape configuration also named Type D [19], is the most typical one. Bone window CT scan may show considerable widening of the JF and high-resolution MR images show significant enhancement of the tumor mass after gadolinium administration. The tumor mass may also display cystic features. Paragangliomas may develop from various points in the petrous bone or along the LCNs in the region of the JF [9]. The venous axis is usually invaded and occluded because the most frequent location of paraganglioma is the jugular bulb region. As stated by Fisch and Mattox [5], the medial wall of the sigmoid sinus is usually spared by the tumor. The full extension of the tumor along the carotid canal may be difficult to identify but this involvement may influence the selection of the approach. Paraganglioma are richly vascularized by feeders coming from the external carotid artery and particularly from the ascending pharyngeal artery. Preoperative embolization of the tumor's feeders may be useful to decrease the blood loss during removal. The preoperative work-up of the patients must include a complete otological and neurological examination, audiological testing, CT, MRI, MR angiogram and digital subtraction angiography.

From the patient's perspective, hearing level, facial nerve status and function of the LCNs are crucial point to select the approach and the therapeutic planning. However, several authors had underlined [27] that cranial nerve impairment may not be present despite microscopic infiltration of tumor among the nerve's fascicles. Hopefully, large tumors are generally associated to LCN deficits that have already been compensated before surgery. In this situation, surgical damage or sacrifice of nerves is well tolerated. However, it may be necessary to leave some tumor against the nerves and discuss adjunctive treatment or careful follow-up. For extensive paragangliomas, it may be scheduled that the IX nerve is difficult to preserve and that the epinerium of the facial nerve may be invaded [5]. General condition, previous treatments like radiation therapy and own opinion of a well-informed patient are essential in the decision-making process.

The team needs to be prepared to this kind of surgery. The collaboration between an ear-head and neck surgeon and a neurosurgeon is requested. They need both to have a perfect knowledge of the anatomy of the normal and pathological skull base. It is also strongly advised to have the whole panel of approaches available in order to provide a tailored surgery. It is also recommended to be able to monitor the electrophysiology of facial nerve and LCNs during the operative time and to offer a postoperative observation in an intensive care unit.

## *The infralabyrinthine transsigmoid transjugular-high cervical approach*

This approach combines several techniques in order to expose the JF and related structures in an extensive manner while preserving the neuro-otologic structures of the petrous bone.

### Dissection of the superficial layers

The patient is positioned supine and the head is turned 70° toward the opposite side. The skin incision is C shaped around the external ear from the temporal fossa to the upper neck, ending in front of the SCM under the angle of mandibula. Skin is elevated and reclined frontward. The external auditory canal is not necessarily divided; It may be the case if there is a need to work in the middle ear cavity in front of the vertical segment of the facial nerve. Temporal muscle is desinserted. Anterior chief of the SCM is desinserted from the mastoid process, showing the splenius capitis. This muscle is also desinserted from the mastoid process. In the depth, the posterior belly of the digastric muscle is identified. During the dissection of the upper neck, under this muscle, the internal jugular vein and the XI nerve are shown. In 80% of cases the XI nerve courses over the IJV posteroinferiorly while it courses under the vein in 20% of cases in the same direction. In front of the IJV, the internal carotid artery runs vertically. At the early step of the operation, there is no need to dissect the vagus nerve in the depth between the IJV and the ICA. Under the mastoid tip, the IJV courses just in front of the lateral process of C1. This process is not directly seen because covered by a group of four muscles as detailed previously and shown in Fig. 10. This is a key landmark for the identification of the inferior part of the operative field and for identification of the vertebral artery before its penetration point in the dura.

## Exposure of the upper pole of the JF

In order to approach the sigmoid sinus and the junction with the jugular bulb, a retrolabyrinthine step is undertaken. This step has been extensively described in previous papers [20]. Briefly, the drilling is conducted gradually toward the depth in front of the sigmoid sinus, exposing the mastoid air cells. Backward it is essential to expose the sinodural angle between the superior petrosal sinus and the sigmoid sinus. The mastoid antrum is identified while the loop of the lateral SCC is approached medially in a more compact yellowish bone. Just under this loop, the facial nerve courses in the Fallopian canal, describing an angle that varies from 95 to 125° between the tympanic and the vertical segment (13 mm). The anatomy and variation of the facial nerve into the petrous bone has been nicely described in the Proctor's textbook [21]. It is not necessary to skeletonize extensively the canal at this time but the nerve is followed as far as the stylomastoid foramen. This foramen is identified in front of the anterior margin of the digastric groove. While drilling the infralabyrinthine air cells, the jugular dome is unroofed using a diamond drill, and cautiously detached from the jugular fossa. At this place and as mentioned above, the wall of the bulb is extremely thin and care should be taken to leave a thin eggshell bone over the dome to protect it.

## Exposure the lateral circumference of the jugular bulb

The occipital bone is also exposed behind the sigmoid sinus and the lateral part of the condyle is drilled under and behind the jugular bulb. It is important to keep in mind the trajectory of the sigmoido-jugular complex and realize that

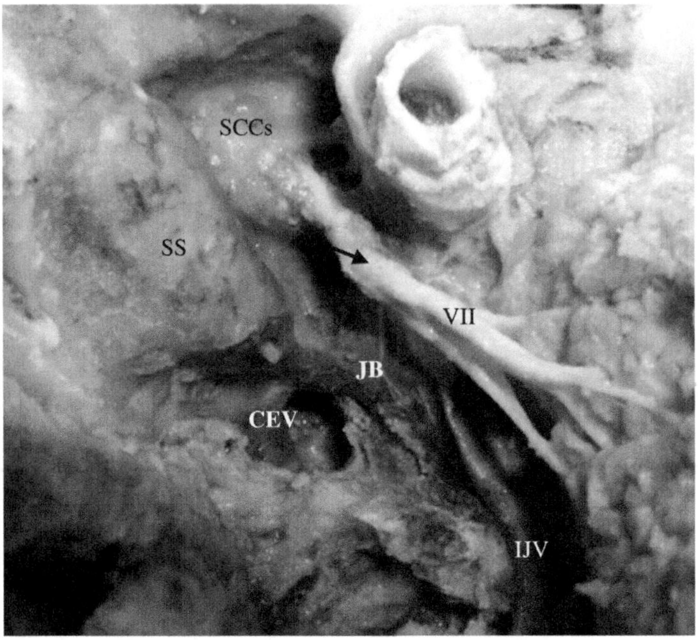


**Fig. 12.** The infralabyrinthine transsigmoid transjugular-high cervical approach is achieved. The approach preserves the intrapetrous neuro-otologic structures. The semicircular canals (*SCCs*) are exposed at the top of the field. The facial nerve (*VII*) is exposed in its vertical segment and can be mobilized along a very short segment in the area of the stylomastoid foramen (*black arrow*). This maneuver allows an optimized exposure of the jugular bulb (*JB*). The venous axis is extensively exposed, from the sinodural angle to the internal jugular vein (*IJV*). *CEV* Condylar emissary vein

this step is conducted in the depth under magnification. The mastoid tip is removed, the digastric muscle is divided and the styloid process identified. It is of importance to note that the facial nerve leave the stylomastoid foramen just laterally to the "pars venosa" of the JF. Thus, in order to control the elements of the JF, particularly the LCNs, the stylomastoid foramen should be opened and the facial nerve identified in its course before entering the parotid gland (Fig. 12). This procedure allows a safe mobilisation of the facial nerve along a restricted segment of its course. Care should be taken to preserve the vascularization of the nerve (see above). In this way, a normal postoperative motor facial function may be expected. Usually, the periosteum of the stylomastoid foramen is tightly attached to the facial nerve; thus the nerve should be elevated with this surrounding tissue, as recommended by Fisch and Mattox [5].

## Exposure of the LCNs inside the jugular foramen

Since the LCNs course anteromedially to the jugular bulb, their intraforaminal segment cannot be exposed if the venous axis is not mobilized. The sigmoid

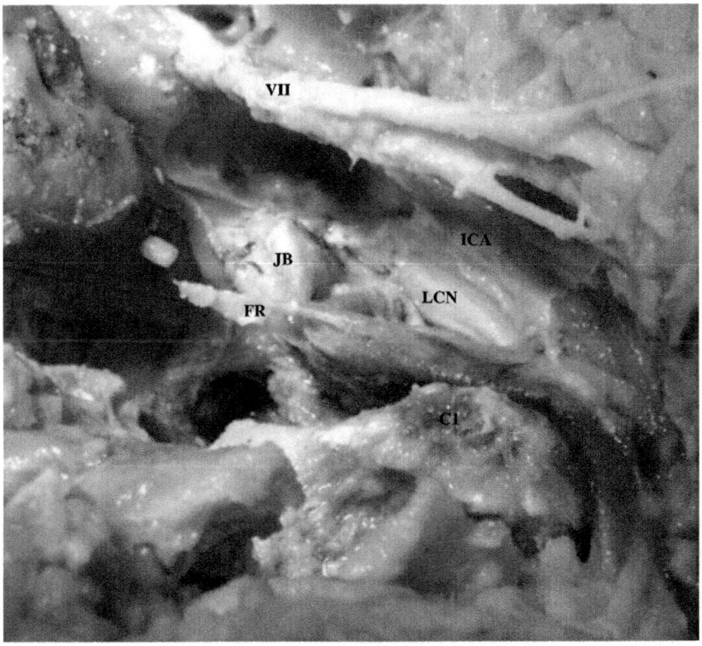


**Fig. 13.** Once the exposure has been achieved, it can be necessary to expose the lower cranial nerves (*LCN*) inside the JF. The IJV is ligated and elevated in a retrograd way. Note the close relationship of the IJV with the lateral mass of the atlas (*C1*). *FR* Fibrous ring, *ICA* Internal carotid artery, *JB* jugular bulb, *LCN* lower cranial nerves

sinus is ligated and divided in its vertical portion after making an incision of the pre- and retrosigmoid dura and put two threads for the ligation. The IJV is also ligated and divided in the neck, under the level of C1, and elevated in a retrograde way as far as it joins the jugular bulb. The jugular bulb is now freed from the jugular fossa (Fig. 13) but achievement of the venous exclusion needs the identification and the occlusion of the aperture of the IPS in the bulb. This venous occlusion is achieved by plugging its aperture with pieces of Surgicel. The permeability of the venous axis and the anatomical variation of the IPS drainage should be adequately assessed by a venous angiogram or MR angiogram before undertaking surgery. The LCNs are now identified and can be dissected in their intraforaminal course depending on the individual pathological anatomy. Since the pre- and retrosigmoid dura has been opened, it is possible to control the intracisternal segment of the LCNs.

## Tumor resection and closure steps

The procedure of tumor resection depends on the insertion and extension of the lesion; it is also greatly influenced by the pathology of the lesion. Careful hemostasis is required because drainage is generally avoided. The posterior tympanotomy is closed using the bone dust that has been harvested in the operative field during drilling, and that is mixed with biological glue. Large strips of abdominal fat cover the cavity of petrectomy and the dura defect in order to avoid cerebrospinal fluid leak.

## Commentaries

This approach has been developed and used by previous authors [6, 22] and is a minimal invasive skull base procedure. The approach is conducted using reliable permanent landmarks and may be routinely performed by any neuro-otologic team. This approach offers multiple corridors to the intra- and extra-dural portions of the JF region, which allows an ideal control of dumbbell shaped tumors. The mobilization of the facial nerve is limited to the region of the stylomastoid foramen and in the distal part of the vertical portion of the facial canal. Thereby, a good facial motor function may be expected after operation. The neuro-otologic structures are preserved inside the petrous bone. The major limitation of this approach is the insufficient exposure of the carotid canal, protympanum and petrous apex.

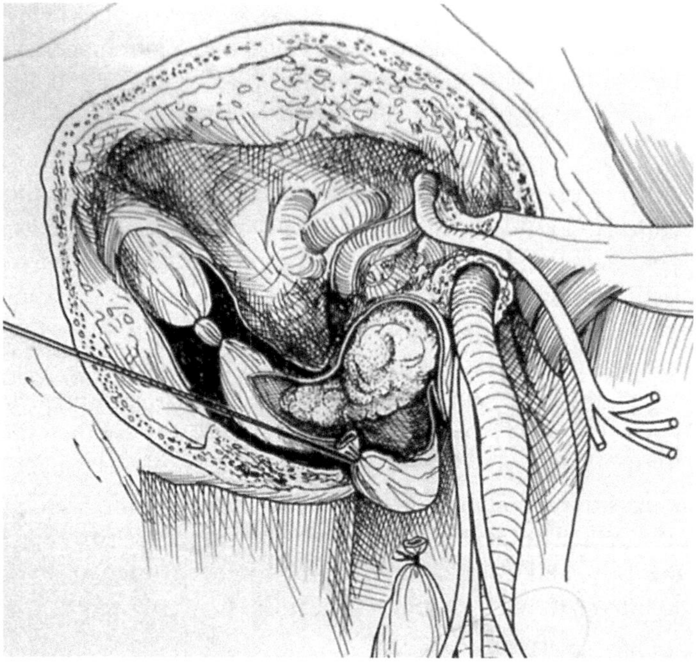

**Fig. 14.** Illustration of an infratemporal Type A approach on the right side. The internal jugular vein and the sigmoid sinus have been ligated and the lumen of the venous channel has been opened, exposing the tumor. Observe the anterior mobilisation of the second and third portion of the facial nerve

### *The Fisch infratemporal fossa approach Type A*

The first steps of this approach are similar to those of the previous approach regarding the skin incision and elevation of fascia and muscles. Blind sac closure of the external auditory canal and total removal of the skin from the external auditory canal are achieved. The facial nerve is identified in the parotid gland and major vessels are exposed in the upper neck. A subtotal petrosectomy is conducted with total mastoidectomy in the way of a retrolabyrinthine approach (Fig. 14). Tympanic and mastoid segment of the facial nerve are identified from the geniculate ganglion to the stylomastoid foramen. The chorda tympani is sectioned and the hypotympanum is exposed. The facial nerve is transposed anteriorly and protected in a new canal that is drilled in the remaining petrous and tympanic bone. These consecutive procedures allow the exposure of the entire carotid canal from the tympanic ostium of the Eustachian tube down to the carotid foramen.

#### Commentaries

In order to control the disease that extends into the middle ear and the carotid canal, it is needed to proceed forward sectioning the external auditory canal, opening the middle ear and mobilizing the facial nerve. This approach preserves the cochlea and posterior labyrinth. Moreover, the mobilization of the facial nerve gives more space available in front of the jugular foramen. In case of additional extension toward the petrous apex, the petroclival area and the parapharyngeal space, it is possible to modify the Type A approach; this modification requires the resection of the superficial lobe of the parotid gland, resection of the TMJ, removal of the styloid muscles and ligaments (Fisch B). Section of the mandibular branch of the trigeminal nerve as described in the Fisch type C approach, should be avoided as possible.

### *The widened transcochlear approach*

Infiltration of the carotid canal, petroclival region and infratemporal fossa justify an extensive approach, which associate at the same time a total petrosectomy as described in the original transcochlear approach described by House and Hitselberger [10] and the dissection of the upper neck. Such combined exposure can be achieved by the widened transcochlear approach as described by Pellet *et al.* [19]. Actually, this approach offers a wider corridor than the Fisch infratemporal Type B approach, but avoids the section of the maxillary branch of the trigeminal nerve.

From an infratemporal fossa Type A, it is possible to proceed toward a widened transcochlear approach (WTCA) because both approaches share the same initial steps. Skin incision, retrolabyrinthine exposure and upper neck dissection are similar. At that time, and before mobilizing the facial nerve,

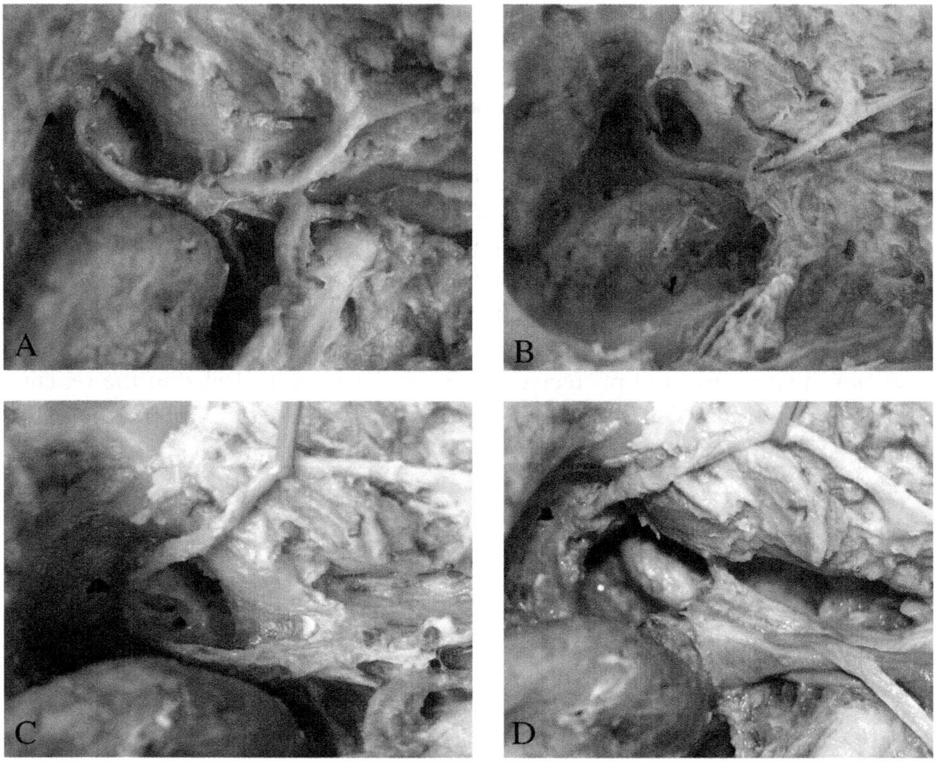


**Fig. 15.** Widened transcochlear approach performed on the right side of an injected specimen. (A) The first steps are equivalent to those that are conducted during an infratemporal Type B approach. (B) The posterior labyrinth (semicircular canals and vestibule) and the cochlea are drilled, in order to expose the first and second portion of the Faloppian canal. (C) The facial nerve has been mobilized from its bony canal and dissected from the stylomastoid foramen. (D) The widened transcochlear approach is now achieved. Note the completeness of the petrosectomy and the wide exposure of the jugular bulb and intrapetrous carotid artery

the semicircular canals are drilled and the vestibule is opened in order to reach the fundus of the IAC. The upper and the lower border of the IAC are then drilled and the surgeon is now in the situation of a translabyrinthine approach. Then, it is time to skeletonize the fallopian canal and mobilize the facial nerve forward, from the geniculate ganglion to the extracranial segment of the nerve (Fig. 15). In some cases it may be useful to mobilize the nerve backward but this step requires the exposure of the geniculate ganglion and section of the superficial petrosal nerve. Once the mobilization of the nerve and the removal of the ossicles have been achieved, the promontory is exposed and the cochlea is entirely drilled. Resection of the cochlea offers significant space above the genu and the horizontal portion of the carotid canal, toward the petrous apex

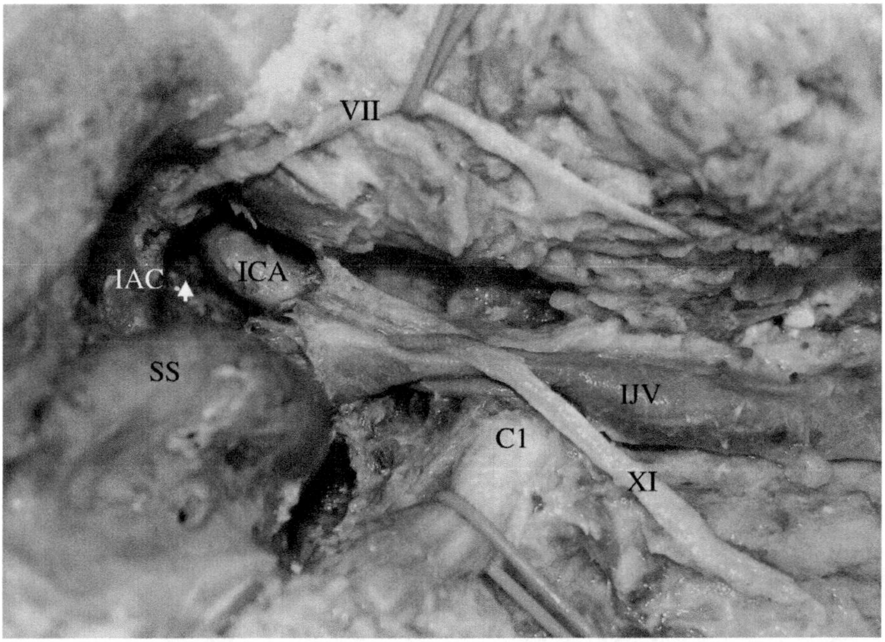


**Fig. 16.** Enlarged view of the Fig. 15. D. *IAC* Internal auditory canal. The white arrow indicates the course of the inferior petrosal sinus after drilling of the petroclival groove

(Fig. 16). The premeatal dura is widely exposed in the triangle delineated by the superior and the inferior petrosal sinuses. The tympanal bone is removed and the ascending branch of the mandibula is pushed forward to widen the corridor in front of the intrapetrous carotid artery.

Due to the wide field that has been exposed and the importance of the bony and dura defect, the closure step needs to be meticulous. As mentioned previously, abdominal fat is a precious material to occlude the cavity but it can be useful to cover the fat with a flap of temporalis muscle that is folded and sutured to the sternocleidomastoid muscle.

## Commentaries

The step of total translocation of the facial nerve implies a postoperative facial deficit that never recovers better than House and Brackman grade III. If the nerve is mobilized backward, it necessitates a section of the superficial petrosal nerves, which compromise permanently the function of the VII bis nerve. Additionally, the intrapetrous neuro-otologic structures are sacrificed by the approach, which implies a hearing loss. The extratime that is needed to achieve the procedure is really significant and justifies a two-surgeons procedure.

## Case illustration

### Case illustration 1

The case of a primarily intracranial lesion with minimal extension into the jugular foramen.

A 30-year-old woman presented with a 6-month history of swallowing disorders and voice modification. She was admitted in neurosurgery following an acute pulmonary infection. She complained of cervical pain, dysphagia, hoarseness and shoulder weakness on the left side. Enhanced MR images (Fig. 17A and B) showed a cystic schwannoma involving the jugular fossa, the cerebellomedullary cistern and cerebellopontine angle on the left side without extension through the jugular foramen. Resection was carried out using a

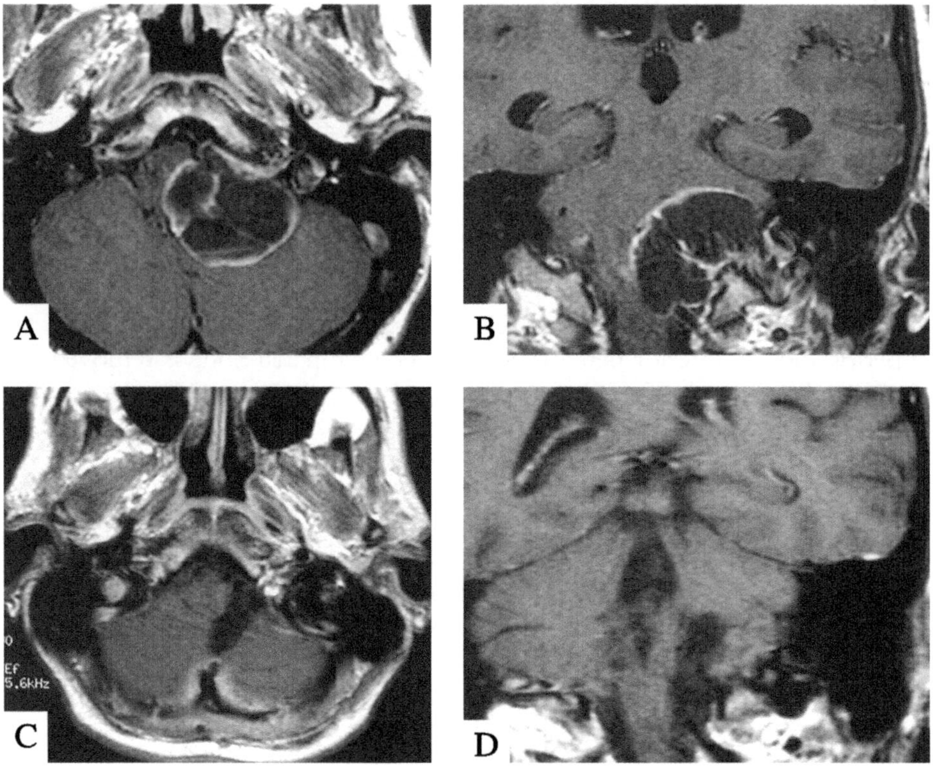


**Fig. 17.** Pre- and postoperative neuroimaging of the case illustration 1. (A) Post-gadolinium T1 image (*axial*) showing a large cystic tumor involving the left cerebello-medullary cistern with mass effect over the medulla. (B) Coronal view using the same sequence. Considering the reduced amount of intraforaminal infiltration, it was decided to operate this patient via a suboccipital retrosigmoid approach. (C and D) post-operative MR images showing the lack of residual tumor

lateral retrosigmoid route. Post-operative MR images (Fig. 17C and D) showed complete resection of the tumor. At the 6-month follow-up examination, the lower cranial nerve dysfunction had significantly improved.

## Case illustration 2

The case of a lesion involving the jugular foramen with minimal intracranial extension.

This 40-year-old male was admitted to our institution for recent onset of hoarseness. He was operated on elsewhere 15-year ago for "partial removal of a posterior fossa schwannoma". Since that time, he complained of some swallowing disorders. The clinical examination showed a laryngeal palsy and a

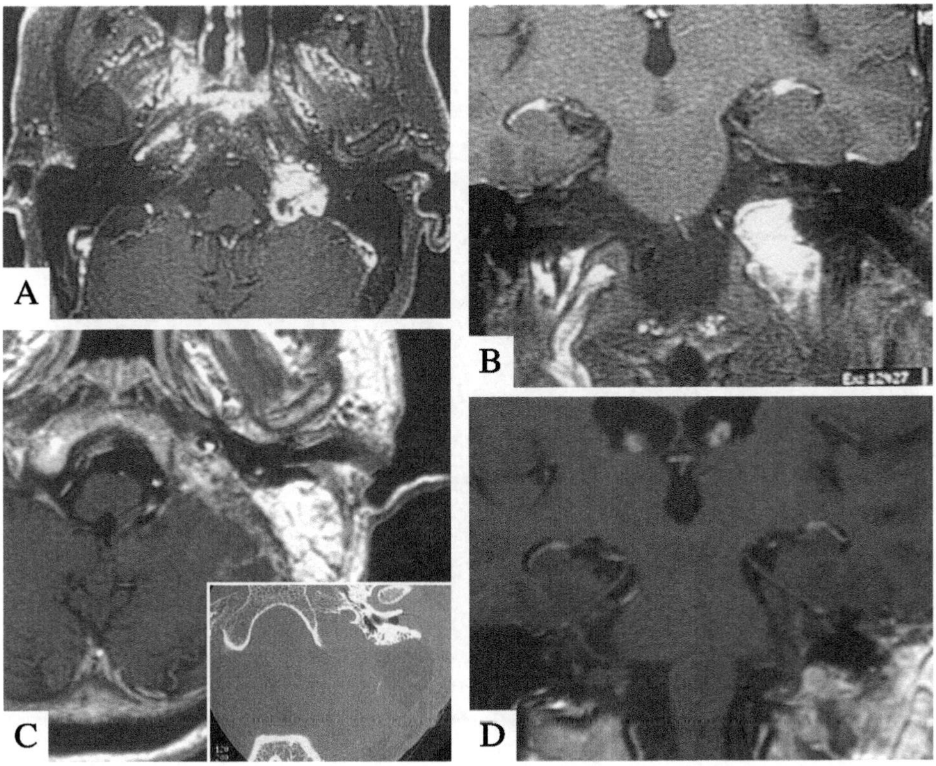


**Fig. 18.** Pre- and postoperative neuroimaging of the case illustration 2. (A) Post-gadolinium T1 image (*axial*) showing an intraforaminal tumor mass on the left side. Note that the intracisternal extension of the lesion is reduced, as confirmed in coronal view (B). This extension justified an infralabyrinthine transigmoid transjugular-high cervical approach. (C and D) Postop imaging confirmed the lack of residual tumor. Post-operative bone window CT scan (*white small screen*) showed the large opening of the jugular foramen

shoulder weakness on the left side. Enhanced MR images showed a jugular foramen schwannoma with minimal intracranial extension and with a small component involving the superior aspect of the posterior parapharyngeal space (Fig. 18A and B). The bony CT scan showed enlargement of the jugular foramen. An infralabyrinthine transigmoid transjugular-high cervical approach was performed and allowed a complete removal of the lesion as shown on MR images (Fig. 18C and D). The cranial nerve dysfunction remained unchanged.

## Case illustration 3

This illustration is about two patients presenting with a very similar clinical history of hypacousia and tinnitus on the right side. In both cases, preoperative examination and neuroradiological work-up concluded to a jugulotympanic paraganglioma (illustration not shown). In both cases it was decided to operate via an infralabyrinthine transigmoid transjugular-high cervical approach. The main difference between the two cases is the distinct course of the eleven

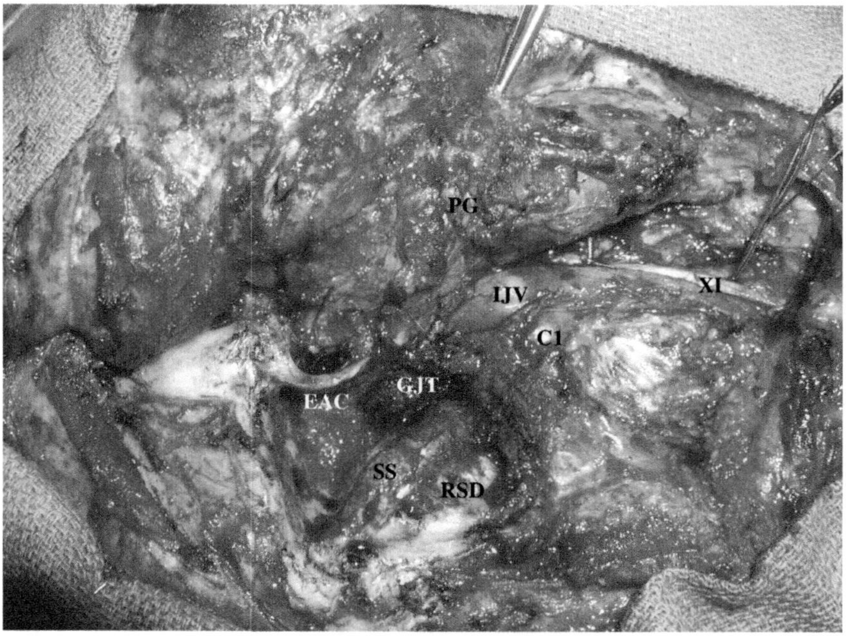


**Fig. 19.** Peroperative view of the case illustration 3. An infralabyrinthine transigmoid transjugular-high cervical approach has been achieved on the right side The glomus jugulare tumor (*GJT*) has been exposed below the posterior labyrinth in the hypotympanum, inside the lumen of the jugular bulb and occluding the internal jugular vein (*IJV*). The external auditory canal (*EAC*) has been cut, the parotid gland (*PG*) has been exposed with the division of the facial nerve. The retrosigmoid dura (*RSD*) has been exposed in order to ligate and divide the sigmoid sinus (*SS*)

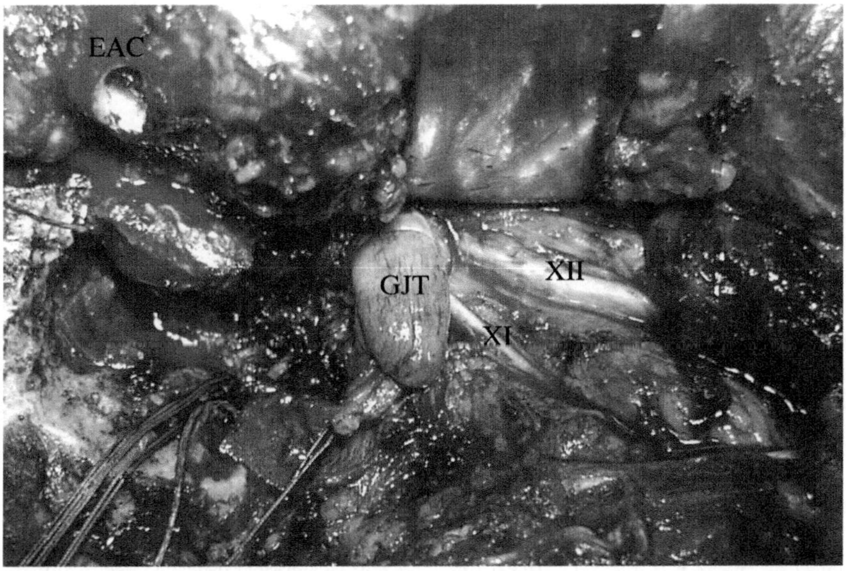


**Fig. 20.** Peroperative view of a right sided jugulotympanic paraganglioma. The tumor origin and tumor extension are similar to what has been observed in the previous case (Fig. 19). At this step, the internal jugular vein has been ligated and opened in order to expose and remove the tumor (*GJT*). Note the position of the eleventh nerve (*XI*) which courses medially to the IJV

nerve; in the first case (Fig. 19), the CN XI courses laterally to the internal jugular vein while it courses medially in the other one (Fig. 20).

## Conclusions

One third of the cranial nerves as well as the major vascular supply and drainage of the brain course through the jugular foramen region. This region may be involved by various diseases which are dominated by the tumors. In order to treat these affections, there is a need to understand the locoregional surgical anatomy of the JF. Surgical approaches are not only influenced by the origin and extensions of the tumor, but also by the clinical condition of the patient, justifying an extensive work-up before treatment. In this paper we have described successively three skull base approaches with a gradual level of exposure and invasiveness. We have shown that the facial nerve and lower cranial nerves are in the close proximity of the operative field and may be jeopardized during exposure or resection of the disease. Thereby, the skull base neurosurgeon needs to be able to master this panel of approaches and to propose an individual tailored surgery. In cases of benign tumors in patients presenting with few symptoms, which is a common situation, we particularly recommend the use of this tailored surgery. The role of radiosurgery in the treatment of residual tumors that infiltrate the LCNs remains to determine but looks promising.

## References

1. Alverina JE, Fraser K, Lanzino G (2006) The occipital artery: a microanatomical study. Neurosurgery 58 Suppl 1: 114–122
2. Ayeni SA, Ohata K, Tanaka K, Hakuba A (1995) The microsurgical anatomy of the jugular foramen. J Neurosurg 83: 903–909
3. Bertalanffy H, Seeger W (1991) The dorsolateral, suboccipital, transcondylar approach to the lower clivus and anterior portion of the craniocervical junction. Neurosurgery 29: 815–821
4. Fisch U (1978) Infratemporal fossa approach to tumours of the temporal bone and base of the skull. J Laryngol Otol 92: 949–967
5. Fisch U, Mattox D (1988) Microsurgery of the skull base. Thieme, Stuttgart, pp 136–173
6. Fournier HD, Laccoureye L, Mercier P (1998) La voie rétroauriculaire transmastoidienne infralabyrinthique. Neurochirurgie 44: 111–116
7. Franklin DJ, Moore GF, Fisch U (1989) Jugular foramen peripheral nerve sheath tumors. Laryngoscope 99: 1081–1087
8. George B, Lot G, Tran Ba Huy P (1995) The juxta condylar approach to the jugular foramen (without petrous bone drilling). Surg Neurol 44: 279–284
9. Glasscock ME, Jackson C, Dickins J, Wiet R (1979) The surgical management of glomus tumors. Laryngoscope 89: 1640–1651
10. House WF, Hitselberger WE (1976) The transcochlear approach to the skull base. Arch Otolaryngol 102: 334–342
11. Hovelacque A (1934) Ostéologie. Doin, Paris 2: 155–156
12. Katsuta T, Rhoton AL, Matsushima T (1997) The jugular foramen: microsurgical anatomy and operative approaches. Neurosurgery 41: 149–202
13. Kawano H, Tono T, Schachern PA, Paparella MM, Komune S (2000) Petrous high jugular bulb: a histological study. Am J Otolaryngol 21: 161–168
14. Lang J (1993) Anatomy of the posterior cranial fossa. In: Sekhar LN, Janecka IP (eds) Surgery of the cranial base. Raven Press, New York, pp 131–146
15. Liscak R, Vladyka V, Wowra B, Kemeny A, Forster D, Burzaco JA, Martinez R, Eustacchio S, Pendl G, Régis J, Pellet W (1999) Gammaknife radiosurgery of the glomus jugulare tumour – early multicentre experience. Acta Neurochir (Wien) 141: 1141–1146
16. Lustig LR, Jackler RK (1996) The variable relationships between the lower cranial nerves and jugular foramen tumors: implications for neural preservation. Am J Otol 17: 658–668
17. Malca SA, Roche PH, Thomassin JMT, Pellet W (1994) An unsual cervical mass tumor: meningioma. A propos of a case of petrous origin. Review of the literature of meningioma presenting as cervical mass. Neurochirurgie 40: 96–108
18. Muthukumar N, Kondziolka D, Lunsford AD, Flickinger JC (1999) Stereotactic radiosurgery for jugular foramen schwannomas. Surg Neurol 52: 172–179
19. Pellet W, Cannoni M, Pech A (1988) The widened trancochlear approach to jugular foramen tumors. J Neurosurg 69: 887–894
20. Pellet W, Cannoni M, Pech A (1989) Otoneurosurgery. Springer, Berlin Heidelberg New York
21. Proctor B (1989) Surgical anatomy of the ear and temporal bone. Thieme, New York

22. Ramina R, Maniglia JJ, Fernandes YB, Paschoal JR, Pfeilsticker LN, Neto MC (2005) Tumors of the jugular foramen: diagnosis and management. Neurosurgery ONS 1 Suppl 57: 59–68
23. Rhoton AL, Buza R (1975) Microsurgical anatomy of the jugular foramen. J Neurosurg 42: 541–550
24. Roche PH, Moriyama T, Thomassin JM, Pellet W (2006) High jugular bulb in the translabyrinthine approach to the cerebellopontine angle: anatomical considerations and surgical management. Acta Neurochir (Wien) 148: 415–420
25. Samii M, Babu RP, Tatagiba M, Sepehrnia A (1995) Sugical treatment of jugular foramen schwannomas. J Neurosurg 82: 924–932
26. Sanna M (1995) Atlas of temporal bone and lateral skull base surgery. Thieme, New York
27. Sen C, Hague K, Kacchara R, Jenkins A, Das S, Catalano P (2001) Jugular foramen: Microscopic anatomic features and implications for neural preservation with reference to glomus tumors involving the temporal bone. Neurosurgery 48: 838–848
28. Van Loveren HR, Sing Liu S, Pensak ML, Keller JT (1996) Anatomy of the jugular foramen: The neurosurgical perspective. Operative technique in otolaryngology head and neck surgery, vol 7, pp 90–94
29. Wen HT, Rhoton AL, Katsuta T de Oliveira E (1997) Microsurgical anatomy of the transcondylar, supracondylar, and paracondylar extensions of the far-lateral approach. J Neurosurg 87: 555–585

## Author index volume 1–33

*Advances and Technical Standards in Neurosurgery*

## Subject index volume 1–33

*Advances and Technical Standards in Neurosurgery*

**Springer**Neurosurgery

## Advances and Technical Standards in Neurosurgery

### Volume 27

2002. XIV, 244 pages. 97 figures, partly in colour.
Hardcover **EUR 114,95**
ISBN 3-211-83605-5

**Advances:** • Multi-Modality Monitoring of Acute Brain Trauma (R. Kett-White, P. J. A. Hutchinson, M. Czosnyka, S. Boniface, J. D. Pickard, P. J. Kirkpatrick) • The Concept of Diffuse Axonal Injury (J. Sahuquillo, A. Poca) • Endoscopic Endonasal Transsphenoidal Surgery (E. de Divitiis, P. Cappabianca) **Technical Standards:** • Surgery of Temporal Lobe Epilepsy (M. Vapalahti) • Surgical Exposure of the Vertebral Artery - Application to Spinal and Skull Base Surgery (B. George) • Neurosurgical Management of Pineal Tumours (Y. Sawamura, N. de Tribolet)

### Volume 26

2000. XVI, 346 pages. 83 figures, partly in colour.
Hardcover **EUR 179,95**
ISBN 3-211-83424-9

**Advances:** • Multiple Subpial Transection (C. E. Polkey) • Hemispheric Disconnection: Callosotomy and Hemispherotomy (J.-G. Villemure, O. Vernet, O. Delalande) • Central Nervous System Lymphomas (H. Loiseau, E. Cuny, A. Vital, F. Cohadon) • Invited Commentary: Treatment of Diseases of the Central Nervous System Using Encapsulated Cells, by A. F. Hottinger and P. Aebischer (Advances and Technical Standards in Neurosurgery Vol. 25) (A. E. Rosser, T. Ostenfeld, C. N. Svendsen) **Technical Standards:** • The Intracranial Venous System as a Neurosurgeon's Perspective (M. Sindou, J. Auque) • Reconstructive Surgery of the Extracranial Arteries ( R. Schmid-Elsässer, R. J. Medele, H.-J. Steiger) • Surgical Treatment of Lumbar Spondylolisthesis (P. W. Detwiler, R. W. Porter, P. P. Han, D. G. Karahalios, R. Masferrer, V. K. H. Sonntag)

*Springer and the Environment*

WE AT SPRINGER FIRMLY BELIEVE THAT AN INTERnational science publisher has a special obligation to the environment, and our corporate policies consistently reflect this conviction.

WE ALSO EXPECT OUR BUSINESS PARTNERS – PRINTERS, paper mills, packaging manufacturers, etc. – to commit themselves to using environmentally friendly materials and production processes.

THE PAPER IN THIS BOOK IS MADE FROM NO-CHLORINE pulp and is acid free, in conformance with international standards for paper permanency.

GPSR Compliance

*The European Union's (EU) General Product Safety Regulation (GPSR) is a set of rules that requires consumer products to be safe and our obligations to ensure this.*

*If you have any concerns about our products, you can contact us on ProductSafety@springernature.com*

In case Publisher is established outside the EU, the EU authorized representative is:

Springer Nature Customer Service Center GmbH
Europaplatz 3
69115 Heidelberg, Germany

**Batch number: 10726302**

Printed by Printforce, the Netherlands